HYPNOSIS and HYPNOTHERAPY with CHILDREN

HYPNOSIS and HYPNOTHERAPY with CHILDREN

G. Gail Gardner, Ph.D.

*Associate Professor of Clinical
Psychology and Pediatrics
University of Colorado Medical School
Denver, Colorado*

Karen Olness, M.D.

*Director, Medical Education and Research
Minneapolis Children's Health Center
Associate Professor of Pediatrics and
Family Practice and Community Health
University of Minnesota
Minneapolis, Minnesota*

Grune & Stratton

A Subsidiary of Harcourt Brace Jovanovich, Publishers
New York   London   Toronto   Sydney   San Francisco

Library of Congress Cataloging in Publication Data

Gardner, G. Gail.
Hypnosis and hypnotherapy with children.

Includes bibliographies and index.
1. Hypnotism—Therapeutic use.   2. Child psychotherapy.
I. Olness, Karen.   II. Title.
RJ505.H86G37   615.8'512'088054   81-6366
ISBN 0-8089-1413-8   AACR2

Grune & Stratton, Inc.
111 Fifth Avenue
New York, New York 10003

Distributed in the United Kingdom by
Academic Press Inc. (London) Ltd.
24/28 Oval Road, London NW 1

Library of Congress Catalog Number 81-6366
International Standard Book Number 0-8089-1413-8

Printed in the United States of America

Contents

Acknowledgments

Over the years, countless people have encouraged us to explore the frontiers of hypnosis and hypnotherapy with children, to document our observations, and eventually to write this book. Among our teachers and mentors, we give special thanks to Erika Fromm, Ph.D., Doris Gruenewald, Ph.D., Josephine Hilgard, M.D., Ph.D., Paul Sacerdote, M.D., Ph.D., and the late Erik Wright, M.D., Ph.D. We have also been encouraged by our many students over the years.

We give thanks and recognition to those who have supported us as teachers of child hypnotherapy, especially Franz Baumann, M.D., who was teaching in our field before we had even discovered it and who is the only pediatrician to have been President of the American Society of Clinical Hypnosis. We would also like to thank Martin T. Orne, M.D., Ph.D., who supported the development of annual workshops on the clinical use of hypnosis with children, sponsored by the Society for Clinical and Experimental Hypnosis. He was also responsible for devoting a special issue of the *International Journal of Clinical and Experimental Hypnosis* to the topic of children.

We say thank you to our children, nieces, and nephews, who have willingly been photographic and research subjects and who have provided us with hours of enjoyable and naturalistic observations as well as ideas for hypnotic techniques. We are also grateful to our patients who have given us new ideas and permitted us to use photographs for teaching hypnotic skills to others.

We gratefully acknowledge the expert secretarial help of Susan Domaschk and Marge Selby and the editing advice from Hakon Torjeson.

Foreword

A book on hypnotherapy with children is welcome because it is long overdue. There has been no general book since the short one by Ambrose in 1961. Much has transpired since then. As gifted clinicians, Dr. Gardner and Dr. Olness have combined their expertness in the fields of child psychology, pediatrics, and hypnotherapy to produce a much-needed and excellent book on hypnosis and hypnotherapy with children. Throughout the book it is abundantly clear that they are skilled clinicians and experienced in a wide range of childhood disorders. From their own practice detailed clinical observations abound. In addition to this rich material they have carefully researched the available literature for significant cases and have presented the more instructive ones in appropriate detail.

Those responsible for the treatment of children are not always familiar with the fact that children are much more responsive than adults to hypnotic procedures. Hence the uncertainty about response to hypnosis is far less of a handicap in the use of hypnosis with children than it is in some instances with adults.

The range of topics reflects a scholarly and well-rounded approach. Particularly interesting is the historical perspective on hypnotherapy with children, which is shown to have been actively pursued over the past two centuries. The book is divided into two parts: Part I describes relevant needs of childhood related to hypnosis and hypnosis with children in general; Part II describes hypnotherapy with children in relation to various psychological, pediatric–medical, and pediatric–surgical problems. The division is both logical and useful.

The sources referred to are widely varied. For example, they include not only the major hypnosis journals but also references to at least 50 journals including those in psychology, pediatrics, and psychiatry as well as those in such specialty journals as anesthesiology, dentistry, hematology, allergy, urology, oncology, and surgery. When the number of books and symposia are added to this list, the range of coverage is impressive. To have information conveniently at hand from all of these sources can prove to be a great advantage to both practitioners and research workers.

Dr. Gardner, the child psychologist, and Dr. Olness, the pediatrician, are committed to the point of view that for a meaningful trial of hypnotherapy to take place two ingredients are essential: first, excellence in training as a clinician ("The hypnotherapist must first be a competent therapist") and, second, excellence in training and experience in hypnosis. Only through this combination can the potential of hypnosis in therapy be fully realized. Skills that the experienced clinician brings to the therapeutic interaction include a knowledge of normal child behavior, a comprehension of the emotional difficulties that children may develop under severe psychological and physical stress, and a thorough understanding of the importance of the patient–therapist relationship. The professional person with a foundation in the theory and practice of hypnosis brings to the interaction a number of skills. Besides such obvious ones as the ability to assess the indications and contraindications for hypnotherapy and the use of appropriate techniques, the book calls attention to other skills important in treatment. First, hypnotherapy must operate in an atmosphere of adequate motivation, confidence, trust, and a generally positive transference. Second, imagination, probably the most significant foundation of hypnotherapy with children, must be used constructively and flexibly by *both* patient and therapist. Third, mastery of the treatment process must reside as much as possible in the patient. Too often hypnosis has been viewed as promoting dependence of the patient on a powerful hypnotherapist, when nothing could be further from the preferred practice. It is recognized now that the patient who is capable of being hypnotized possesses the *talent* for hypnosis, while the hypnotherapist acts as the coach who can assist in mobilizing and directing such talent toward therapeutic goals. The end-product then belongs to the patient who has learned how to integrate the processes whereby his or her talent and the therapist's direction become fused under the designation of self-hypnosis. In many clinical cases cited by the authors, this process is begun as early as the first session. Naturally there are certain conditions under which self-hypnosis may be much too difficult or perhaps impossible to achieve, but in general the patient who has learned self-hypnosis achieves independence early in the treatment process.

The authors recognize that while the number of carefully designed research studies has been growing, much remains to be done. Useful as individual case reports are for the concreteness with which they depict the practical procedures in dealing with a patient, scientific advance requires more studies that include a number of well-defined cases treated under controlled conditions. Through intensive research in laboratories connected with universities and foundations during the last 25 years, hypnotic science has moved steadily ahead so that today the essence of hypnosis and its parameters are better understood. Clinical insights provided by individual case reports now suggest directions along which it will be fruitful to proceed. It goes without saying that this overview of hypnotherapy with children by Gardner and Olness will prove of great value in both stimulating and guiding such an effort.

As a psychiatrist who has been engaged in hypnotic research and therapy with both adults and children for a number of years, I believe that this thoughtful book will prove of value to a wide range of professional people. It is well directed toward psychologists, pediatricians, psychiatrists, and other professional practitioners. It can profitably be read by researchers and therapists, whether they are involved with hypnosis, or considering such involvement, at the level of the child, the adolescent, or the adult.

Josephine R. Hilgard, M.D., Ph.D.
Department of Psychiatry
Stanford Medical School
Department of Psychology
Stanford University
Stanford, California

Introduction

More than a decade ago, we separately became interested in the possibilities of using therapeutic hypnosis with children, one of us as a clinical child psychologist, the other as a pediatrician. We were impressed with the lack of knowledge in the area of child hypnosis, not only among child health professionals but also among hypnotherapists, most of whom worked only with adults. At various times we were told (1) that children are not hypnotizable, (2) that something had been written about child hypnosis but few people knew what or by whom, and (3) that there was no information about child hypnotherapy because hypnotherapy is not an appropriate treatment for children.

Neither of us gave up. We scoured the literature, found a few people who did use hypnotherapy successfully and appropriately with children, discarded all the wrong information we had been given, and began to use hypnotherapy with our child patients. We soon met and began teaching together. Interest and knowledge expanded, both in the United States and in other countries. Eventually we decided that the available information warranted a comprehensive text on the topic, and thus we collaborated to write this book.

We now sometimes hear that child hypnotherapy is a recent development. This is not true; it is only the breadth of interest that is recent. Hypnotherapy has been used with children for more than 200 years. In 1959, Weitzenhoffer published "A Bibliography of Hypnotism in Pediatrics" containing 86 references—many in French and German—spanning 1886 to 1959. In 1980, Gardner published a bibliog-

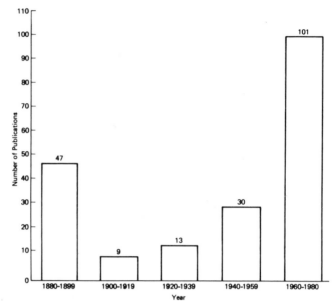

Figure 1. *Number of publications concerning child hypnosis in each 20-year period from 1880 to 1980.*

raphy of 114 references dating from 1955 to 1980, almost entirely limited to publications in American journals. As shown in Figure 1, there was a flurry of interest in the field in the late 19th century, followed by a decline for more than 50 years, and then a tremendous revival in the 1960s and 1970s.

The growth of interest in child hypnotherapy is also reflected in expanded opportunities for training in this subspecialty. For example, in 1971 one of us was invited to lecture for an hour on child hypnosis as part of an advanced-level workshop sponsored by the Society for Clinical and Experimental Hypnosis. In 1976, the same society initiated a full 3-day workshop on clinical hypnosis with children, and this workshop has been conducted annually since then. The International Society of Hypnosis and the American Society of Clinical Hypnosis have similarly increased emphasis on children in their workshops. Seminars on hypnosis, including child hypnosis, are now included in many medical school curricula and in graduate school programs in clinical psychology.

In line with the heightened interest in child hypnotherapy, we discuss three broad topics in this book. First, we review the early history of therapeutic hypnosis with children, emphasizing the 19th century literature so as to collect in one place those intriguing reports that predated modern scientific methods. Second, we discuss issues related to child hypnosis, by which we mean a child can enter that altered state of consciousness that most people define as hypnosis. Here we review in detail the normative studies of the 1960s and 1970s, which uniformly conclude that, in general, children have a higher level of hypnotic responsiveness than adults. We review and discuss a wide range of variables cited, either in research studies or in the course of clinical observation and theoretical speculation, as possible correlates of hypnotizability in children. This section concludes with a survey of hypnotic induction techniques appropriate for children of different ages and abilities. Third, we review the broad topic of hypnotherapy with children, with chapters devoted to the treatment of psychological, medical, and surgical problems. Here we include both a critical review of the literature and a sample of our own clinical experience.

From the outset, we want to distinguish between child hypnosis and child hypnotherapy, terms much too often confused. *Hypnosis is an altered state of consciousness.* No scientist claims fully to understand its parameters, but most people in the field agree that it is a state of consciousness different both from the normal waking state and from any of the stages of sleep. It resembles in some ways, but is not identical with, various kinds of meditative states, especially with respect to characteristics of narrowly focused attention, primary process thinking, and ego receptivity (Fromm, 1977, 1979). There are also characteristic alterations in cognition associated especially with deeper levels of hypnosis, and these forms of "trance logic" may be elicited by careful experimental methods (Orne, 1959). The lighter levels of hypnosis are sometimes indistinguishable from simple physical and mental relaxation. In some cases, therefore, it is really inappropriate to use the term "hypnosis" at all; in other cases, hypnotic phenomena may be elicited that cannot be explained by relaxation alone; in still other cases, the distinction is very difficult, casting doubt on the validity of research conclusions.

Hypnotherapy is a treatment modality in which the patient is in the altered state of hypnosis at least part of the time. The patient in hypnosis is then treated with any of a number of methods ranging from simple suggestion to psychoanalysis. Strictly speaking, no patient is treated by "hypnosis," that is, by the mere fact of having entered a certain altered state of consciousness, although this confusion of terms is very common in the literature. A patient who merely goes into hypnosis may experience reduced tension and even reduced tension-related pain, but there is no specific therapeutic intervention. Hypnotherapy, by definition, implies therapeutic intervention either by a therapist or by the patient. In the latter case, the term "self-hypnosis" is so widespread that we have chosen to retain it rather than coin a new term. We acknowledge the inconsistency.

Inasmuch as there is disagreement, confusion, and imperfect knowledge about hypnosis, these problems are greatly multiplied in the case of hypnotherapy. There are very few cases of "successful hypnotherapy" in which one can be absolutely certain that the results are due to hypnotherapy and not to something else; some would say there are no such cases at all. On the other hand, some people are overly enthusiastic and make claims about hypnotherapy far in excess of the bounds of scientific responsibility. We take a middle position on this issue. We believe that when some patients are treated for some problems while in the state of hypnosis, changes occur that would not have occurred had the patients been in the normal waking state. Otherwise we would not be practicing hypnotherapy. We recognize that our belief may be challenged. The sophistication of outcome studies of hypnotherapy lags behind that of psychotherapy, a field in which there is still contention as to its benefits. We fully expect that future research will prove some of the statements we make in this book wrong. We do not claim to be writing the *dernier cri* in our subspecialty. On the contrary, we look forward to the time when more careful clinical reports and more sophisticated research will permit us to revise this book in the direction of greater certainty, allowing us to make a greater contribution to the children with whom we work. For the present, if we raise at least as many questions as we answer, we will have fulfilled our purpose.

We emphasize that this book is not intended to be a "how-to-do-it" guide for persons with no previous training in hypnotherapy. One does not learn these skills from a textbook any more than one learns psychotherapy or pediatrics by reading a book. We hope our readers will avail themselves of opportunities for training in hypnotherapy

---

*Detailed information about training opportunities in hypnosis and hypnotherapy may be obtained from the following organizations:

American Society of Clinical Hypnosis
2250 East Devon Avenue, Suite 336
Des Plaines, Illinois 60018
(312) 297–3317

Society for Clinical and Experimental Hypnosis
129-A Kings Park Drive
Liverpool, New York 13088
(315) 652–7299

International Society of Hypnosis
111 North 49th Street, Box 144
Philadelphia, Pennsylvania 19139

and its subspecialty, child hypnotherapy. Of course, not all training opportunities are of the same quality. We recommend workshops and courses sponsored by the Society for Clinical and Experimental Hypnosis, the American Society of Clinical Hypnosis, and the International Society of Hypnosis* as well as courses offered by approved medical and graduate schools. We intend this book to complement these courses, providing a degree of thoroughness and detail that is best appreciated at a leisurely pace.

The recommended workshops are limited to persons already trained in the health professions: physicians, psychologists, dentists, clinical social workers. We cannot overemphasize the point that a hypnotherapist first must be a competent therapist, and a person doing research in hypnosis must first have a solid background in research techniques. Our book is directed to child health professionals who assume primary responsibility for child patients and to researchers in related areas. We hope that it will provide our colleagues with new ideas and will stimulate creative approaches to understanding children and helping them develop their potential to the fullest extent.

REFERENCES

Fromm, E. An ego-psychological theory of altered states of consciousness. *The International Journal of Clinical and Experimental Hypnosis*, 1977, *25*, 372–387.

Fromm, E. The nature of hypnosis and other altered states of consciousness: An ego psychological theory. In E. Fromm and R. E. Shor (Eds.), *Hypnosis: Developments in research and new perspectives* (2nd ed.). Hawthorne, N.Y.: Aldine, 1979.

Gardner, G. G. Hypnosis with children: Selected readings. *The International Journal of Clinical and Experimental Hypnosis*, 1980, *28*, 289–293.

Orne, M. T. The nature of hypnosis: Artifact and essence. *Journal of Abnormal and Social Psychology*, 1959, *58*, 277–299.

Weitzenhoffer, A. M. A bibliography of hypnotism in pediatrics. *The American Journal of Clinical Hypnosis*, 1959, *2*, 92–95.

PART I
Hypnosis with Children

1

Scenes of Childhood

To help the reader more fully understand our approach to hypnotherapy, we present some themes of child development that form the rationale for our methods with children.

THE URGE FOR EXPERIENCE

Beginning at birth, babies seek stimulation. In the first days of life, they prefer to focus their gaze on something and prefer a more complex visual stimulus (e.g., a striped pattern) to a simple one (e.g., a solid red square). Most of all, they enjoy gazing at a human face. Very soon, children define all objects as things-to-find-out-about, and they make maximal use of sensory and motor development to experience themselves and their world. They do this first with mouths and eyes, then with hands, and finally with their whole bodies. If the results of such experiences are generally pleasurable, they continue to explore in more complex ways, using to their own advantage such developing ego functions as motility and coordination, language, perceptual skills, memory, ability to distinguish between reality and fantasy, and social skills. Temperamental and environmental factors combine to shape and often to put limits on the child's urge for experience, but only rarely can these cancel the urge altogether. For example, in the case of the frightened child who retreats to a corner on the first day of school, a patient teacher usually finds that the child prefers to

3

stand facing the room rather than facing the wall. For such children, visual exploration often leads to good school adjustment as efficiently as motor exploration for other children. As Fromm (1972) pointed out, it is very important not to confuse behavioral passivity with ego passivity.

THE URGE FOR MASTERY

Right on the heels of the urge for experience comes the urge for mastery, both of the self and of the environment. Objects and people become things-to-do-something-with. Ego activity and behavioral activity join forces, sometimes to the dismay of parents who find the contents of the cupboard in a heap on the floor. It is sheer pleasure to share with children in the mastery process. One of us once watched a bright 2-year-old playing with number blocks of varying lengths and said to the child, "Did you know that two twos make four?" The little girl repeated "two twos make four?", picked up two "two blocks," aligned them with a "four block," and sat on the floor utterly delighted with her accomplishment. As children grow older, they continue to experience the same drive for mastery, unless this aspect of ego functioning is seriously derailed by environmental or physical handicaps. Murphy and associates have published excellent research on the various pathways by which children achieve fulfillment of the urge for mastery (Murphy, 1962; Murphy & Moriarty, 1976).

THE URGE FOR SOCIAL INTERACTION

Children are social creatures. Even at birth, their favorite visual stimulus is a human face. Children develop language not only for its own reward of mastery but because it vastly increases possibilities for social interaction. The endless "why" questions of the toddler are often less a request for information than for social play, just as endless requests for peek-a-boo or chase-around-the-tree serve to exercise social as much as sensory and motor needs. Social interaction is more than social control, more than merely a way to have needs satisfied; it is a pleasure in itself. Children progress from interaction with parents to interaction with peers, and in this way develop social skills that may provide pleasure for the rest of their lives. Again, ego development can be derailed, but most children manage to remember that at least some relationships are safe and may be both a means to pleasure and pleasurable themselves. Although some children may be slow to warm up in new relationships, very few choose to remain isolated.

THE URGE FOR THE INNER WORLD OF IMAGINATION

Just as children enjoy increasing the range of their experiences in and with the outer world, they also delight in the realms of inner experience: fantasy, imagery, imagination. These functions serve useful purposes. Children may survey several possible actions in fantasy and then select the best apparent behavioral choice, thus saving time and energy. They may use fantasy to modify unpleasant situations, to gratify unmet needs, or to prepare for creativity and achievement (J. R. Hilgard, 1970; Olness, 1978). But imaginative involvements may be pleasures in their own right. For example, one of us once asked a group of 15 4-year-olds to report dreams. After the first child described what was probably a nocturnal "monster" dream, the rest excitedly jumped in with variations. It was obvious that, for the most part, these other reports were not dreams but instead were entries in a competition to see who could create the wildest monster story; all had happy masterful endings, again following the lead of the first child who managed to throw her dream monster out the window. Inasmuch as we now recognize a basic need for nocturnal dreams, we could posit a similar need for waking reverie and fantasy. In fact, we wonder whether Western culture's devaluation of fantasy during adolescence may not contribute to some of the conflict and strife typical of that developmental period.

THE URGE FOR WELLNESS

Under most circumstances, children choose to be healthy rather than sick, comfortable rather than distressed. Children like to be well. When physically stressed, the body automatically adapts in an effort to restore integration. Thus, platelets and white cells rush to the site of a wound to stop bleeding and prevent infection. Likewise, when psychologically distressed, the individual uses various defense mechanisms and coping devices to handle the situation as adaptively as possible. Maladaptive behavior serves a purpose, conscious or unconscious or both. But almost always there is some part of the person that would gladly trade maladaptive behavior for behavior that serves the same purpose in a more constructive and truly self-satisfying way. In the case of maladaptive behavior in children, there is the added advantage of a higher degree of ego resiliency and flexibility than is often seen with adults. Children have still another advantage in their search for wellness, namely their generally greater comfort in seeking help and allowing a certain degree of adaptive regression that is inherent in a helping relationship.

IMPLICATIONS FOR HYPNOTHERAPY

In our therapeutic work, we recognize that we are not treating problems; we are treating children who happen to have problems. No matter how severe the problems of our child patients, we address ourselves to their strivings for experience, for mastery, for social interaction, for the inner world of imagination, and for wellness. Thus we gain an ally in that part of the child that wants to experience life to the fullest, and this alliance becomes the basis of treatment.

When we select hypnotherapy as the treatment of choice for a particular child's problem, we emphasize specific therapeutic techniques that enhance and strengthen healthy strivings. Induction techniques are selected partly on the basis of experiential satisfaction. Treatment is conducted in the context of a safe, comfortable relationship in which the child capitalizes on imagery skills to enhance feelings of control and mastery and to recover a state of wellness to the greatest extent possible. Treatment should not require passive submission but rather active and joyful participation. In the final analysis, we see ourselves as guides, coaches, teachers. It is the children who heal themselves.

REFERENCES

Fromm, E. Ego activity and ego passivity in hypnosis. *The International Journal of Clinical and Experimental Hypnosis*, 1972, *20*, 238–251.

Hilgard, J. R. *Personality and hypnosis: A study of imaginative involvement*. Chicago: University of Chicago Press, 1970.

Murphy, L. *The widening world of childhood: Paths toward mastery*. New York: Basic Books, 1962.

Murphy, L. B., & Moriarty, A. E. *Vulnerability, coping, and growth: From infancy to adolescence*. New Haven: Yale University Press, 1976.

Olness, K. Little people, images, and child health. Presidential Address, Northwestern Pediatric Society, Minneapolis, September 28, 1978.

2

Early Uses of Hypnosis with Children

The use of hypnoticlike techniques with children goes back to ancient times. Both the Old and New Testament contain accounts of ill children responding to healing methods based on suggestion and faith (I Kings XVII:17–24; Mark IX:17–27). Children in primitive cultures have employed trance phenomena in initiation rites and other ceremonies (Mead, 1949).

FRANZ ANTON MESMER (1734–1815)

The modern history of hypnosis begins with Mesmer, an Austrian physician whose interest in the healing power of magnetic influence was a logical extension of attention to magnetic forces among astronomers and physicists of that time. In 1766, Mesmer wrote a dissertation entitled "The Influences of the Planets on the Human Body" (cited in Tinterow, 1970).

During the next decade, Mesmer developed his theory of animal magnetism. Briefly, the theory held that all objects in the universe are connected by and filled with a physical fluid having magnetic properties. When this fluid is out of balance in the human body, disease occurs. Certain techniques can be employed to restore the fluid to proper equilibrium and thus heal the patient. Mesmer's techniques included staring into his patients' eyes and making various "passes" over their bodies, using his own "magnetic influence" to promote a cure.

While living in Vienna, Mesmer (cited in Tinterow, 1970) reported his use of animal magnetism to cure several patients, including children and adolescents. Though details of his methods with specific patients are sketchy, verbal instructions and suggestions seem to have been minimized in favor of the "passes" that supposedly restored the patient's own magnetic fluid to proper balance.

One of Mesmer's patients was Miss Ossine, an 18-year-old girl whose problems included tuberculosis, melancholia, fits, rage, vomiting, spitting up blood, and fainting. She recovered after treatment with animal magnetism. Another patient, also 18 years old at the time of treatment, was Miss Paradis, who had been blind since age 4 and who suffered melancholia, "accompanied by stoppages in the spleen and liver" that often brought on fits of delirium and rage. Most significant is Mesmer's awareness of the extent to which parental interference can sabotage treatment. Following restoration of the girl's sight by animal magnetism, a public dispute developed over whether she could really see or was just faking. Moreover, the father became fearful that his daughter's disability pension might be stopped. He terminated her treatment, whereupon she soon relapsed into frequent seizures and later into blindness. The father then changed his mind and asked that Mesmer resume treatment. Intensive treatment for 15 days again controlled the seizures and restored the girl's vision, after which she returned home. Subsequently, the family claimed that she had again relapsed. Mesmer thought the girl was being forced to imitate her maladies, but he could not obtain further follow-up.

At the same time, Mesmer described his treatment of Miss Wipior, age 9, who had a tumor on one cornea, rendering her blind in that eye. He stated that animal magnetism resulted in partial removal of the tumor so that the child could read sideways. He anticipated a full cure, but circumstances interrupted the treatment.

Following his work with these and other patients, Mesmer became discouraged by his colleagues' repeated charges that animal magnetism was no more than quackery. In 1778, he moved to Paris where he initially enjoyed good favor and, in 1779, published his famous "Dissertations on the Discovery of Animal Magnetism." His fame spread rapidly and he began treating patients in large groups, using more and more dramatic methods. His colleagues again charged quackery, and local scientific societies refused to acknowledge his discoveries. Once more discouraged, Mesmer left Paris, but "mesmerism" continued to flourish in the hands of his disciples, especially Charles d'Eslon.

THE FRANKLIN COMMISSION

In 1784, King Louis XVI appointed a commission to investigate mesmerism and, particularly, the claims of the disciple, d'Eslon (cited in Tinterow, 1970). The president of the commission was Benjamin Franklin, then the American Ambassador to France. Other distinguished members included the chemist Lavoisier and the physician Guillotin. The commissioners agreed that some patients were cured by mesmerism, but they questioned the underlying theory of the existence of magnetic fluid.

In experiments designed to test the theory, the commissioners took pains to include several children, particularly from the lower classes, so as to minimize the effects of prior knowledge and expectation. One of these was Claude Renand, a 6-year-old boy with tuberculosis. Unlike other patients, who had usually experienced pain, perspiration, and convulsions during mesmeric treatment, little Claude reported no sensation at all. Another child subject was Geneviève Leroux, age 9, suffering convulsions and chorea; she, too, felt no sensation. Procedures used with these and other subjects included passes made with iron rods and hand or finger pressure on various body parts, sometimes for several hours. An assistant played rapid piano music for the purpose of enhancing the likelihood of a "convulsive crisis."

Since Mesmer had claimed that he could transfer magnetic influence to inanimate objects and that patients could then be healed merely by touching these objects, the Commission tested this aspect of the theory, again with a naive child as subject. On the extensive grounds of Franklin's estate outside Paris, d'Eslon magnetized a certain apricot tree. A 12-year-old boy, known to be susceptible to the more common methods of animal magnetism, remained indoors, unaware of which tree was magnetized. The commissioners reported their observations in detail.

The boy was then brought into the orchard, his eyes covered with a bandage, and successively taken to trees upon which the procedure had not been performed, and he embraced them for the space of two minutes, the method of communication which had been prescribed by M. d'Eslon.

At the first tree, the boy, being questioned at the end of a minute, declared that he had perspired in large drops, he coughed, spit, and complained of a slight pain in his head; the distance of the tree which had been magnetized was about twenty-seven feet.

At the second tree he felt the sensations of stupefaction and pain in his head; the distance was thirty-six feet.

At the third tree, the stupefaction and headache increased considerably, and he said that he believed he was approaching the tree which had been magnetized. The distance was then about thirty-eight feet.

In line with the fourth tree, one which had not been rendered the object of the procedure, and at a distance of about twenty-four feet from the tree which had, the boy fell into a crisis, he fainted, his limbs stiffened, and he was carried on to a plot of grass, where M d'Eslon hurried to his side and revived him.

The result of this experiment is entirely contrary to the theory of animal magnetism. M. d'Eslon accounted for it by observing that all the trees, by their very nature, participated in the magnetism, and that their magnetism was reinforced by his presence. But in that case, a person, sensitive to the power of magnetism, could not hazard a walk in the garden without the risk of convulsions, an assertion which is contradicted by the experience of every day. The presence of M. d'Eslon had no greater influence here than in the coach, in which the boy came along with him. He was placed opposite the coach and he felt nothing. If he had experienced no sensation even under the tree which was magnetized, it might have been said that at least on that day he had not been sufficiently susceptible. However, the boy fell into a crisis under a tree which was not magnetized. The crisis was therefore the effect of no physical or exterior cause, but is to be attributed solely to the influence of imagination. The experiment is therefore entirely conclusive. The boy knew that he was about to be led to a tree upon which the magnetical operation had been performed, his imagination was struck, it was increased by the successive steps of the experiment, and at the fourth tree it was raised to the height necessary to produce the crisis. [quoted in Tinterow, 1970, pp. 108–109]

The commissioners thus rejected the theory of animal magnetism and concluded that the results of these and other experiments "are uniform in their nature, and contribute alike to the same decision. They authorize us to conclude that the imagination is the true cause of the effects attributed to the magnetism" (quoted in Tinterow, 1970, p. 114).

JOHN ELLIOTSON (1791–1868)

Charges and countercharges raged between Mesmer's disciples and others who agreed with the Franklin Commission report. The controversy between proponents of animal magnetism and those of imagination spread to England where the defense of animal magnetism was led by John Elliotson, a distinguished physician whose achievements included introducing the stethoscope to his country. Hoping to convince his colleagues, Elliotson decided in 1842 to edit a journal, *The Zoist*, concerned with information about cerebral physiology and mesmerism. The 13 volumes of this journal, published from 1842 to 1856, contain several references to the use of mesmerism in the management of childhood problems. Apparently Elliotson lacked the scientific sophistication of the 1784 Commission, for much of his argument in support of the theory rested on evidence that patients could be cured after mesmerism, a point never contested by the Commission. Like Mesmer and d'Eslon, Elliotson was denounced by the medical profession and the practice of mesmerism was prohibited in many English hospitals. The doctor and his pupils reported many successful cases in *The Zoist*, being unwilling to submit these papers to traditional medical journals where they would not have been accepted. Failures were not reported.

Elliotson (1843a) reported an 18-year-old boy with rheumatism and delirium with convulsions, probably associated with fever. The boy made little progress during the first month of medical treatment, which included bleedings, opium, purgatives, head shaving and application of lotions to the scalp, quinine, musk, creosote, iron, prussic acid, and arsenic. His behavior was so violent that he was tied with ropes across his bed and further restrained by three strong men. At this point, Elliotson visited the patient. In the first session, 45 minutes of mesmeric passes had no effect. Elliotson turned the case over to one of his former pupils. The following evening's session lasted over 2 hours; the doctor noted that the convulsive attack—which usually occurred in the evening—ended a bit sooner than usual. Medication was continued in reduced doses. Mesmeric treatment continued each evening, with gradual improvement noted. After 1 week, the doctor reported that the boy was becoming attached to him. To our knowledge, this is the earliest reference to the transference aspects of the hypnotherapeutic relationship. The transference was reported almost in passing, and its role in the curative process was not fully recognized. Eleven days after mesmeric treatment began, the patient's violent attacks ceased, and treatment stopped. He continued to sleep poorly for several weeks, a problem which Elliotson attributed to premature termination of treatment.

In the same paper, Elliotson reported successful mesmeric treatment in 8 cases of chorea, of which 6 were children ranging in age from 9 to 17 years. Duration of treatment ranged from 1 day to 2 months. With the exception of iron, other medications were discontinued, most of them doing more harm than good.

In 1843, Elliotson published a book entitled *Numerous Cases of Surgical Operations Without Pain in the Mesmeric State*, describing both his own work and that of his colleagues. Here he mentioned several cases of painless dental extractions in children. He reported that after 5 minutes of mesmeric passes a colleague had opened a large abscess behind the ear of a 12-year-old boy. The patient was comfortable throughout the procedure. He also reported a colleague's operation on a 17-year-old girl to release knee contractures while she was in a mesmeric trance. She experienced no pain and was unaware that the procedures had been accomplished until she saw spots of blood on the sheets of her hospital bed.

Elliotson concluded from his clinical experience that his favorable results were attributable to mesmeric passes, and he continued to deny most vehemently that imagination played any role in the cures. He apparently never saw that his methods could not provide any evidence in favor of one theory or the other.

JAMES BRAID (1795–1860)

Braid was an English surgeon, a contemporary of Elliotson, who began investigating mesmerism as a complete skeptic. Unlike Elliotson, when he saw that such phenomena as induced catalepsy and analgesia were real, he elected to avoid diatribes and to be open-minded with regard to the underlying theoretical explanation, though he leaned toward imagination as a good possibility.

In 1843, Braid wrote of his techniques:

> I feel we have acquired in this process a valuable addition to our curative means; but I repudiate the idea of holding it up as a universal remedy; nor do I even pretend to understand, as yet, the whole range of diseases in which it may be useful. . . . Whether the extraordinary physical effects are produced through the imagination chiefly, or by other means, it appears to me quite certain, that the imagination has never been so much under our control, or capable of being made to act in the same beneficial and uniform manner, by any other mode of management hitherto known. [Braid, 1843/1960]*

However, Braid rejected the idea that imagination alone could produce trance.

Both for theoretical and for practical reasons, Braid discarded the whole idea of animal magnetism, and he avoided the word mesmerism. Thinking of trance phenomena as some sort of nervous sleep, he coined the term "hypnosis" from the Greek word "hypnos," meaning sleep. He abandoned use of passes and, instead, required his subjects to fix their gaze on an object and concentrate attention on a single idea (monoideism). Braid's elucidation of the psychological aspects of hypnosis were a major contribution, and his theories were subsequently adopted by Broca, Charcot, Liébault, and Bernheim.

---

*From *Neurypnology; or the Rationale of Nervous Sleep* by J. Braid. Revised as *Braid on Hypnotism*, New York: Julian Press, 1960. (Originally published, 1843.) With permission.

Braid was impressed by the ease and rapidity with which trance could be induced, and he took careful notice of instances in which some individuals went into a trance state without any formal induction. In an 1855 work, he reported an anecdote in which an elderly man discovered a boy who had climbed up into one of his apple trees and was in the midst of stealing an apple.

At this moment the gentleman addressed the boy in a *stern* manner, declaring that he would *fix him there* in the position he was then in. Having said so, the gentleman left the orchard and went off to church, not doubting that the boy would soon come down and effect his escape when he knew the master of the orchard was gone. However, it turned out otherwise; for, on going into the orchard on his return from church, he was not a little surprised to find that the boy had been spell-bound by his declaration to that effect—for there he still remained, *in the exact attitude in which he left him, with his arm outstretched, and his hand ready to lay hold of the apple.* By some farther remarks from this gentleman the spell was broken, and the boy allowed to escape without further punishment. [Braid, 1855]

In this and other anecdotes, Braid recognized the power mind has over body, and he pointed out that children were frequently "sensitive" in this regard. He failed to recognize these instances as spontaneous hypnosis, describing them instead as waking phenomena. Holding to the idea that hypnotic phenomena were produced by formal visual and mental fixation, he said, "In cases of children, and those (adults) of weak intellect, or of restless and excitable minds, whom I could not manage so as to make them comply with these simple rules, I have always been foiled, although most anxious to succeed" (Braid, 1843/1960). He made this comment in spite of the fact that, in the same paper, he reported inducing light hypnosis with arm catalepsy in 32 children at once by making them stand and sit over a period of 10 to 12 minutes. It seems that, like Mesmer and Elliotson before him, Braid made the mistake of defining hypnotic phenomena by the techniques he used to produce them.

Braid seemed tantalizingly close to the step of recognizing the independence of trance phenomena from particular induction methods. He fully recognized that the operator involved in trance production did not communicate any magnetic, electric, or other force from his own body, but rather acted as an engineer, using various modes to direct vital forces within the patient's body. He recognized the importance of the patient's faith and confidence in the process. He even recognized the possibility of self-hypnosis, using it to manage his own pains. But it would be several more years before his speculations about the role of imagination in hypnosis would be deliberately applied to child patients.

JEAN-MARTIN CHARCOT (1835–1893)

Charcot, a distinguished French neurologist, began his investigations of hypnosis at the School of the Salpêtrière in 1878. His descriptions of hypnosis in neurological terms gave it a new measure of scientific respectability. By 1882, the subject appeared regularly in the best medical journals as well as in the lay press. Scientific journals devoted entirely to hypnosis sprang up in both France and Germany (Tinterow, 1970).

In spite of—or perhaps because of—Charcot's having his own clinic with ample numbers of assistants to work with patients, he really did little to advance understanding of hypnosis, especially in the case of children. He conceived of hypnosis as a pathological state, a form of hysterical neurosis, able to be produced more easily in women than in men. He considered all children insusceptible. According to a biography by Guillain (cited in Tinterow, 1970), Charcot failed to check the work of his assistants and never personally hypnotized a single patient. Having developed a theory, he unwittingly restricted his experimental work in such a way that the data could only support his ideas. Late in his life, in the face of increasing criticism, he saw the need to revise his theory, but by this time he was quite ill, and he died without beginning the actual work of revision.

AUGUSTE AMBROSE LIÉBAULT (1823–1904) AND HIPPOLYTE BERNHEIM (1840–1919)

At about the same time that Charcot founded the School of the Salpêtrière, Liébault founded another French school devoted to the investigation of hypnosis, the School of Nancy. He was soon joined by Bernheim, and together they developed theories and gathered data that opposed those of Charcot and have since proved to be more accurate. Specifically, they conceived of hypnosis as an entirely normal phenomenon based chiefly on suggestion and imagination, thus clarifying and extending the earlier speculation of Braid. In 1888, Bernheim wrote, "I define hypnotism as the induction of a peculiar psychical condition which increases the susceptibility to suggestion. Often, it is true, the sleep that may be induced facilitates suggestion, but it is not the necessary preliminary. It is suggestion that rules hypnotism" (cited in Tinterow, 1970, p. 454). He concluded that hypnosis occurs as a result of various induction methods "acting upon imagination."

As might be expected on the basis of their theories, Liébault and

Table 2-1
Norms of Hypnotizability

Age (years)	Somnambulism (percentage)	Less Deep Hypnotism (percentage)	Refractory (percentage)
0–6	26.5	73.7	–
7–13	55.3	44.4	–
14–20	25.2	64.2	10.3
21–27	13.2	77.4	9.1
28–34	22.6	71.2	5.9
35–41	10.5	81.1	8.2
42–48	21.6	65.9	12.2
49–55	7.3	87.9	4.4
56–62	7.3	78.0	14.4
63+	11.8	74.3	13.5

Adapted from Bramwell, 1903/1956.

Bernheim found that most children were quickly and easily hypnotized, so long as they were able to pay attention and understand instructions. Their method consisted of eye fixation with repeated suggestions for eye closure and sleep. They did not insist on sleep if the subject showed no such inclinations, but they manually pushed down the eyelids if the subject's eyes remained open more than a few minutes.* Any resistance was met by more forceful commands.

More than their predecessors, Liébault and Bernheim recognized individual differences in response to hypnotic suggestions. Hypnosis was not an all-or-none phenomenon, but could be manifested at varying degrees of depth. The deepest level, somnambulism, and each of the lighter levels had characteristic features, although there were individual differences in response within each level as well as between levels. Once they made these advances toward greater scientific sophistication, the next step was to carry out normative studies on a large scale. According to Bramwell (1903/1956), Liébault compiled data from 755 subjects and found no differences in hypnotizability between males and females. Beaunis restated the data in order to focus on age differences across the whole range from young children to the elderly. As shown in Table 2-1, the highest percentage of somnambules oc-

---

*Although American children today often fail to follow suggestions for eye closure, we must remember that Liébault and Bernheim used more authoritarian methods than most clinicians use now and that their child subjects grew up in a more authoritarian culture than American children today. Hence the differences in compliance are understandable.

curred in children 7 to 14 years of age. No subject in this age group or in the group of children younger than 7 was entirely refractory.

J. MILNE BRAMWELL (1852–1925)

Bramwell was an English psychotherapist who began to use hypnosis in 1889. In 1903, he published *Hypnotism: Its History, Practice, and Theory*, a comprehensive review which was widely quoted as the major text in the field for many years. From vignettes of his own cases and those of his colleagues, we get a good idea of the range of childhood disorders treated with hypnotherapy at the turn of the century. These disorders included: behavior problems (e.g., stealing, lying, masturbation, insolence); chorea; eczema; enuresis; headaches; hyperhidrosis (excessive sweating); nailbiting; night terrors; seizures; and stammering (Bramwell, 1903/1956). The success rate was reportedly very high, but we are not sure whether all failures were reported. The children described ranged in age from 3 to 19.

THE BEGINNING OF CHILD HYPNOTHERAPY IN AMERICA

So far as we know, the first publication concerning child hypnosis in a major American journal was a paper in *Science* entitled "Suggestion in Infancy" (Baldwin, 1891). The author discussed the idea that the rise of interest in hypnosis had opened the way for increased understanding of infant behavior beyond mere physiological or reflex reactions. Such behavior could now be understood in terms of environmental influences, especially what he called ideomotor suggestions. For example, he described his use of reward and punishment to extinguish scratching behavior in a 3-month-old infant. He also discussed the child's development of imitative behavior, beginning at about 8 months. Baldwin did not use hypnosis per se but rather understood the possibility of understanding hypnotic phenomena as a point of departure for the study of consciousness, an idea that has only recently come back into sharp focus (E. R. Hilgard, 1977).

Lightner Witmer, who coined the term "clinical psychology" and opened the first American psychological clinic in 1896 at the University of Pennsylvania, published a sharply critical paper about hypnosis in the 1897 volume of *Pediatrics*. He discussed his alarm that pedagogical uses of hypnosis were often considered a panacea. By his use of the term "pedagogical," he meant not only the use of hypnosis in formal education; he also included any hypnotic treatment in which suggestions were given chiefly for the purpose of educating the patient, e.g., to expend constructive effort in work or to desist from objectionable habits. Like Charcot, Witmer thought that "the susceptibility to hypnotic influence is itself a stigma of neuroticism, perhaps of hysteria" (p. 26). He believed that hypnosis weakened the will and fostered impulsivity, adding that "mental tonic is what such persons need, not such mental perversion as hypnotism is" (p. 27).

In the same volume of *Pediatrics*, Mason (1897) replied to Witmer with matching vehemence in support of pedagogical hypnosis, especially in the case of children. He described the beneficial effects of hypnosis for a wide variety of pediatric problems. He denied that he considered it a panacea, or that it weakened the patient's will or capacity for independent judgment. Countering Witmer's notion of hypnosis as a phenomenon seen chiefly in hysterics, Mason cited Bernheim's hypnotic research with large numbers of normal subjects.

Citing his own case records, Mason reported successful hypnotherapy with a 15-year-old girl suffering from lack of concentration and poor memory for schoolwork, a 7-year-old boy who was too frightened to cooperate with necessary medical treatment, a 5-year-old girl suffering frequent night terrors, and a 16-year-old boy referred because of masturbation and cigarette smoking. In each case "the treatment was essentially educational—the dismissal of the abnormal, hurtful or evil ideas and tendencies and the restoration or introduction of new, normal and helpful ones in their place" (p. 104). Treatment time varied from one session to a long series of visits.

By 1900, both in America and in Europe, interest in child hypnosis was waning and would not revive again for nearly half a century. Then it got off to a slow start, not becoming a major research area until the late 1950s and early 1960s. During the two World Wars, interest in adult hypnosis increased briefly, as a result of pressure to get disabled soldiers back on the battlefield quickly. But, during these periods, little was learned that was relevant to the treatment of children. When interest in child hypnosis increased again in the 1950s, researchers and clinicians began essentially where they had left off half a century before.

CONCLUSIONS

Early reports of hypnotherapy with children were primarily anecdotal, often in the context of emotional appeals to support or refute current theories and speculations about various aspects of human behavior. Nevertheless, by the end of the 19th century, those who had studied the field carefully already knew that children were suitable hypnotic subjects, that the peak of hypnotizability occurred in middle childhood, and that hypnotic techniques were applicable to a wide variety of childhood medical and psychological problems.

REFERENCES

Baldwin, J. M. Suggestion in infancy. *Science*, 1891, *17*, 113–117.

Braid, J. The physiology of fascination and the critics criticized. Manchester, Grant & Co., 1855.

Braid, J. *Neurypnology; or the rationale of nervous sleep*. Revised as *Braid on hypnotism, 1889*. New York: Julian Press, 1960. (Originally published, 1843.)

Bramwell, J. M. *Hypnotism: Its history, practice and theory*. Reissued with new introduction. New York: Julian Press, 1956. (Originally published, 1903.)

Elliotson, J. Cases of cures by mesmerism. *The Zoist*, 1843, *1*, 161–208. (a)

Elliotson, J. *Numerous cases of surgical operations without pain in the mesmeric state*. Philadelphia: Lea and Blanchard, 1843. (b)

Hilgard, E. R. *Divided consciousness: Multiple controls in human thought and action*. New York: John Wiley & Sons, 1977.

Mason, R. O. Educational uses of hypnotism: A reply to Prof. Lightner Witmer's editorial in *Pediatrics* for January 1, 1897. *Pediatrics*, 1897, *3*, 97–105.

Mead, M. *Male and female: A study of the sexes in a changing world*. New York: William Morrow, 1949.

Tinterow, M. M. *Foundations of hypnosis: From Mesmer to Freud*. Springfield, Ill.: Charles C Thomas, 1970.

Witmer, L. The use of hypnotism in education. *Pediatrics*, 1897, *3*, 23–27.

3

Norms of Hypnotizability in Children

The question of degrees of hypnotizability in children is not new. In the 1880s, Liébault (cited in Tinterow, 1970) struggled with it in his studies of hypnotizability that included subjects from early childhood to over 60 years of age. In the 1930s, Clark Hull (1933) and his students, especially Messerschmidt (1933a, 1933b), studied children's responses to waking suggestibility items. Although they did not equate suggestibility with hypnotizability, the two traits were positively correlated.

The results of the early studies were quite similar to more recent studies. That is, early research concluded that hypnotizability and suggestibility are quite limited in young children, increase markedly in the middle childhood years from about 7 to 14, and then decrease somewhat in adolescence, becoming quite stable throughout early and midadulthood, then tailing off again in the older population.

With all normative studies reaching essentially the same conclusion, one is tempted to review them rather briefly and then move on to other issues. The major problem is that these research findings are at variance with a growing body of clinical data indicating that children of preschool age, and perhaps even younger, do in fact respond positively to what is described as the therapeutic use of hypnosis. The issues involved in this controversy are complex. Thus, we choose to confront them head-on, in order to leave the reader with some measure of confusion in place of what appears on the surface to be an easy answer. We begin with a critical review of recent normative studies and then deal with the special problem of hypnotizability in young children.

RECENT NORMATIVE STUDIES

Stukát (1958) and Barber and Calverley (1963) administered tests of suggestibility to children at various ages. Since they did not claim to be using hypnotic techniques, we will not review their studies in detail. It should be noted that their findings for suggestibility are similar to studies measuring hypnotizability. This is seen in Figure 3-1, which compares their results with normative data for hypnotic susceptibility in children. Once can conclude either that the traits measured by the three scales are highly correlated or that suggestibility, as measured by these tests, and hypnotic susceptibility are essentially the same trait.

Commenting on Tromater's (1961) review of early studies of child-

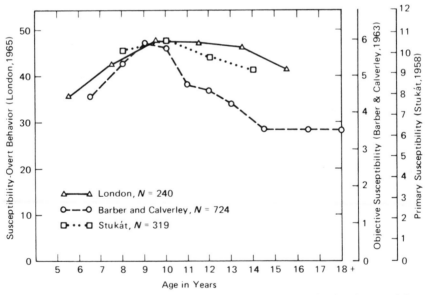

Figure 3-1. *Changes in suggestibility with age. Barber and Calverley's and Stukát's suggestibility scales (not involving hypnosis) correlate highly with hypnotic performances. London did use hypnotic techniques. (Redrawn from "Hypnosis and Childlikeness" by E. R. Hilgard, in J. P. Hill (Ed.),* Minnesota Symposia on Child Psychology *(Vol. 5), Minneapolis: Lund Press, 1971. With permission.)*

hood hypnotizability, London (1962) observed that early efforts to assess hypnotizability in children were in general agreement that children, as a group, are more susceptible than adults and that there is a curvilinear relationship between age and susceptibility, with a peak in the 8- to 12-year age range. London (1962) noted methodological problems in these early studies, especially the lack of an operational definition of susceptibility and imprecise measuring devices, and he set out to remedy these problems.

London developed a test called the Children's Hypnotic Susceptibility Scale (1963) that was based on the items in the Stanford Hypnotic Susceptibility Scale, Form A (SHSS, Form A) (Weitzenhoffer & Hilgard, 1959). The Children's Scale (CHSS) is included in its entirety in Appendix A. It contains 22 items in two parts, of which Part I is parallel in content to SHSS, Form A. Part II contains some more difficult items such as visual hallucinations and thirst and taste hallucinations. Administration of the scale requires 45 to 60 minutes for each child.

Because some children in the pilot studies (London, 1962) appeared to be faking or "playing along" with the instructions, the subjects received two scores for each item, one based on their overt behavioral response (OB) and the other based on the examiner's impression of the extent of the subjects' subjective involvement (SI), that is, whether they appeared to be (1) faking or role playing, (2) partially involved or (3) deeply involved in the item. The product of these two scores yielded a total score (TOT). Usually, the score ultimately derived for each subject is the total for Part I and Part II combined. Sometimes the emphasis is on a part score. For example, if one wants to make comparisons with the SHSS, Form A, a 12-item test scored on the basis of the subject's overt behavior, then one would score the CHSS only for Part I, which contains the 12 parallel items, and only for overt behavior. Interscorer reliability, based on a pilot sample of 36 children, ranged from .90 to .96 for the various part and combined scores. Retest reliability, based on overt behavior scores of 39 children retested after 1 week, was .92, indicating consistent performance in children similar to that found for adults.

Using data from 57 children, London (1962) found that children were more often successful on almost all CHSS items, as compared with adults on the SHSS, lending further credence to the notion that children are more susceptible. London was unable to establish a significant curvilinear relationship between age and susceptibility, although there was a trend in that direction. He predicted that the trend would become statistically meaningful when the sample size was increased, but he thought the curve would remain a shallow one, indicating that the relationship between susceptibility and age cannot be accounted for simply on the basis of age. He noted that "there is probably more variability among children at any given age than between children of any two successive ages" (p. 87).

To study the possibility that role playing might account for high scores among some children, London (1962) selected a new sample of 40 children, age 5 to 11 years, the group in which role playing tended to occur. After performing six "playlets," he engaged each subject in a simulation task, following the motivation instructions for adults designed by Orne (1959). In his classic studies of hypnotic simulation, Orne compared nonhypnotizable subjects who were told to simulate hypnosis with highly hypnotizable subjects and found that even well-trained examiners could not tell which subjects belonged to which group. London's instructions to each child in his simulation study were as follows:

> We are going to be alone in this room for a couple more minutes and then I am going to get Mrs. X. When she comes in, she will think that I have hypnotized you, and that you are in a deep hypnotic trance. Do you know what that means? Well, what I want you to do is make her think that you are really hypnotized, and to do everything she tells you as if you were hypnotized. The things will be very easy for you, and the only thing you need to know is that, when she comes in, your eyes should be closed, and always keep them closed unless she tells you to open them.
>
> Now, she may be a little bit suspicious that you aren't hypnotized because she knows that there will be one or two kids in here who are just faking, and she will wonder a little if it is you. If she thinks that you are faking, she will stop what she is doing right away—but as long as she keeps on going, you will know that you are fooling her into thinking you are hypnotized. [p. 87]*

For the children in this limited age range, there was a linear relationship between age and simulation ability. The simulation scores on the CHSS, Part II were lower than those for hypnotic subjects below age 8 but merged thereafter. In other words, simulation was obvious below age 8, but indistinguishable from hypnotic performance at higher ages. Noting that the youngest subjects were poor simulators and that older adolescents tend to be too honest to simulate on hypnotic susceptibility tests, London was left with the conclusion that "children in the middle group achieve peak scores because they can communicate simulated performances with the same effectiveness that

---

*Reprinted from the April 1962 *International Journal of Clinical and Experimental Hypnosis.* Copyrighted by the Society for Clinical and Experimental Hypnosis, April, 1962.

they do real performances and we cannot tell them apart" (p. 90). This does not mean that all children in this group simulate, and those that do may do so only on selected items. Yet, when these children do simulate, it is not likely to be noticed, even by trained examiners. London concluded that the evidence for curvilinearity is weak, and is even further weakened by the insensitivity of the CHSS to the simulation of individual items.

London noted that the subjects in these studies were chiefly from upper-middle-class backgrounds but did not speculate about the impact of social class distribution on his results.

London (1965) standardized his scale on a group of 240 children, ages 5 to 16, with 10 boys and 10 girls at each year level. These subjects came from a group of 303 children whose parents responded to a form letter. Again the sample was markedly skewed toward the upper-middle-class professional and managerial level. For this new sample, interscorer reliability for the Full Scale CHSS ranged from .88 to .97 for the three obtained scores (overt behavior, subjective involvement, and total). Test–retest reliability (N = 50) after 1 week ranged from .75 to .84.

As in the pilot studies, there was a modest curvilinear relationship between age and susceptibility, with the peak in the 9- to 12-year range (Fig. 3-2). And again the standard deviations were large at all ages. London noted that "the extent of susceptibility or the lack of it

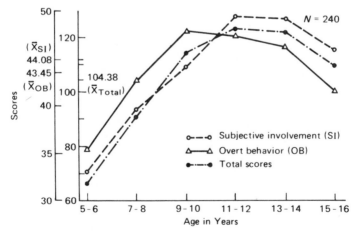

Figure 3-2. *Mean Full Scale susceptibility scores, by age group, of the standardization sample (N=240) for the CHSS. (Redrawn from "Developmental Experiments in Hypnosis" by P. London, Journal of Projective Techniques and Personality Assessment, 1965, 29, 189–199. With permission.)*

among different children within a single age group is more impressive than are changes across ages" (p. 195).

The mean score of the standardization sample of 240 children (8.16) was significantly larger than the mean score of college students (5.25) in the normative data for the SHSS, Form A. When scores were grouped into high, medium, and low categories for children, the largest group fell in the range of high susceptibility; for adults, the largest group fell in the range of low susceptibility. These data again support the notion that children are more susceptible to hypnosis than adults (London & Cooper, 1969).

Cooper and London (1971) reported longitudinal data for a subset of the standardization sample. The intercorrelations across time periods, ranging from 1 week to 2 years, were significantly positive, but by no means perfect. Moreover, the correlations for younger children were lower than those for older children. These results are similar to those obtained in the measurement of intelligence, namely, that it is harder to predict from obtained scores to future scores for younger children than for older children. Results of this longitudinal study were similar to those of the cross-sectional studies, leading the authors to conclude that changes in susceptibility do occur with age and that these changes are extremely stable.

Morgan and E. R. Hilgard (1973) reported a massive study of age differences in hypnotic susceptibility for 1232 subjects, ranging in age from 5 to 78 years. Again the subjects clustered in the middle socioeconomic class. The results for children, based on a slightly modified SHSS, Form A, were similar to those cited earlier, with a peak in the preadolescent years and a gradual decline thereafter. Morgan and Hilgard did not comment on the issue of simulation.

There were no significant sex differences in hypnotic susceptibility in any of these studies or in the report of Cooper and London (1966), which specifically addressed this issue.

The most recent normative study (Morgan & J. R. Hilgard, 1979) came to the same conclusions regarding age and hypnotizability as the earlier studies. Its significance lies in the fact that the score is based on a short scale, The Stanford Hypnotic Clinical Scale for Children (SHCS-Child) that can be administered in 20 minutes. This scale is presented in Appendix B. The brevity of the scale makes it feasible to use in a primarily therapeutic setting, thus providing a beginning means to address the question of whether the child whose condition improves in the process of hypnotherapy actually improves because of hypnotherapy.

Over the years, many clinicians have argued that the use of a scale to measure hypnotizability was, at best, irrelevant and, at worst, improper. They argued that clinical and laboratory hypnosis are two different entities with little or no connection. Then they argued that, even if a scale could measure the kind of hypnotizability that is observed in a clinical setting, patients subjected to such a scale would experience frustration and failure that would both interfere with rapport and compromise therapeutic progress. Contrary to the assumptions of the first argument, Hilgard and Hilgard (1975) have found that adult subjects who score higher on a hypnotizability scale tend to respond more effectively to suggestions for pain control, both in experimental and in clinical settings. Contrary to the assumptions of the second argument, Morgan and J. R. Hilgard (1979) did not find any marked concerns about failure in the context of their permissive induction and suggestions. If a child began to apologize for a failed item, the examiner immediately countered with, "We are just as interested in what people don't experience as we are in what people do experience." Children in the clinical setting were told, "Not everybody does the same things. We have to find those things that are best for you, some you will find much more interesting than others. There will be some that we can build on" (Morgan & J. R. Hilgard, 1979, p. 154).

The Morgan and Hilgard (1979) study makes another major contribution to the field of hypnosis. Unfortunately the authors make no mention of it, and we would like to take this opportunity to give them the credit they deserve. For the first time in the series of studies reported here, the term "susceptibility" has been omitted and the term "responsivity" used in its place. This shift reflects a growing awareness that the capacity to experience hypnosis is chiefly a skill or talent of the subject and not a phenomenon created by the hypnotist. The hypnotist is a teacher or guide rather than a controlling force. Thus the term "hypnotic virtuoso" describes the behavior of the subject, not the hypnotist. The change in terminology reflects the change over the last few decades from an authoritarian to a permissive approach in hypnosis and hypnotherapy. We are in full agreement that the locus of control should be and is in the subject. Therefore, in this book, we use the term "responsiveness" or its equivalent except when referring to historical matters.

The SHCS-Child includes one form for children 6 to 16 years old and another form for children 4 to 8 years old. The form for older children is based on an eye closure-relaxation induction followed by seven test items. The form for younger children is based on an active imagination induction, since young or immature children often respond negatively to suggestions for eye closure. This form contains six test items. In both forms, the items are intrinsically interesting to children, allow some success at all ages, and have direct relevance for choice of therapeutic techniques. The test correlated .67 with the longer Stanford Hypnotic Susceptibility Scale, Form A, modified slightly for use with children.

In the early stages of its development, the SHCS-Child consisted of only one form, utilizing an eye closure-relaxation induction. The second form (active imagination) was created when the authors discovered that the younger children failed most or all items in the relaxation condition but passed some of the same items in the imagination condition. At that time, exhibiting a degree of flexibility not seen in earlier studies, the authors modified the induction for younger children so that they could pass more items. The awareness of this need for flexibility now takes us into a new area, guaranteed to confuse more than to clarify what has already become a muddied field in the area of norms of hypnotizability in children.

HYPNOSIS AS A FUNCTION OF INDUCTION AND MEASUREMENT TECHNIQUES

Historically, the measurement of hypnotic susceptibility (responsivity) has consisted of a hypnotic induction emphasizing relaxation and eye closure followed by a number of test items reflecting various phenomena that most people agree typify hypnotic behavior. Subjects who score very low on these scales are said not to be hypnotizable. Moreover, some researchers (e.g., Barber, 1979) have taken the position that, if there is no formal hypnotic induction, the subject cannot be said to be in hypnosis at all.

We disagree with Barber's position. As yet, there is no absolute knowledge of the boundaries that define hypnosis. But we take the position that certain kinds of behavior can be described as hypnotic behavior. These behaviors include, but are not limited to, the behaviors elicited by standard scales of hypnotizability. And it is important to note that people vary in terms of their ability to experience different hypnotic phenomena. For example, two individuals with identical scores on a hypnotizability scale may have passed different kinds of items in order to obtain those scores.

We also believe that people vary in terms of the antecedent conditions that are necessary in order to experience hypnosis. In this regard, we find it refreshing that Morgan and J. R. Hilgard (1979) directed their research to show that some children respond positively to test items following one kind of induction but not another. Figure 3-3

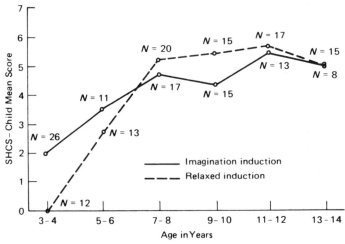

Figure 3-3. *Mean scores by age on seven items of the SHCH-Child. Imagination induction is compared with relaxation induction. (Redrawn from "The Stanford Hypnotic Clinical Scale for Children" by A. H. Morgan and J. R. Hilgard,* The American Journal of Clinical Hypnosis, *1979, 21, 148–155. With permission.)*

shows the mean scores for their subjects following eye closure-relaxation and imagination inductions.

When children obtain different scores following different induction procedures, one might ask which scores are the "true" scores. We answer simply whichever scores are higher. That is, the purpose of a scale of hypnotic responsiveness is to allow the subjects to demonstrate their skills. But the findings of Morgan and J. R. Hilgard suggest that, in measuring hypnotizability, we have put some children in a position, through inappropriate induction techniques, where they do not do what they really can do. We then come to the false conclusion that they really cannot do it.

The situation is analogous to forcing a child into a sitting position and then measuring height by the distance of the child's head from the floor. Or, we could picture tying a child's hands behind his back, and then concluding that he is not mature enough to tie his shoes. We can only wonder what the normative data of London and Cooper and others would look like—particularly for younger children—if they modified the hypnotic induction in such a way as to maximize the child's ability to respond to the test items.

If the nature of hypnotic induction can affect scores on a responsivity scale, then the nature of the test items themselves will clearly also affect the scores. Logically, some items will be passed at virtually all ages, some at one age but not another, and some items might not be passed by children of any age. The test score will depend on which kinds of items and how many of each kind and which difficulty levels are included. As with intelligence, ultimately the meaning of hypnotizability is reduced to what precisely is tested by the test.

E. R. Hilgard and colleagues (Hilgard, Weitzenhoffer, Landes, & Moore, 1961) recognized the need for an operational definition when they wrote that "what we shall mean by hypnotic susceptibility for the purpose of our investigations is a relatively persistent tendency to yield the phenomena historically recognized as belonging to the hypnotic trance, *when the opportunity to yield these phenomena is given under standard conditions*" (p. 1). Adult scales of hypnotizability sample a variety of hypnotic phenomena, with items placed roughly in order of difficulty and high scorers considered more "susceptible" than low ones.

In the case of children, degrees of item difficulty are not the same as those for adults or even for children of different ages. Therefore we must at least pause before we conclude that, on a particular scale of children's hypnotic responsiveness, a specific score necessarily means the same thing that it does on an adult scale. We must question whether the broad-sample-of-hypnotic-phenomena approach is as appropriate for children as it is for adults. That is, some so-called traditional hypnotic phenomena may be traditional for adults but not for children or for certain groups of children because of developmental issues. To use another analogy, we do not administer to young children the same types of intelligence test items we use for adults on, say, the Stanford Binet, recognizing that certain language and abstract reasoning skills are simply not developed in the young child. That is, we define intelligence somewhat differently for young children than for adults.

Moreover, if we want the concept "hypnosis" to mean roughly the same thing for children as for adults, then we should be reasonably confident that a given item is tapping the same thing for children as for adults as well as tapping the same thing for children of different ages. Such item equivalence is probably not the case in some instances, as evidenced by data relating age to item difficulty on scales of hypnotic responsiveness in children.

London and Cooper (1969) reported item difficulty for their standardization sample of 240 children for the Children's Hypnotic Susceptibility Scale (CHSS), and they compared percent passing each item with the equivalent data for adults on the SHSS, Form A. In Table 3-1 we have adapted these data, and rank ordered each item in terms of relative difficulty for children and for adults.

Table 3-1
Item Difficulty for Children on the CHSS and
for Adults on the SHSS, Form A

Item	Rank Order of Difficulty*	
	Children	Adults
Auditory hallucination	1.0	6.0
Postural sway	2.0	3.0
Hands together	3.0	2.0
Hand lowering	4.0	1.0
Finger lock	5.0	8.0
Posthypnotic suggestion	6.5	5.0
Amnesia	6.5	8.0
Arm rigidity	8.0	8.0
Verbal inhibition	9.0	11.0
Eye catalepsy	10.0	10.0
Arm immobilization	11.0	12.0
Eye closure	12.0	4.0

Adapted from London and Cooper, 1969.
*1 = easiest item; 12 = hardest item.

When these data are studied, the most striking finding is that eye closure is the most difficult item of all for children, while it is relatively easy for adults. We suspect that, in the case of children, suggestions for eye closure trigger negative attitudes and concerns about sleep and that these issues preclude the sort of detached interest in motor phenomena that most likely predominates for adults. If the item is tapping something in children that has little or nothing to do with hypnosis, then it really does not belong in the test.

Moore and Cooper (1966) commented on the difficulty with eye closure for children as compared to adults. They noted that the CHSS employs a Chevreul pendulum for this item with the instruction to hold the chain, look at the ball, and try to prevent it from moving. The parallel adult item (SHSS, Form B) required the subject merely to look passively at a fixed target. They concluded that "for children, it may be that the interesting activity of trying to hold the attractive plastic ball stationary is less conducive to eye closure than focusing the gaze on a target some distance away" (p. 320). If this is true, then again the two items are not measuring the same thing.

To give another example, children find the auditory hallucination item very easy (89 percent pass) whereas for adults it is moderately difficult (35 percent pass). In this case, we have a notion that the item

Table 3-2

Relative Item Difficulty on the CHSS across Age Levels (N = 240)

Item	Age (years)*					
	5–6	7–8	9–10	11–12	13–14	15–16
Amnesia	1.0	11.5	13.0	10.0	16.0	12.0
Auditory hallucination	2.0	2.0	2.0	1.5	1.0	4.5
Hands together	3.5	6.0	5.0	12.5	4.5	3.0
Cold hallucination	3.5	4.0	5.0	7.0	8.0	6.0
Postural sway	5.0	9.0	8.5	3.5	2.5	1.5
Television	6.5	6.0	3.5	5.5	8.0	10.0
Visual hallucination	6.5	1.0	1.0	1.5	4.5	8.5
Finger lock	8.0	8.0	8.5	12.5	6.0	12.0
Hand lowering	9.0	3.0	11.5	10.0	8.0	4.5
Taste hallucination	10.0	6.0	5.0	3.5	10.0	15.5
Arm rigidity	11.0	11.5	10.0	16.0	19.0	19.5
Verbal inhibition	13.0	15.5	16.0	18.0	13.5	19.5
Smell hallucination	13.0	10.0	17.0	8.0	16.0	8.5
Dream	13.0	13.0	3.5	5.5	2.5	1.5
Posthypnotic suggestion II	15.0	15.5	14.5	21.0	18.0	17.0
Arm immobilization	16.0	18.0	19.5	17.0	13.5	19.5
Eye closure	17.5	21.0	22.0	22.0	21.0	15.5
Posthypnotic suggestion I	17.5	15.5	11.5	10.0	11.0	12.0
Eye catalepsy	19.5	15.5	14.5	20.0	16.0	22.0
Anesthesia	19.5	19.5	19.5	19.0	20.0	19.5
Regression	21.5	19.5	21.0	14.5	12.0	7.0
Posthypnotic suggestion III	21.5	22.0	18.0	14.5	22.0	14.0

Adapted from London and Cooper, 1969.
*1 = easiest item; 22 = hardest item.

probably is measuring the same for children as for adults, with children simply being more skilled at this particular task.

Moore and Lauer (1963) studied item difficulty for a sample of 48 children, age 6 to 12, and compared their data to adult scores, with essentially the same results as London and Cooper's (1969) sample.

Questions about the meaning of test items become even more interesting when we look at the data in Table 3-2, showing the relative difficulty of each item for children at different ages. Although we have not attempted any statistical analysis of these data, we are struck by several instances in which there are marked shifts in difficulty level from one age group to another. For example, it is astonishing that the amnesia item is the easiest of all for the 5- to 6-year-olds, while it is moderately difficult for children at all other ages and for adults. We strongly suspect that, while the item taps problems of memory retrieval for subjects beyond age 6, it taps problems of memory storage in the very young child. Since memory storage is not really what the item is designed to measure, it should probably not be in the test for this young age group.

All this goes to say that we agree with E. R. Hilgard and colleagues (1961). If a scale purports to sample hypnotic phenomena, then it should do that and not something else. We would therefore anticipate some sort of revision of the CHSS in the same way and for the same reasons that intelligence tests or aptitude tests are subjected to item analysis and revised according to the data obtained.

After having dealt with some of the more formal problems involved in test construction, we now turn to the relevance of a hypnotic responsiveness scale for a therapeutic situation. Morgan (1974) and Morgan and J. R. Hilgard (1979) both address this issue. Morgan noted that the factor analytic studies on the SHSS, Form A yielded three main factors: factor I included challenge items (e.g., arm immobilization, finger lock); factor II included direct suggestion items (e.g., hand lowering, eye closure); factor III included cognitive items (e.g., fly hallucination, posthypnotic amnesia). Morgan noted that challenge items are relatively difficult for children and place the locus of control outside the child. Moreover, such items may encourage young children to balk because they have not yet resolved developmental issues in which oppositional behavior is a major response style. Morgan concluded that use of such items is probably undesirable in a treatment situation. On the other hand, direct suggestion items are easy for children, are readily converted to autosuggestions, and may therefore be especially appropriate in the context of treatment. Likewise, cognitive items are easy and also may provide information which is useful in treatment. Morgan and J. R. Hilgard (1979) applied these conclusions advantageously in the development of their short clinical scale for children. In other words, general hypnotic responsivity is not the same as the particular kind or kinds of responsivity that may be appropriate and relevant in a clinical situation. One should be able to predict something about treatment response from the latter but not necessarily from the former.

HYPNOSIS AND THE YOUNG CHILD

Several clinical reports have claimed the effectiveness of hypnotherapy with preschool children for such diverse problems as easing induction of anesthesia (Antitch, 1967; Cullen, 1958), alleviating distress and reducing pain (Gardner, 1978; LaBaw, 1973; Olness, in press), controlling enuresis and encopresis (Olness, 1975, 1976), and adjusting to contact lenses (Olness & Gardner, 1978). Yet the available scales indicated that 5- and 6-year-old children are not very responsive as compared with older children. The recent short clinical scale (Morgan & J. R. Hilgard, 1979) reaches down to age 4, and we have virtually no information about children age 3 and younger. It is generally assumed that children too young for the scales would score even lower than the 5-year-olds for whom data are available. Since we must assume that subjects who are not hypnotizable could not profitably utilize hypnosis in the course of treatment, we must either conclude that the claims for hypnotherapeutic efficacy are based on some aspect of the therapeutic relationship or process other than hypnosis, or we must revise our assumptions about hypnotizability.

Gardner (1977) reviewed the question of hypnosis with infants and preschool children in some detail, noting that the primary problem is how one defines hypnosis.

> The tendency has been to look at a score on a scale, or to consider a response to some sort of formal hypnotic induction, or at least to assess the subject's verbal report of his own experiences. These criteria are not applicable to very young children; we have no scales below age 5, generally recognized formal induction methods do not exist below about age 4, and the youngsters do not have adequate verbal fluency to describe their experiences in acceptable detail.
>
> In the absence of the usual criteria for defining hypnosis, one must rely on observations of certain behaviors of the young child which are similar to behaviors associated with hypnosis in adults. These include (1) quiet, wakeful behavior, which may or may not lead to sleep, following soothing repetitive stimulation which is a primary characteristic of most formal induction procedures, (2) involvement in vivid imagery during induction in children beyond infancy, (3) heightened attention to a narrow focus with concomitant alterations in awareness, (4) capacity to follow post-hypnotic suggestions as evidenced by behavior which deviates from what is known to be the child's usual behavior in a particular situation. [pp. 158-159]*

Gardner (1977) reviewed clinical evidence supporting the notion that small children develop reliable ways of quieting themselves, such as rocking or talking rhythmically. She noted that parents also find reliable ways of calming their young children. Specific examples include stroking some part of the body, playing music, turning on a vacuum cleaner, and putting an electric shaver near the child. She has

---

*From "Hypnosis with Infants and Preschool Children" by G. G. Gardner, *The American Journal of Clinical Hypnosis*, 1977, *19*, 158-162. With permission.

since found that the sound of a small hair dryer has the same quieting effect on a fretful infant. She described young patients who responded positively to rhythmic stimulation. She noted studies of hypnosis (Morgan, 1973; Ruch, 1975) in which the authors suggest that hypnotic talent may be present from a very young age or even from birth, and she also reported pertinent studies in child development that show children as young as 2 having the capacity for fantasy and rapport and the desire for mastery intrinsic to the hypnotic situation. She suggested developing a scale that might tap hypnotic potentialities in very young children, adding that hypnotherapy might be more appropriate for this age group than hitherto recognized.

A test of hypnotic responsiveness may be conceptualized as a work sample; for any subject, one must be sure that the work sample is relevant to available behavior and abilities. Rather than insisting that hypnotic responsiveness is present only if a large number of hypnotic phenomena can be elicited, it might be more useful in the case of very young children to start from a position closer to Bartlett's (1968) definition of hypnosis as "a control of the normal control of input (information) for the purpose of controlling output (behavior)" (p. 69). Some hypnosis researchers seem to be moving in this general direction.

For example, J. R. Hilgard and Morgan (1978) noted the following:

First, for the young child, approximately the age group of four to six, with as always a few exceptions, it is inappropriate to rely upon formal hypnotic procedures. These procedures involve two major elements: (a) the implied difference between voluntary and involuntary action, and (b) the expectation of distraction through self-controlled fantasy. Instead, this group is more responsive to a kind of *protohypnosis*, in which the distraction has at first been set up in the external situation. That is, the very young child is better able to be distracted by listening to a story or by participating in a verbal game with a friendly adult than by removing himself from the scene through his own fantasy or through reliving an earlier game or experience on his own. Gradually the content of the external stimulation can be altered in such a way that the child achieves the control. From the beginning, the primary goal is to give the control to the child. This technique of distraction works with children who are unable to use formal hypnosis; such a group also includes some of the older children. [p. 286]*

In a later paper, the same authors concluded that "the child under 6 is hypnotizable, but not according to the same practices commonly used with older children" (p. 154).

---

*From "Treatment of Anxiety and Pain in Childhood Cancer through Hypnosis" by J. R. Hilgard and A. H. Morgan, in F. H. Frankel and H. S. Zamansky (Eds.), *Hypnosis at its Bicentennial: Selected Papers*, New York: Plenum Press, 1978. With permission.

In the 1978 paper, J. R. Hilgard and Morgan noted the rather poor response of the youngest children to hypnotic suggestions for pain and anxiety control during such major medical procedures as spinal taps and bone marrow aspirates. We would add that, even if these results follow from the use of fully appropriate induction techniques and suggestions, the fact that the young subjects did not respond much to hypnosis for this purpose does not mean they might not respond positively in some less threatening situation. General hypnotic responsiveness and responsiveness in a particular laboratory or clinical setting may be two very different things.

In the case of young children, the field is wide open for advances in the study of hypnotic responsivity and its clinical applications.

CONCLUSIONS

We have strayed far from the simple curvilinear relationship, with its peak in the middle childhood years that is often assumed to describe accurately the norms of hypnotizability in children. Major problems include the difficulty in identifying instances in which subjects in middle childhood simulate hypnosis, use of samples limited to the middle socioeconomic class, very large standard deviations, weaknesses in test construction, frequent use of induction techniques that may interfere with hypnotic responsiveness, use of items to measure hypnotizability that may actually be measuring something quite different, and lack of data and methods of assessing hypnotizability in very young children.

The truth is that we really cannot say very much with confidence concerning hypnotic responsiveness in children. While there is obviously a tremendous need for more research, we believe we can conclude two things. First, most studies err on the side of underestimating children's hypnotic talent. Second—and this conclusion derives from the first—the lack of solid evidence concerning children's hypnotic responsiveness does not imply that we should abandon our clinical efforts to help children through hypnotherapy. On the contrary, in a context of proper modesty, we should continue and expand clinical efforts and thereby enlarge the data bank. Many children do respond to hypnotherapy, and many reports conclude that the crucial element in treatment is hypnosis and not something else. In a field where the state of the art is not as primitive as it is in child hypnosis, such an argument would, at best, be considered very weak. In this field, however, it seems to be the only reasonable place to stand for the time being.

REFERENCES

Antitch, J. L. S. The use of hypnosis in pediatric anesthesia. *Journal of the American Society of Psychosomatic Dentistry and Medicine*, 1967, *14*, 70–75.

Barber, T. X. Suggested ("hypnotic") behavior: The trance paradigm versus an alternative paradigm. In E. Fromm and R. E. Shor (Eds.), *Hypnosis: Developments in research and new perspectives* (2nd ed.). Hawthorne, N.Y.: Aldine, 1979.

Barber, T. X., & Calverley, D. S. "Hypnotic-like" suggestibility in children. *Journal of Abnormal and Social Psychology*, 1963, *66*, 589–597.

Bartlett, E. E. A proposed definition of hypnosis with a theory of its mechanism of action. *The American Journal of Clinical Hypnosis*, 1968, *11*, 69–73.

Cooper, L. M., & London, P. Sex and hypnotic susceptibility in children. *The International Journal of Clinical and Experimental Hypnosis*, 1966, *14*, 55–60.

Cooper, L. M., & London, P. The development of hypnotic susceptibility: A longitudinal (convergence) study. *Child Development*, 1971, *42*, 487–503.

Cullen, S. C. Current comment and case reports: Hypno-induction techniques in pediatric anesthesia. *Anesthesiology*, 1958, *19*, 279–281.

Gardner, G. G. Hypnosis with infants and preschool children. *The American Journal of Clinical Hypnosis*, 1977, *19*, 158–162.

Gardner, G. G. The use of hypnotherapy in a pediatric setting. In E. Gellert (Ed.), *Psychosocial aspects of pediatric care*. New York: Grune & Stratton, 1978.

Hilgard, E. R. Hypnosis and childlikeness. In J. P. Hill (Ed.), *Minnesota Symposia on Child Psychology* (Vol. 5). Minneapolis: Lund Press, 1971.

Hilgard, E. R., & Hilgard, J. R. *Hypnosis in the relief of pain*. Los Altos, Calif.: William Kaufman, Inc., 1975.

Hilgard, E. R., Weitzenhoffer, A. M., Landes, J., & Moore, R. K. The distribution of susceptibility to hypnosis in a student population: A study using the Stanford Hypnotic Susceptibility Scale. *Psychological Monographs*, 1961, *75*, (8, Whole No. 512).

Hilgard, J. R., & Morgan, A. H. Treatment of anxiety and pain in childhood cancer through hypnosis. In F. H. Frankel and H. S. Zamansky (Eds.), *Hypnosis at its bicentennial: Selected papers*. New York: Plenum Press, 1978.

Hull, C. L. *Hypnosis and suggestibility: An experimental approach*. New York: D. Appleton-Century, 1933.

LaBaw, W. L. Adjunctive trance therapy with severely burned children. *International Journal of Child Psychotherapy*, 1973, *2*, 80–92.

London, P. Hypnosis in children: An experimental approach. *The International Journal of Clinical and Experimental Hypnosis*, 1962, *10*, 79–91.

London, P. *Children's Hypnotic Susceptibility Scale*. Palo Alto, Calif.: Consulting Psychologists Press, 1963.

London, P. Developmental experiments in hypnosis. *Journal of Projective Techniques and Personality Assessment*, 1965, *29*, 189–199.

London, P., & Cooper, L. M. Norms of hypnotic susceptibility in children. *Developmental Psychology*, 1969, *1*, 113–124.

Messerschmidt, R. Responses of boys between the ages of five and sixteen years to Hull's postural suggestion test. *Journal of Genetic Psychology*, 1933, *43*, 405–421. (a)

Messerschmidt, R. The suggestibility of boys and girls between the ages of six and sixteen years. *Journal of Genetic Psychology*, 1933, *43*, 422–437. (b)

Moore, R. K., & Cooper, L. M. Item difficulty in childhood hypnotic susceptibility scales as a function of item wording, repetition, and age. *The International Journal of Clinical and Experimental Hypnosis*, 1966, *14*, 316–323.

Moore, R. K., & Lauer, L. W. Hypnotic susceptibility in middle childhood. *The International Journal of Clinical and Experimental Hypnosis*, 1963, *11*, 167–174.

Morgan, A. H. The heritability of hypnotic susceptibility in twins. *Journal of Abnormal Psychology*, 1973, *82*, 55–61.

Morgan, A. H. Hypnotizability in children as a function of the nature of the suggestion item. Paper presented at the 82nd American Psychological Association Convention, New Orleans, 1974.

Morgan, A. H., & Hilgard, E. R. Age differences in susceptibility to hypnosis. *The International Journal of Clinical and Experimental Hypnosis*, 1973, *21*, 78–85.

Morgan, A. H., & Hilgard, J. R. The Stanford Hypnotic Clinical Scale for Children. *The American Journal of Clinical Hypnosis*, 1979, *21*, 148–155.

Olness, K. The use of self-hypnosis in the treatment of childhood nocturnal enuresis: A report on forty patients. *Clinical Pediatrics*, 1975, *14*, 273–279.

Olness, K. Autohypnosis in functional megacolon in children. *The American Journal of Clinical Hypnosis*, 1976, *19*, 28–32.

Olness, K. Imagery (self-hypnosis) as adjunct therapy in childhood cancer: Clinical experience with 25 patients. *Journal of Pediatric Hematology-Oncology*, in press.

Olness, K., & Gardner, G. G. Some guidelines for uses of hypnotherapy in pediatrics. *Pediatrics*, 1978, *62*, 228–233.

Orne, M. T. The nature of hypnosis: Artifact and essence. *Journal of Abnormal and Social Psychology*, 1959, *58*, 277–299.

Ruch, J. C. Self-hypnosis: The result of heterohypnosis or vice-versa? *The International Journal of Clinical and Experimental Hypnosis*, 1975, *23*, 282–304.

Stukát, K. G. *Suggestibility: A factorial and experimental analysis.* Stockholm: Almquist & Wiksell, 1958.

Tinterow, M. M. *Foundations of hypnosis: From Mesmer to Freud.* Springfield, Ill.: Charles C Thomas, 1970.

Tromater, F. T. Some developmental correlates of hypnotic susceptibility. Unpublished master's thesis, University of Illinois, Urbana, 1961.

Weitzenhoffer, A. M., & Hilgard, E. R. *Stanford Hypnotic Susceptibility Scale, Forms A and B.* Palo Alto, Calif.: Consulting Psychologists Press, 1959.

4

Correlates of Childhood Hypnotic Responsiveness

Researchers and clinicians have wrestled with the problem of determining why children, as a group, are more responsive to hypnosis than adults. Some suggested answers are based on research; others are derived from theories of child development; still others are derived from informal observations of children. We will discuss a wide variety of possible correlates, evaluating the available data. A few correlates have already been discussed and we mention them briefly for the sake of completion.

VARIABLES

Age

The relationship between age and hypnotic responsivity is very complex. The repeated finding of a modest curvilinear relationship, with its peak in middle childhood, may or may not be entirely accurate. Some of the correlates postulated below derive from the assumption that the results of the normative studies are truly a reflection of reality.

Sex

We have noted that there are no significant differences in hypnotic responsiveness between boys and girls at any age. Therefore, it is reasonable to combine data for both sexes in discussing research and clinical findings.

Nature of the Induction and of the Suggestion Item

Children of different ages respond best to different kinds of inductions, and specific items may measure different dimensions at one age than at another. The reader will have to bear this in mind in evaluating clinical findings presented in later chapters.

Genetics

Morgan, E. R. Hilgard, and Davert (1970) studied hypnotic responsiveness of 76 pairs of twins, together with their parents and siblings close in age, using the SHSS, Form A (Weitzenhoffer & E. R. Hilgard, 1959). Morgan (1973) later increased the twin sample to 140 pairs, including the original 76. Since larger samples yield more reliable data, we will report data only from the more recent study. The twins' age range was 5 to 22 years. Zygosity of the twin pairs was based primarily on the mothers' reports, this method having been found to correlate very highly with serological methods. Both members of a twin pair were hypnotized simultaneously, in separate rooms, in order to avoid experimenter bias or communication between the twins. Parents also completed a questionnaire, rating each child for similarity to father and to mother on 11 personality and temperamental variables.

The correlations for monozygotic twins were statistically significant both for males ($r = .54$) and for females ($r = .49$). Correlations for dizygotic twins and for sibling nontwin pairs were not different from zero ($r = .08 - .25$). Moreover, the correlation for monozygotic pairs ($r = .52$) was significantly higher than the correlation for like-sexed dizygotic pairs ($r = .18$). These data, together with a computed heritability index of .64 and a low but significant correlation between midparent and mean child susceptibility, were consistent with the interpretation of a genetic contribution.

Personality resemblance, as rated by the parents, was positively related to hypnotizability scores for either sexed child and the like-sexed parent. No such interaction existed for either sexed child and the opposite-sexed parent. Morgan (1973) interpreted these results as suggesting an environmental contribution to hypnotizability, based mainly on identification with the like-sexed parent and modeling of that parent's behavior. She concluded that "hypnotizability thus appears to be the product of both a genetic predisposition and subsequent environmental influences, as well as their interaction" (p. 61).

Cognitive Development

London (1965) correlated hypnotizability scores on the CHSS (London, 1963) with intelligence test scores for a group of 42 children, age 8 to 12, taken from his standardization sample and for a group of 54 children, age 6 to 12, participating in the Fels Institute Longitudinal Study. For the first group, IQ scores were extrapolated from scores on the Vocabulary subtest of the Wechsler Intelligence Scale for Children (WISC) (Wechsler, 1949). For the Fels group, complete WISC scores were available. The relationship between hypnotizability and intelligence was positive but modest. Comparing the difference in the correlation coefficients for the two samples, London concluded that the Fels sample data ($r = .25$) were probably more accurate than the standardization sample ($r = .43$).

Jacobs and Jacobs (1966) studied hypnotizability of 64 school children, age 4 to 17, who were referred because of poor school achievement associated with a variety of factors including manifest brain injury, mental retardation, delinquency, behavior disorders, and psychoses. No standardized scale of hypnotizability was utilized. The subjects were considered to be in hypnosis "when eye closure with rhythmic eyeball movements, increased and forceful swallowing, masked facies, regular slow respiration and muscular relaxation were obtained, followed by a catalepsy of the eyelids or the extremities" (p. 270).

Sixty of the children were given one or more of several individual intelligence tests, either privately or by a school psychologist. The IQ distribution was skewed toward the lower end, with 5 subjects scoring from 50 to 70 and 5 subjects below 50. Only 3 subjects scored above 130. Visual inspection of the data indicated that those with the highest IQs achieved a trance state more often than those rated below average or inferior in intelligence. No tests of statistical significance were performed. The large incidence of severe neurological and emotional disorders and the likelihood that the children came from a wide range of social class backgrounds make it impossible to compare these data meaningfully with the London (1965) data.

Brunnquell (1979) suggested that the responses to different hypnotic induction techniques by children of different ages could be understood in terms of theories of cognitive development proposed by Piaget and Werner. For example, young children tend to have idiosyncratic perceptions that do not match adult views, and they may therefore be expected to respond to suggested hypnotic imagery in idiosyncratic ways; the child hypnotherapist must be aware of these tendencies. Brunnquell also noted that children's tendencies to respond easily to hypnotic suggestions might be related to their natural tendency to merge motor, affective, and cognitive behavior, as when they assume that a hostile thought is equivalent to a hostile act. It is easy to see how a child would have little difficulty with ideomotor suggestions, for example, thinking about a body movement or sensation and then having it actually occur. An adult would normally have to work harder to achieve this sort of syncretic functioning.

Electroencephalographic (EEG) Patterns

Children's EEG patterns have been studied in hopes of finding some relationship to hypnotizability. Cooper and London (1976) and London (1976) studied a sample of 35 normal children, age 7 to 16. Hypnotic susceptibility was significantly correlated with alpha duration ($r = .29$) when the children's eyes were open. Although the alpha duration increased as expected when the children were told to close their eyes, the relationship between alpha and hypnotizability vanished ($r = -.09$). The authors noted that alpha represents a relatively alert state of consciousness in children, and they surmised that

since it is well known also that young children do not like to keep their eyes shut for long, the relatively higher incidence of alpha duration in the Eyes Closed condition of this study may represent exactly the opposite of what it would represent in an adult study; namely, that the children are *more* alerted when their eyes are closed than when they are opened. [p. 146]*

They concluded that it might have been more appropriate to study theta waves. The data were further confused by the finding that the magnitude of the correlations varied markedly from one experimenter to another.

Jacobs and Jacobs (1966) found, in a group of children with poor school achievement, that children with markedly abnormal EEGs showed poor responsiveness to hypnotic induction. As noted in the section on intelligence, many of their subjects manifested mental re-

---

*Reprinted from the April 1976 *International Journal of Clinical and Experimental Hypnosis.* Copyrighted by the Society for Clinical and Experimental Hypnosis, April, 1976.

tardation and frank brain damage, thus making the data even more difficult to interpret.

Response to Thermal Biofeedback Training

Several studies of adults have found no relationship between scores on various hypnotizability scales and response to biofeedback training for control of peripheral skin temperature (Engstrom, 1976; Frischholz & Tryon, 1980; Roberts et al., 1975). Engstrom (1976), however, found that when subjects attempted to change skin temperature using hypnosis alone, with no biofeedback, low hypnotizable subjects failed while highly hypnotizable subjects succeeded.

Children are reported to respond to thermal biofeedback training (Hunter, et al., 1976; Lynch, et al., 1976). We know of no studies of children in which success in such training has been correlated with hypnotic responsiveness.

Dikel and Olness (1980) studied control of peripheral skin temperature in children, age 5 to 15, who had previous successful experiences using self-hypnosis for a variety of clinical problems. Most children succeeded at this task. There were no differences in temperature control between children who used hypnotic imagery alone and those who combined hypnosis with biofeedback training. Moreover, neither of these two groups differed from a third group, with no previous hypnosis training, that achieved temperature control using biofeedback alone. Since some children in the third group reported using spontaneous thermal imagery (e.g., putting their hands into snow) similar to the imagery offered to the first two groups by the experimenters, it seemed possible that the third group had actually used hypnotic techniques in spite of the effort to control for this variable. A few children who achieved little temperature change using hypnosis alone were much more successful when biofeedback was added; although the authors did not measure hypnotic responsiveness, it is possible that these subjects were at the lower end of that continuum. Subjects who responded minimally to biofeedback alone were not offered the opportunity to see whether they might do better with hypnosis training.

King and Montgomery (1980) discussed complex methodological problems in evaluating the results of thermal biofeedback training. Given the additional complexities of measuring hypnotic responsiveness in children, we anticipate that it will be some time before there is clarification of the relationship between the two skills. Our hunch is that the two skills are unrelated in children as well as in adults. We wonder whether children whose locus of control is external may respond better to biofeedback training, whereas those who tend more toward internal locus of control may be able to change skin temperature more easily with hypnosis. There may also be other unexplored moderating variables that determine whether biofeedback or hypnosis is most effective for individual patients with migraine headaches or other problems related to skin temperature and blood flow. We are still a long way from this type of prescriptive therapy.

Achievement Motivation

In 1966, London despaired of ever finding personality variables that would correlate with hypnotizability in children. Later reports (Cooper & London, 1976) were somewhat more optimistic with respect to achievement motivation. In the study of 35 children, in which EEG data were also reported, the subjects were asked to solve puzzles 1 week after the CHSS was administered. They were asked to try to get the solution independently, although they could request parental help if they wished. Children with the highest hypnotic susceptibility scores tended to wait the longest before requesting help, indicating higher achievement motivation. These findings were hypothesized to reflect variations in child-rearing practices, especially with respect to independence training.

The research on hypnotizability and achievement motivation is consistent with clinical impressions that children's natural desire for mastery of skills and for understanding of, and participation in, their environment is directly related to their responsiveness to hypnosis (Erickson, 1958; Gardner, 1974a). Clinicians capitalize on these qualities when they introduce hypnosis to a child as "something new you can learn how to do—not everybody knows how to do it, just as not everybody knows how to ride a bike."

Role Playing

London (1962) observed that some subjects seemed to be faking on the CHSS, especially those in the 8- to 12-year age group. This observation was supported by the ability of children in this age group to simulate hypnosis when instructed to do so.

In further examination of these findings, especially in the context of Sarbin's (1950) role theory of hypnotic susceptibility, Bowers and London (1965) compared the abilities of 40 children, age 5 to 11, on two role-playing tasks. One was a measure of dramatic acting skill; the other was a hypnotic simulation test. When age and intelligence were held statistically constant, there was no correlation between the two measures.

Madsen and London (1966) then explored the relationship of these two skills to hypnotic susceptibility scores on the CHSS. The subjects were 42 middle-class children age 7 to 11 years. The dramatic acting test measured the extent to which the children could portray the cultural stereotype of such familiar roles as mother, bully, teacher, and sheriff. The hypnotic simulation test was the one described in the earlier London (1962) studies. All subjects were given the CHSS, followed 1 week later by the two role-playing tests. Hypnotizability scores were significantly correlated with scores on the simulation test, but there was no relationship between CHSS scores and dramatic acting ability. Thus, role playing is a complex behavior, made up of several skills that may or may not be related to each other and to other variables.

Madsen and London (1966) noted that children who scored low on the CHSS scored about five points higher on the simulation test given 1 week later. For high scorers on the CHSS, the later simulation score was essentially unchanged. They postulated a possible rehearsal effect for the low susceptible children and designed another study to test that hypothesis.

In the second study (London & Madsen, 1968), 34 children, age 7 to 11, were given the same tests as in the first study, but this time the order was reversed, with the CHSS following the role-playing tests. Unlike the earlier (1966) study, there was no significant correlation between hypnotic simulation and hypnotic susceptibility. In other words, if the subjects were familiarized with the various phenomena on the CHSS, they could role play the part of a hypnotized person with some proficiency. But they could not simulate a set of behaviors about which they knew very little. With respect to overt behavior scores, prior simulation experience had virtually no effect on the later CHSS scores. However, to the surprise of the experimenters, prior simulation experience led to a significant decrease on CHSS subjective involvement scores measuring the degree to which the experimenters thought the subjects were really involved in the items.

The experimenters concluded that attempting deliberately to act like a hypnotized person inhibits ability to become deeply involved in a similar task. To put it in another framework (Fromm, 1977), approaching a task in the context of ego activity may interfere with later ability to perform that task in a more ego-receptive mode.

Imaginative Involvement

Several studies of child development have clearly established that children in the 2- to 5-year age range not only are capable of imagery and fantasy but spend a great deal of their time in various types of imaginative behavior (Gould, 1972; Murphy, 1962; Singer, 1973, 1974).

The idea that imagination is an important factor in hypnotic responsiveness is at least as old as the commission that investigated Mesmer's theories in 1784. The positive relationship between various kinds of imaginative involvement and hypnotizability in adults is now well established, particularly as a result of careful investigations by J. R. Hilgard (1970). In her elaborate study of young adults, she not only found that highly hypnotizable subjects engaged in a variety of imaginative involvements as adults, but also that these subjects—in contrast to those who were low on susceptibility tests—more frequently engaged in imaginative experiences in childhood, according to their own reports. In the highly hypnotizable subjects, imagination was typically related to stimuli outside the person rather than autistic or inner-stimulated imagination. Parents either reinforced fantasy or at least did not interfere with it.

Many child clinicians are convinced that the readiness with which children respond to hypnosis is related to their imaginative skills and involvements (Ambrose, 1961; Boswell, 1962; Erickson, 1958; Gardner, 1974a; Jacobs, 1962; Olness & Gardner, 1978). Gardner (1974a) has described several aspects of cognitive and emotional development in children that are probably related both to imaginative involvement and to hypnotizability. These include (1) capacity for intense concentration, immersion, focused attention on a limited stimulus field, and full absorption in the immediate present; (2) a tendency toward concrete, literal thinking; (3) limited reality testing, love of magic, and readiness to shift back and forth between reality and fantasy; (4) intensity of feeling states, often in an all-or-nothing way; and (5) openness to new ideas and delight with new experiences in a context of felt safety and trust.

Some writers have offered explanations of changes in hypnotic responsiveness with age largely in terms of development and decline of imaginative skills. E. R. Hilgard (1971) made the following interpretation:

> Hypnosis reaches its height in the preadolescent period because by that time language and experience have stimulated imagination and given it content, so that those characteristics described as childlikeness have had a full opportunity to bloom. . . . [In late adolescence] reality-orientations conflict with the free enjoyment of a life of fantasy and adventure, and for many people this means a reduction in their hypnotizability. [p. 38]*

---

*From "Hypnosis and Childlikeness" by E. R. Hilgard, in J. P. Hill (Ed.), *Minnesota Symposia on Child Psychology* (Vol. 5), Minneapolis: Lund Press, 1971. With permission.

J. R. Hilgard (1970) commented similarly on declining hypnotizability with age:

one may hazard the guess that the conditions of increasing rational sophistication and the needs for competency and achievement bring with them a decline in wonderment; these changes with age somehow counteract the imaginative involvements so important in hypnosis and substitute for them interactions on a reality level that make hypnosis increasingly difficult. [p. 189]*

Despite the weight of evidence based on research with adults and clinical experience with children, there has been almost no research on the relationship between imaginative involvement and hypnotizability in children. In London's (1966) study of a large number of personality variables in relation to childhood hypnotizability, he included information about the children's tendency to be imaginative and to engage in an active fantasy life, obtaining his data through interviews with parents of 111 children. Specific questions concerned imaginary playmates, extent of dreaming, whether the child talked to him- or herself much, and whether the child played imaginative games either alone or with other children. None of these items—alone or in combination—correlated with CHSS scores, although they correlated positively with each other. There was, however, a certain moderating effect of imagination on age and susceptibility. That is, there was a significant correlation between age and susceptibility for children low in imagination, but there was no age-susceptibility relationship for children whose imagination scores were high. Considering the very large number of variables studied, London was hesitant to make very much of these findings.

In view of the research on adults and the clinical data for children, it is rather surprising that no one has attempted to correlate direct measurements of imaginative involvement in children with their scores on measures of hypnotic responsiveness.

Attitudes toward Adults

Gardner (1974a) has hypothesized that children may be especially responsive to hypnotic suggestions because they are generally predisposed to trust adults, responsive to social influence and authority, and comfortable about engaging in help-seeking behavior. Most children feel safe when they experience regressive aspects of hypnosis in the presence of a presumably competent adult. In most cases they do not

---

*Reprinted from *Personality and Hypnosis: A Study of Imaginative Involvement* by J. R. Hilgard by permission of The University of Chicago Press. © 1970 by The University of Chicago.

experience the degree of anxiety about control that often interferes with hypnotic responsiveness in adults. There has been no research to test these hypotheses.

Parent–Child Interaction

Several psychoanalytic writers (Ambrose, 1963, 1968; Boswell, 1962; Call, 1976; Krojanker, 1969) focus on transferential and regressive aspects of the hypnotic relationship. In this context, it becomes possible to specify the kinds of parent–child relationships most conducive to hypnotic responsiveness in the child. For example, Call (1976) noted that

what is elicited during hypnotic induction is the child's subjectively experienced relationship with the powerful, internalized, omnipotent (because of the child's relative helplessness) parent imago. During this regression, no clear distinction exists between self and parent figure. The child is united with the omnipotent figure of the past, i.e., experiences with the omnipotent parent imago as a part of one's self. It is within this perspective that the phenomena characteristic of the hypnotic state should be viewed, i.e., the child's psychic experience, not the externally observed adultomorphized "reality." . . . It would be consistent to expect that the child who has, in the past, experienced himself in relation to a well-defined, powerful, omnipotent parent would be more hypnotizable than would say a child whose earlier experience with parent figures had been fragmented or ill-defined, or had been dominated by laissez-faire parental influences. [pp. 151–152]*

Results of two retrospective studies of young adults (Hilgard & Hilgard, 1962; J. R. Hilgard, 1970), found that subjects who identified with work habits and attitudes of neither parent were low in hypnotizability. The same was true for identification with parental temperament. In both studies, highly hypnotizable subjects identified most strongly with the opposite-sexed parent. The families of highly hypnotizable subjects were characterized by a combination of warmth and strict discipline, a setting in which the children knew what was expected and in which the likelihood of clear identifications and strong ego development was optimized. J. R. Hilgard hypothesized that the hypnotizable subject may later incorporate the hypnotist in the same way that the parents were incorporated, with a certain readiness to conform to authority even if it seems rather illogical.

---

*Reprinted from the April 1976 *International Journal of Clinical and Experimental Hypnosis*. Copyrighted by the Society for Clinical and Experimental Hypnosis, April, 1976.

In a longitudinal study, children who had initially been studied in kindergarten were tested for hypnotizability and related behaviors when they reached their senior year in high school (Nowlis, 1969). The results indicated that "a rather stern, restrictive, and punitive home environment at the time the children were in kindergarten was related to higher susceptibility to hypnotic-like experience when the children reached the twelfth grade in high school" (p. 114). In these comparisons, "hypnotic-like experience" was measured by Shor's Personal Experiences Questionnaire, Form L (Shor, 1960; Shor, Orne, & O'Connell, 1962), an inventory of trancelike experiences in everyday life that predicts hypnotizability but is not itself a test of hypnotizability. On an actual hypnotizability scale, the Harvard Group Scale of Hypnotic Susceptibility, Form A (Shor & Orne, 1962), only one antecedent child-rearing variable was significantly related to hypnotizability, namely, pressure for conformity with table standards. In view of the many variables studied, the author concluded that this one finding should probably be attributed to chance.

In the only study in which parent–child relationships and childhood hypnotizability have been studied concurrently, Cooper and London (1976) found that parents of highly hypnotizable subjects tended to rate themselves as more strict, anxious, and impatient than parents of low hypnotizable subjects. When these parents offered help to their children on a puzzle task, the suggestions given by parents of highly susceptible children were more abstract and constructive than the suggestions given by parents of low susceptible children. Cooper and London suggested caution in interpreting these results because of the large number of variables studied.

Despite methodological differences and difficulties in the studies of J. R. Hilgard (1970), Nowlis (1969), and Cooper and London (1976), the results of all three point in the same direction, leading to a position of greater credence than would have been possible from any of the studies taken alone.

FACTORS THAT MAY COMPROMISE HYPNOTIC RESPONSIVENESS

In an extensive review of correlates of hypnotic responsiveness in childhood, it is necessary to go beyond the developmental issues that have concerned us so far. We will discuss several variables not directly related to hypnotic talent but that may enhance or impede hypnotic responsiveness.

Misconceptions about Hypnosis

We have found that many children approach hypnotherapy with a great deal of misinformation. Typically, they believe that they will somehow be put to sleep, be under the absolute control of the hypnotist, and not remember anything that transpires during the hypnotic session. While sometimes children get these notions from parents and other adults, more often the "information" comes from television. For example, we saw one children's program that portrayed a mad scientist who used a shiny ring to bring various people under his spell. When his victims wore the ring, they walked around in an obvious trancelike state, followed his instructions including embarrassing and antisocial behavior while muttering "Yes, master," and had no memory of their behavior when the trance was lifted by taking off the scientist's ring.

Fortunately, the effect of such programs is usually more positive than negative with respect to children's willingness to experience hypnosis. They are more intrigued by the "magic" portrayed than they are concerned about being controlled or made to engage in unacceptable behavior. However, for therapeutic as well as educational reasons, it is wise to preface a hypnotic induction with a didactic session in which misconceptions are clarified. We know of one 12-year-old boy who initially refused hypnosis on religious grounds because he thought it involved some sort of demons or witchcraft. Only after being assured that neither he nor the therapist were possessed by demons did he consent to hypnotic induction.

Some children refuse therapeutic hypnosis despite all efforts at clarification; in a few cases, the children have even demonstrated that they are hypnotizable but still refuse to apply their skills to a particular problem. Reasons for resistance are not always clear, but may include (1) being unwilling to give up a symptom because of secondary gains; (2) equating hypnosis with loss of autonomy and choice; (3) equating freedom from pain and anxiety with death, in severe illness; (4) being unwilling to give up a symptom that serves a major defensive function against debilitating depression or psychosis; (5) experiencing anxiety with certain induction techniques which compromise coping mechanisms, for example, resisting dissociative imagery because of a need for cognitive mastery during medical procedures; and (6) having had a previous negative experience with another hypnotherapist. When the therapist understands the resistance, sometimes further clarification or modification of technique will be helpful; at times the therapist will decide that hypnotherapy is contraindicated. Occasionally the therapist will be unable to understand the resistance, and the child will remain refractory to hypnosis.

Some children are reluctant to express their fears and misgivings, and one must apply the same patience and skill that one uses when introducing other unfamiliar treatment methods. Generally speaking, children are enthusiastic about experiencing hypnosis.

Attitudes of Significant Adults

Some child clinicians despair of attempting hypnotherapy with children because of presumed negative attitudes on the part of patients' parents, teachers, clergy, and other adults from whom children get their concept of reality and of appropriate behavior.

Educators and Child Health Professionals

Woody and Herr (1966) surveyed 102 psychologists in various academic and clinical settings. The 84 subjects who responded generally said they were uncertain as to the propriety of psychologists in a public school system using hypnosis as a therapeutic or diagnostic technique. They were more positive when asked about the use of hypnosis at the college level.

Many adults have more positive attitudes about child hypnosis. Traphagen (1959) reported predominately positive attitudes among several professional groups including teachers (70 percent) and psychiatrists (67 percent). There were fewer positive responses from social workers (43 percent) and from administrators of schools and agencies (33 percent). Gardner (1976) found a high frequency of positive responses among pediatric nurses (98 percent), with frequencies lower but still predominately favorable among pediatricians (78 percent), child psychologists (76 percent), and child psychiatrists (62 percent). In both studies, responses were often based on little actual knowledge of hypnosis and its potential clinical applications.

Unfortunately, relatively positive professional attitudes toward hypnosis tend not to be translated into the development of training opportunities in applied child hypnosis. In a survey of predoctoral programs in medicine, dentistry, and clinical psychology (Parrish, 1975), hypnosis training was available in only 4 of 21 internship centers specializing in the treatment of children. In 83 general internship centers, 55 (66 percent) offered training in hypnosis; the report did not state how many of these included training in child hypnosis.

Misconceptions, negative attitudes, and a lack of information about hypnosis among child health professionals not only limit the number of children who might be referred for hypnotherapy; they also can sabotage ongoing hypnotherapy done by a qualified professional with a motivated and capable child. It is disheartening to give a post-surgical child patient hypnotic suggestions for increased food intake only to discover that someone else has put the emesis basin closer to the child than the dinner tray! In an effort to remedy this problem, Olness (1977) has instituted a series of inservice hypnosis education programs at a children's hospital. She offers lectures about suggestion and hypnosis not only to the pediatricians, nurses, and medical students, but also to administrative, secretarial, and housekeeping personnel. Her results have been encouraging.

Parents

Traphagen (1959) found a preponderance of positive attitudes toward hypnosis among parents (65 percent), higher than she expected. We find positive attitudes among most parents of our prospective child hypnotherapy patients. Some parents are interested to discover that they have unwittingly been using hypnoticlike techniques with their children. For example, Katie Y., age 12, frequently gagged or vomited when taking oral medication. Her mother spontaneously developed the idea of helping her child by describing in detail her favorite foods while she swallowed her pills. When we pointed out the similarity to hypnosis, Katie quickly learned to use the favorite food imagery independently and easily resolved her problem with the medication. Even when parents are at first reluctant, it is usually possible to help them shift to a more positive stance toward hypnosis. Gardner (1974b) described techniques designed to help parents who are reluctant about hypnosis to move from being obstacles to becoming allies in their children's treatment. The approach includes three basic steps: educational, observational, and experiential. Details of each of these steps follow.

It is usually best to begin with a relatively didactic discussion with the parents, especially eliciting and responding to their specific questions and concerns. Hypnosis can be defined as basically a state of mind, usually combining relaxation with concentration on a desired point of focus so that other undesired thoughts or feelings then fade into the background. Such shifts of attention are easily demonstrated by asking the parents to focus on sounds which were not previously noticed, such as the typing in the reception area or the soft hum of the air conditioner. The heightened attention which characterizes hypnosis is then described in the context of everyday events such as a mother's ability to waken to her infant's cry while sleeping through other louder but insignificant noises. In answering other questions concerning hypnosis generally, Wolberg's (1965) mimeographed materials for use with his patients may be helpful.

This general discussion easily leads to the specific issue of why hypnosis may be appropriate for a particular child. Thus, the mother may be told that the goal is to help the child focus on comfort so that pain will ease, on feelings of well-being so that anxiety will diminish, or on pleasant hunger in order to counteract nausea and vomiting. A few basic principles of induction techniques, such as relaxation training and guided imagery, can then be explained, emphasizing the need to tailor the induction to the needs of each child, and providing some understanding of simple physiological and psychological principles that account for the success of the techniques. Throughout, the parents' specific questions are answered, and misconceptions are clarified, including such things as the distinction between hypnosis and sleep and concerns about spontaneous hypnosis or greater susceptibility to charlatans. The goals are (a) to teach the parents that hypnosis can be described in simple, everyday terms without resorting to concepts suggesting magic or witchcraft and (b) to help the parents understand that hypnosis may be a specifically useful treatment modality for their child. This writer finds that, after this discussion, almost all parents are willing to let their children have a trial of hypnotherapy. For those who are not, the issue is not pushed any further.

If the parents become enthusiastic about the possible value of hypnotherapy for the child, they have already accomplished a major step toward becoming a hypnotherapeutic ally. Usually children look to their parents for guidance and assurance when facing new situations, and if the parents communicate a confident attitude toward hypnosis, the child is much more likely to be trusting and cooperative.

For those parents who permit hypnotherapy for their children, the second phase of parent training consists of having them observe their children in hypnosis. Observation is usually postponed, however,—and especially in older children—until after the initial induction, since this is often the point of maximum concern for both the child and the hypnotherapist regarding whether a state of hypnosis can be achieved and whether it will be effective for the problem at hand. This writer finds that having any third party present, e.g., parent, doctor, or nurse, increases the likelihood of anxiety about successful performance. This anxiety may then seriously interfere with success, since it draws attention away from the task and replaces desired relaxation with tension. However, occasionally the parents may be invited to observe the first session if the child is particularly anxious and wants his parents to stay with him.

When rapport is established between the therapist and the child, and when it is clear to both that the child can use hypnosis to alleviate his problem, the parent is then invited to observe a hypnotic session. Ideally this is done after the child has been taught self-hypnosis (easily mastered by most children eight years of age or older), because then the parents see that the child can be in control both of induction (usually simple techniques such as eye-fixation, visual imagery, or reverse hand-levitation) and dehypnotization (usually counting silently to five).

An important part of the observation session is to have the parent watch the therapist communicate with the child in hypnosis, requiring the child to give both nonverbal and verbal responses and then to transfer hypnotic rapport to the parents and have them also communicate verbally and nonverbally with the child. This exercise helps assure the parent that the child is in contact with his surroundings and in control of the hypnotic state as much as necessary. Parents who initially went along with the idea because of desperation or "blind faith" now have keener understanding and are able to be even more supportive, both in sessions with the therapist and when the child is asked to practice self-hypnosis for use with a chronic condition or for repeated painful procedures or unpleasant experiences where the therapist may not always be available. With a little further training, they are also now in a position to help their child deepen or maintain a hypnotic state or achieve the initial induction when the child may be too anxious or in too much discomfort to concentrate effectively alone.

The parents' effectiveness as hypnotherapists is usually enhanced by the third phase of parent training, namely, having them experience hypnosis themselves. This step further dispels the idea of hypnosis as magic, removes any remaining doubts and fears, and allows review of details not previously discussed. Often this occurs informally as a natural consequence of the observational phase. That is, the parents spontaneously report feelings of relaxation compatible with light hypnosis while watching their child in hypnosis. The dynamics of this phenomenon are not clear, though this writer has seen it with adults watching other adults as well as with adults watching children. Usually the observer is a "participant observer" in the sense of having warm, tender feelings for and/or identifications with the subject. There may also be an element of contagion of the trusting relationship between the subject and therapist. Once, when both parents observed a hypnotic session with a six-year-old nauseated girl, suggestions were given that she could feel quiet and a bit sleepy and that soon she would experience nice hungry feelings so that it would feel good to take fluids and medicine. Not only did the suggestions prove effective for the child, but mother later reported that she became pleasantly sleepy, while father said he developed marked hunger and went out for a snack! Both parents described their experience with amusement, commenting also that they were glad to know something of what their child experienced. Another parent, after experiencing a formal induction, reported that experiencing hypnosis herself really convinced her that a person in hypnosis is "awake and aware" and that this allowed her to feel more secure when she helped her son use self-hypnosis.

For parents who experience a formal induction, there is usually only one hypnotic session, focusing mainly on aspects of induction, deepening, and dehypnotization, often in the presence of the child so as to maximize mutual trust and confidence. The experiential phase of training may be omitted, if it is not anticipated that the parents will actually assume the role of hypnotherapist or if the child will not be asked to use self-hypnosis or if the parents resist the idea of experiencing hypnosis themselves, even though they accept it for their child. In most cases, only one parent goes through this phase, and this writer uses formal parent induction in less than half the cases of child hypnotherapy. [pp. 45–47]*

Since publishing the 1974 paper on parental attitudes, Gardner has continued the educational and observational steps of parent training but has decreased the frequency of having parents actually experience formal hypnotic induction. Moreover, when parents do request formal hypnotic induction for themselves, Gardner now insists that the child not be present, at least initially. This change developed when it became clear that some parents—even in brief hypnosis—might use the opportunity to experience grief or other feelings whose full expression might be inappropriate in front of the child.

Situational Variables

Sometimes a child's physical or psychological condition precludes use of hypnosis, at least for the present time. Such conditions include unconsciousness, anxiety or pain to such an extreme degree that the child is unable to focus any attention on the hypnotherapist, and extreme debilitation with inability to move from a passive to an active stance. Occasionally time limitations preclude effective use of hypnosis, although we have been impressed with how much can be accomplished in a very short period when circumstances seem suboptimal, for example, in an emergency situation when everyone, including the patient, is markedly anxious.

CONCLUSIONS

Gardner and Hinton (1980) reviewed correlates of hypnotic responsiveness in children. Considering the great diversity of possible correlates, they noted the lack of any serious attempt to ground the findings in the context of a cohesive theory. Even the comments of psychoanalytic writers have been limited in scope. In light of recent advances in theoretical conceptualizations of hypnosis (e.g., Fromm,

---

*From "Parents: Obstacles or Allies in Child Hypnotherapy?" by G. G. Gardner, *The American Journal of Clinical Hypnosis*, 1974, *17*, 44–49. With permission.

1977; Fromm & Gardner, 1979; Fromm & Hurt, 1980), we anticipate that future research will more clearly identify correlates of childhood hypnotic responsiveness and evaluate their relative significance in a more orderly way.

REFERENCES

Ambrose, G. *Hypnotherapy with children* (2nd ed.). London: Staples, 1961.

Ambrose, G. Hypnotherapy for children. In J. M. Schneck (Ed.), *Hypnosis in modern medicine* (3rd ed.). Springfield, Ill.: Charles C Thomas, 1963.

Ambrose, G. Hypnosis in the treatment of children. *The American Journal of Clinical Hypnosis*, 1968, *11*, 1–5.

Boswell, L. K., Jr. Pediatric hypnosis. *The British Journal of Medical Hypnotism*, 1962, *13*, 4–11.

Bowers, P., & London, P. Developmental correlates of role playing ability. *Child Development*, 1965, *30*, 499–508.

Brunnquell, D. Hypnosis and developmental theory. Paper presented at the annual meeting of the American Society of Clinical Hypnosis, San Francisco, November, 1979.

Call, J. D. Children, parents, and hypnosis: A discussion. *The International Journal of Clinical and Experimental Hypnosis*, 1976, *24*, 149–155.

Cooper, L. M., & London, P. Children's hypnotic susceptibility, personality, and EEG patterns. *The International Journal of Clinical and Experimental Hypnosis*, 1976, *24*, 140–148.

Dikel, W., & Olness, K. Self-hypnosis, biofeedback, and voluntary peripheral temperature control in children. *Pediatrics*, 1980, *66*, 335–340.

Engstrom, D. R. Hypnotic susceptibility, EEG alpha, and self-regulation. In G. E. Schwartz & D. Shapiro (Eds.), *Consciousness and self-regulation* (Vol. 1). New York: Plenum, 1976.

Erickson, M. H. Pediatric hypnotherapy. *The American Journal of Clinical Hypnosis*, 1958, *1*, 25–29.

Frischholz, E. J., & Tryon, W. W. Hypnotizability in relation to the ability to learn thermal biofeedback. *The American Journal of Clinical Hypnosis*, 1980, *23*, 53–56.

Fromm, E. An ego-psychological theory of altered states of consciousness. *The International Journal of Clinical and Experimental Hypnosis*, 1977, *25*, 372–387.

Fromm, E., & Gardner, G. G. Ego psychology and hypnoanalysis: An integration of theory and technique. *Bulletin of the Menninger Clinic*, 1979, *43*, 413–423.

Fromm, E., & Hurt, S. W. Ego-psychological parameters of hypnosis and altered states of consciousness. In G. D. Burrows and L. Dennerstein (Eds.), *Handbook of hypnosis and psychosomatic medicine*. New York: Elsevier/North-Holland Biomedical Press, 1980.

Gardner, G. G. Hypnosis with children. *The International Journal of Clinical and Experimental Hypnosis*, 1974, *22*, 20–38. (a)

Gardner, G. G. Parents: Obstacles or allies in child hypnotherapy? *The American Journal of Clinical Hypnosis*, 1974, *17*, 44–49. (b)

Gardner, G. G. Attitudes of child health professionals toward hypnosis: Implications for training. *The International Journal of Clinical and Experimental Hypnosis*, 1976, *24*, 63–73.

Gardner, G. G., & Hinton, R. M. Hypnosis with children. In G. D. Burrows and L.

Dennerstein (Eds.), *Handbook of hypnosis and psychosomatic medicine.* New York: Elsevier/North-Holland Biomedical Press, 1980.

Gould, R. *Child studies through fantasy: Cognitive-affective patterns in development.* New York: Quadrangle Books, 1972.

Hilgard, E. R. Hypnosis and childlikeness. In J. P. Hill (Ed.), *Minnesota symposia on child psychology* (Vol. 5). Minneapolis: Lund Press, 1971.

Hilgard, J. R. *Personality and hypnosis: A study of imaginative involvement.* Chicago: University of Chicago Press, 1970.

Hilgard, J. R., & Hilgard, E. R. Developmental-interactive aspects of hypnosis: Some illustrative cases. *Genetic Psychology Monographs,* 1962, *66,* 143–178.

Hunter, S. H., Russell, H. L., Russell, E. D., & Zimmerman, R. L. Control of fingertip temperature increases via biofeedback in learning-disabled and normal children. *Perceptual and Motor Skills,* 1976, *43,* 743–755.

Jacobs, L. Hypnosis in clinical pediatrics. *New York State Journal of Medicine,* 1962, *62,* 3781–3787.

Jacobs, L., & Jacobs, J. Hypnotizability of children as related to hemispheric reference and neurological organization. *The American Journal of Clinical Hypnosis,* 1966, *8,* 269–274.

King, N. J., & Montgomery, R. B. Biofeedback-induced control of human peripheral temperature: A critical review of the literature. *Psychological Bulletin,* 1980, *88,* 738–752.

Krojanker, R. J. Human hypnosis, animal hypnotic states, and the induction of sleep in infants. *The American Journal of Clinical Hypnosis,* 1969, *11,* 178–179.

London, P. Child hypnosis and personality. *The American Journal of Clinical Hypnosis,* 1966, *8,* 161–168.

London, P. Hypnosis in children: An experimental approach. *The International Journal of Clinical and Experimental Hypnosis,* 1962, *10,* 79–91.

London, P. Developmental experiments in hypnosis. *Journal of Projective Techniques and Personality Assessment,* 1965, *29,* 189–199.

London P. *Children's Hypnotic Susceptibility Scale.* Palo Alto, Calif.: Consulting Psychologists Press, 1963.

London, P. Kidding around with hypnosis. *The International Journal of Clinical and Experimental Hypnosis,* 1976, *24,* 105–121.

London, P., & Madsen, C. H., Jr. Effect of role playing on hypnotic susceptibility in children. *Journal of Personality and Social Psychology,* 1968, *10,* 66–68.

Lynch, W. C., Hama, H., Kohn, S., & Miller, N. E. Instrumental control of peripheral vasomotor responses in children. *Psychophysiology,* 1976, *13,* 219–221.

Madsen, C. H., Jr., & London, P. Role playing and hypnotic susceptibility in children. *Journal of Personality and Social Psychology,* 1966, *3,* 13–19.

Morgan, A. H. The heritability of hypnotic susceptibility in twins. *Journal of Abnormal Psychology,* 1973, *82,* 55–61.

Morgan, A. H., Hilgard, E. R., & Davert, E. C. The heritability of hypnotic susceptibility of twins: A preliminary report. *Behavior Genetics,* 1970, *1,* 213–224.

Murphy, L. *The widening world of childhood: Paths toward mastery.* New York: Basic Books, 1962.

Nowlis, D. P. The child-rearing antecedents of hypnotic susceptibility and of naturally occurring hypnotic-like experience. *The International Journal of Clinical and Experimental Hypnosis,* 1969, *17,* 109–120.

Olness, K. In-service hypnosis education in a children's hospital. *The American Journal of Clinical Hypnosis,* 1977, *20,* 80–83.

Olness, K., & Gardner, G. G. Some guidelines for uses of hypnotherapy in pediatrics. *Pediatrics,* 1978, *62,* 228–233.

Parrish, M. J. Predoctoral training in clinical hypnosis: A national survey of availability and educator attitudes in schools of medicine, dentistry, and graduate clinical psychology. *The International Journal of Clinical and Experimental Hypnosis*, 1975, *23*, 249–265.

Roberts, A. H., Schuler, J., Bacon, J. G., Zimmerman, R. L., & Patterson, R. Individual differences and autonomic control, absorption, and the unilateral control of skin temperature. *Journal of Abnormal Psychology*, 1975, *84*, 272–279.

Sarbin, T. R. Contributions to role-taking theory: I. Hypnotic behavior. *Psychological Review*, 1950, *57*, 225–270.

Shor, R. E. The frequency of naturally occurring "hypnotic-like" experiences in the normal college population. *The International Journal of Clinical and Experimental Hypnosis*, 1960, *8*, 151–163.

Shor, R. E., & Orne, E. C. *The Harvard Group Scale of Hypnotic Susceptibility, Form A*. Palo Alto, Calif.: Consulting Psychologists Press, 1962.

Shor, R. E., Orne, M. T., & O'Connell, D. N. Validation and cross-validation of a scale of self-reported personal experiences which predicts hypnotizability. *Journal of Psychology*, 1962, *53*, 55–75.

Singer, J. L. *The child's world of make-believe: Experimental studies of imaginative play*. New York: Academic Press, 1973.

Singer, J. L. *Imagery and daydream methods in psychotherapy and behavior modification*. New York: Academic Press, 1974.

Traphagen, V. A survey of attitudes toward hypnotherapy with children. *The American Journal of Clinical Hypnosis*, 1959, *2*, 138–142.

Weitzenhoffer, A. M., & Hilgard, E. R. *Stanford Hypnotic Susceptibility Scale, Forms A and B*. Palo Alto, Calif.: Consulting Psychologists Press, 1959.

Wechsler, D. *Wechsler Intelligence Scale for Children*. New York: The Psychological Corporation, 1949.

Wolberg, L. R. Hypnosis in short-term therapy. In L. R. Wolberg (Ed.), *Short-term psychotherapy*. New York: Grune & Stratton, 1965.

Woody, R. H., & Herr, E. L. Psychologists and hypnosis: Part II. Use in educational settings. *The American Journal of Clinical Hypnosis*, 1966, *9*, 254–256.

5

Hypnotic Induction
Techniques for Children

Children respond to a large number of hypnotic induction techniques, each with countless variations. Any induction method may also be used as a deepening method, and methods may be combined in almost any order. The choice of an appropriate induction for any given child depends on the needs and preferences of the child and on the experience and creativity of the therapist. Success is certain to be limited if a therapist is competent only in the use of one or two induction techniques for children or attempts to utilize techniques suited for adults without adding modifications that may be necessary for child patients.

Any health specialist who undertakes hypnotic induction with children must first have considerable knowledge of child development and expertise in working with children in the context of his or her primary profession (e.g., pediatrics, child psychology, or psychiatry). One also needs to know something about the social and cultural backgrounds of child patients, general likes and dislikes, and themes of interest related to story books, television programs, and current movies. For individual patients, successful hypnotic inductions are often based on knowledge of particular likes and dislikes, comfort areas, language preferences, past experiences, and aspirations about the future. Sometimes unexpected resistance to one technique demands a rapid shift to another. In short, a child hypnotherapist must first be a competent child therapist, and the same requirements apply to researchers studying hypnotic phenomena in children.

Compared with adults, children are more likely to wiggle and move about, open their eyes or refuse to close them, and make spontaneous comments during hypnotic inductions. Although these behaviors may indicate resistance, this is not necessarily the case. Most often the child is simply adapting the induction to his or her behavioral style, and the wise hypnotherapist also adapts accordingly. Many children have negative attitudes about going to sleep or, having been told that a favorite pet has been "put to sleep," equate being put to sleep with being put to death. Therefore, we usually avoid such words as "sleepy," "drowsy," and "tired" in our inductions. Likewise, since some children—especially 4- and 5-year-olds—resist closing their eyes and may even be frightened by the idea, we do not stress eye closure as important to induction, although we sometimes tell children that they may be able to concentrate better if they close their eyes. In all instances the choice is theirs. We adapt our language to the children's levels of understanding, neither talking down to them nor using overly complex language.

The induction techniques that we will describe are all permissive in nature, emphasizing children's involvement and control and encouraging their active participation in the process of experiencing and utilizing the hypnotic state. We avoid authoritarian methods widely used in the past, including such phrases as "You will" or "I want you to do this now." Such methods, in which the hypnotherapist uses a controlling or commanding manner, may indeed result in successful induction for some children, although less so now than in earlier times or in cultures in which children expect adults to be very strict and authoritarian.

Moreover, when hypnotic induction is employed in the context of medical or psychological therapy, we believe that authoritarian methods are contraindicated, especially the use of challenges (e.g., "You will not be able to open your eyes no matter how hard you try"). The purpose of therapy is always to increase the child's control of a desired feeling or behavior, and any induction that emphasizes loss of control can only inhibit therapeutic progress. We do not mean to imply that the therapist avoids any structuring of the situation or dilutes the patient's perception of him or her as a competent, helping person. We do, however, emphasize the distinction between being authoritative and being authoritarian.

Although we shall describe several specific hypnotic induction techniques, our list is by no means a complete compendium. Nor is this chapter intended as a substitute for direct training with experts in the field. We suspect that many professionals who give up hypnotherapy do so because they never acquired a solid base of personal training. Appropriate avenues of training are discussed in the Introduction.

While some children expect and benefit from relatively formalized induction techniques, many respond equally well or better to a more simple, casual approach. In some cases it may be sufficient to say, "Just think about how you feel when you are building a block house at home; just let yourself feel that way now."

Erickson (1958) was particularly aware that children frequently go into hypnosis without any formal induction. This phenomenon can present problems to researchers who define hypnosis as whatever occurs following a hypnotic induction. However, the criteria for determining the presence or absence of hypnosis can only be based on patient or subject behaviors known to be characteristic of the state of hypnosis and not on behaviors of the person doing the induction.

The choice of induction techniques depends not only on patient variables, but also on the style and preferences of the therapist. A hypnotherapist is not likely to be successful using a method with which he or she is uncomfortable. Moreover, hypnotherapists should always be alert to the possible value of new methods along with inevitable changes in cultural trends such as norms for social behavior, child-rearing methods, and educational approaches. New developments in science and the arts that shape children's interests and attitudes will also have relevance for hypnotic induction techniques. It may turn out that some methods currently in general use will be outdated or inappropriate for children of future generations.

Some of the techniques we describe have been invented by our child patients or by children in our families or their friends. For techniques in use for a long time, and with several variations, we have been unable to trace their originators, and we apologize to these unsung heroes.

In the course of any hypnotic induction, we give positive feedback to the child's responses, and we communicate expectations of success by focusing on possibilities and avoiding words such as "try" that imply that failure may be the outcome. Since we believe our patients will benefit most from hypnotherapy if they enjoy the induction, we work in ways that are enjoyable to us as well, using humor where appropriate and never taking ourselves too seriously.

THE PREINDUCTION INTERVIEW

Depending on the needs of the child, the preinduction interview may be quite brief or very extensive. In emergency situations it may be deferred entirely. The interview usually includes discussion of the reasons for utilizing hypnosis in relation to a particular problem, review of the child's ideas about hypnosis, clarification of misconceptions, and full reply to questions. If details of the child's likes and dislikes, significant experiences, fears, hopes, and comfort areas have not already been obtained, these areas are also discussed at this time.

A SAMPLE OF HYPNOTIC INDUCTION TECHNIQUES FOR CHILDREN

The following descriptions of these techniques consist of the actual words we might say to a child. Obviously our own phrasing varies from child to child, as it does also from one therapist to another. We emphasize again that these are samples and that variations are both necessary and appropriate.

Visual Imagery Techniques

Favorite place. "Think about a favorite place where you have been and where you like to be. It might be easier if you close your eyes, but you can leave them open if you like or leave them open until you close them." For children who cannot think of a real favorite place, ask them to think of an imaginary one. It sometimes helps to ask children to tell the therapist their favorite place; the therapist can then enhance the imagery by adding specific details. Important information about the child is sometimes obtained, similar to the information obtained from psychological projective tests that elicit fantasy. When children offer more than one favorite place and indicate no preference, the therapist may enhance rapport by suggesting the one with which he or she is most familiar. The therapist may also suggest the situation involving the patient most actively, especially if the goals of treatment include enhanced competence and active mastery of a problem. The imagery need not be at all related to the problem. "See yourself, feel yourself in that favorite place which you have chosen. Look around and see the shapes and colors, hear the sounds. Let yourself really be there now. It's good for everybody to be in a favorite place sometimes, a place where you like to be, a place where you like how you feel. You can feel those good feelings now. Take some time to enjoy it. When you feel as if you are really there, let me know by lifting one finger to say yes." If the child looks troubled, the therapist should inquire as to the difficulty. Comment that not everyone likes to go to a favorite place and suggest a different method. Occasionally a child who successfully images a favorite place may then have an unexpected negative reaction—for example, sadness because a grandparent who also enjoyed that place has died. Depending on the goals of treatment, the therapist may choose either to shift to another method or to help the child explore the emotional reaction. Prior to the beginning of the induction the child can be told that he or she can talk in hypnosis, especially if a hypnotic interview is part of the treatment plan.

Multiple animals. "Do you like animals? Good. Which do you like best? Fine. Just imagine that you can see yourself sitting in a very nice place with a puppy [or whatever animal the child has chosen]. It might help to close your eyes. Feel that puppy's soft fur and see its color. Now, just for fun, pretend it is another color or striped or polka dotted. Let it be any way you like, and the puppy is happy too. You can change the color anytime you choose. And you can imagine a second puppy just like the first, the same colors, the same soft fur. Two puppies, and you can see yourself playing with them. Now, you may choose to make three puppies and change their color back to the first color or to another. You can tell me about the puppies if you like."

Flower garden. "You said you like flowers. Just let yourself imagine being in a beautiful, big flower garden with all your favorite flowers. You may have your favorite toy or stuffed animal with you. See the bright colors. Smell the sweet smells. If you like, you can touch the petals and feel how soft they are. Imagine that it's all right for you to pick as many flowers as you want from this big flower garden. You can keep them for yourself. Or you can pick some for someone special. Feel your arms widening around a bigger and bigger bouquet until you have all you want. If you take them to a special person, you can see how happy that person looks when you give the flowers. You can feel happy too."

Favorite activity. "Tell me something you like to do. [The child answers.] Good. Just imagine that you can see yourself doing that. Let yourself really enjoy it." This method emphasizes the active participation mentioned in the favorite place technique. Some children actually engage in physical activity appropriate to the imagery, such as strumming their fingers as if playing a piano.

Cloud gazing. "What are some colors you like? Good. Let yourself imagine some beautiful clouds in the sky and see them change into one of your favorite colors. Good. Now let them change into another color. Or perhaps several nice colors. The clouds may change shape too, as you continue to watch them. It will be interesting to see what they become. You can be part of those clouds, if you like, feeling very comfortable, very good." This technique may not be appropriate for a child who has been told that death means "going up to heaven to live with God." Use special caution if there has been a recent death of a family member, friend, or pet, or if the child has an illness which may result in death.

Letters. "You have told me that you like to write. Let yourself see a blackboard or a piece of paper with an A on it. Now watch the A turn into a B. Then let the B turn into a C. See as many letters as you like. When you are feeling very comfortable, very good, let me know by lifting one finger." One can do the same with numbers. If the child looks troubled, consider the possibility that letters and numbers may have symbolic meaning—for example, letters as grades or numbers as ages. One may get spontaneous age regression or age progression with the number method, and this may or may not be desirable, depending on the therapeutic goals.

Television (or movie). "You told me you like to watch TV and that your favorite program is _____." For children who name a particularly violent program as their favorite, some therapists prefer to inquire about other interests and use a different method. It is probably better to inquire casually for other interests than to ask the child for a less violent program since the child may interpret the latter as rejection. "Just imagine yourself getting ready to watch your favorite TV program. Where is the TV set you are watching? Good. Just get comfortable and, when you are ready, turn on the set. Listen to the click as you turn to the channel you want. Now you can see your favorite program. When the sound and the picture are just right for you, let me know by lifting one finger. Good. Just continue watching and listening, feeling very comfortable, very good." If the child is undergoing a medical treatment procedure, the therapist may give repeated suggestions for continued watching. If the therapist intends to give hypnotic or posthypnotic suggestions, these may often be interspersed in the context of the program. For example, if the child has resisted taking oral medication, the therapist can suggest that the TV hero or heroine is happy to take medicine that will cure illness. Or the child can be asked for a favorite food, then given the suggestion that the TV character is eating that food and wants to share it with the child. The medication is then hallucinated as the favorite food. Most children have no problem merging themselves into a TV program. We have seen desperately ill children accept oral medications in the context of these suggestions. In psychotherapeutic treatment the therapist may use the TV technique to explore problem areas or to help the child toward constructive resolution. In this and virtually all other hypnotic induction techniques, there is really no sharp distinction between induction and therapeutic work. Even when an induction technique is used without any therapeutic suggestions, the child's experience of the induction itself will be either therapeutic or countertherapeutic. Of course the same is true for all aspects of the doctor–patient interaction in hypnotherapy as well as in other forms of treatment.

Auditory Imagery

Favorite song. "You said that you like to sing. Where do you like to do that best? Good. Imagine that you are there now, singing your favorite song. Sing the song through in your mind. Enjoy doing it very well, making just the sounds you like. When you have come to the end of the song, let me know by lifting one finger. Or you can sing it again if you like." The patient may be asked to tap out the beat with one or more fingers. When the tapping ceases, the therapist knows the patient has ended the song.

Playing a musical instrument. If the patient enjoys playing a musical instrument, the therapist can adapt the Favorite Song technique accordingly.

Listening to music. "You said you like music. What kind of music do you like to listen to? Exactly what piece of music would you like to hear now? Good. Just imagine yourself hearing that very clearly now, as loud or soft as you like. You may imagine watching the musicians too. You can let me know when the music has ended." For some children actually listening to a tape recording may be better than imagining it. We have occasionally asked patients to bring in taped music or have brought in a tape ourselves of a patient's favorite music (Gardner & Tarnow, 1980).

Movement Imagery

Flying blanket. This method, invented by one of Olness's children, should not be used if the patient is afraid of flying or of heights. "Imagine that you are going on a picnic, going with your favorite people to a special place for a picnic. You have your favorite things to eat and drink. You can see and smell and taste them. Enjoy playing games with your family and friends. Then when you are finished eating and drinking and playing games, you may see a blanket spread out there on the ground. It's your favorite color, smooth and soft. You may sit on it or lie on it. Pretend it's a flying blanket and you are the pilot. You are in control. You can fly just a few inches above the ground, just above the grass or higher, even above the trees if you want. You're the pilot. You can go where you want and as fast or as slowly as you wish, just by thinking about it. You can land and visit your friends or you can land at the zoo or anywhere you like. You're the pilot and you're in charge. You might fly by a tree and see birds in a nest. You can speed up and slow down. Enjoy going where you want. Take all the time you need to feel very comfortable. When you are ready, you can find a nice comfortable landing spot and land your flying blanket. When you have landed, let me know by lifting one finger."

Driving or riding. "Do you like to do things like ride a bicycle or ride a horse? Good. Which do you like best? Fine. Just get comfortable and imagine that you are doing that now. You are just where you want to be, and it's a perfect day. Imagine going exactly where you wish at the speed you wish. You are in control and you can go wherever you like. Enjoy what you see. Enjoy the feeling. Enjoy being able to go at any speed you like. And each time you change speed or direction, let that be a signal to get even more comfortable than you were before. When you are very very comfortable, you can gradually slow down. Find a good stopping or resting place and rest, very comfortably." For children who are frightened of passivity, it may be best to omit the suggestion to slow down and stop. Therapeutic suggestions may be given while the trip is in progress.

Sports activity. "You told me you like to play football. Imagine yourself at the age you are now or older, playing on your favorite football team, wearing its uniform, playing the position you like. Let yourself get very comfortable as you imagine a game with your team winning. You are helping your team win. Feel your control as your muscles move the way you tell them, running or throwing or kicking. Enjoy being with the winning team and continue until the game is won. Let me know when the game is over by lifting one finger." This method may be especially suited for children for whom enhanced muscular control is a therapeutic goal, provided they do not have excessively negative attitudes about their sports ability.

Bouncing ball. "Sometimes it's fun to think of going wherever you want. Pretend you're a bouncing ball, maybe a big one, and you can be any color you want, even striped or with polka dots. It might be easier if you shut your eyes. Be that bouncing ball and bounce wherever you want. Bounce, bounce, bounce. You can go wherever you wish. You can bounce up a tree and along a branch. You can bounce over your house or over the hospital. You can bounce along a path in the woods or on a sidewalk. If you like to swim you can bounce and float, bounce and float. If anything is bothering you, you can let it bounce right off. Keeping bouncing until you find the right place for you to stop and when you've stopped, let me know."

Playground activity. "I know you like to go to the playground and play on the swing and the slide. You can pretend you are there now. Imagine yourself getting on the swing and starting to swing back and forth. Just a little at first, then more, back and forth just as fast or slow as you like. Back and forth. Back and forth. Feeling very good. So easy. And when you are ready to go to the slide, just let the swing slow down and imagine yourself at the top of a nice, long, smooth slide, a slide that is just right for you. As you go down that slide, you can feel more and more comfortable. Feel your body going gently down and down. So smooth. So easy. Down and down. When you reach the bottom, you may find something you like very much. So comfortable. When you reach the bottom, you can just enjoy what you find there. Lift one finger when you get to the bottom. If you like, you can tell me what you find there."

Story-Telling Techniques

With young children or those who are too anxious to participate much in other imagery techniques, the therapist may decide to make up a story suited to the child's needs and interests. This technique may be especially useful with small children who are undergoing painful or frightening medical procedures. The story may be an entirely new fantasy production or it may be a variation of a TV program or other theme with which the child is familiar. The therapist may take full responsibility for the story or may ask the child to contribute ideas to the extent that he or she is able. This method provides an opportunity for the therapist to engage the child in humorous fantasy, a good antidote for anxiety. For example, the therapist might begin by telling a familiar story and then substitute doctors, nurses, or family members for the original characters. Most young children delight in these antics, although a few will insist that the story be told "the right way." Although some might consider story telling a distraction technique rather than a hypnotic technique, we have seen narrowed focus of attention and altered sensation that typically characterize the hypnotic state. Of course the therapist can also intersperse into the story suggestions for comfort, analgesia, and calm. We do not offer any examples here since this method is almost entirely a function of the therapist's own creativity and ingenuity.

Ideomotor Techniques

These methods are distinguished from movement imagery techniques because the latter do not necessarily involve any actual movement by the child, though movement may occur. Ideomotor techniques ask the child to focus mentally on the idea of a particular movement and then to let the movement occur without conscious muscle activity. Such methods are especially valuable when the therapist wishes to communicate the idea that the child can gain increased control over pain and other physical responses that previously seemed beyond control. They may also facilitate the idea that one's attitudes can affect the healing process and that willingness or openness to change can replace complete passivity in treatment. These methods are most often suited for children of at least school age, but sometimes younger children may benefit.

Hands moving together. "Hold your arms straight out in front of you, your palms facing each other, about a foot apart [Fig. 5-1 (left)]. Good. Now imagine two powerful magnets, one in each palm. You know how magnets attract each other. Just think about those two very strong magnets and you may notice that your hands begin to move closer together all by themselves, without your doing anything [Fig. 5-1 (right)]. Good. Notice that the closer the magnets are together, the stronger they pull. And the stronger they pull, the closer your hands move together. Soon they will touch. When that happens, just let go

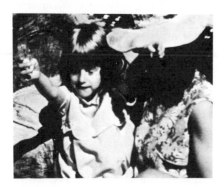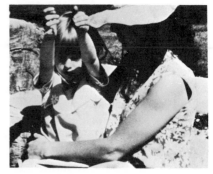

Figure 5-1. *Hands-moving-together technique. (Left) Initial position. (Right) Progressive movement of hands toward each other.*

of those imaginary magnets, let your hands and arms drift down to a comfortable position, take one deep breath and let yourself relax all over."

Hand levitation. "Let your hand and arm just rest comfortably on the arm of the chair. Notice the texture of the fabric beneath your fingers. Now imagine that there is a string tied around your wrist and that big, bright helium-filled balloons are tied to the other end of the string, the kind of balloons that float up all by themselves. Lots of balloons, your favorite colors, just floating, so light, so easy. Effortless. As you focus on the lightness of those balloons, you may notice how that hand begins to feel light too" (Fig. 5-2). Note the shift from "your hand" to "that hand" in order to facilitate dissociation. "Soon one of the fingers may begin to feel especially light. One of the fingers may begin to lift up." Notice carefully which finger moves and comment accordingly. "Good. I see that finger moving. I wonder what will move next. Yes. Now another finger is moving. Now the whole hand. Just focus on the balloons and on the feeling of lightness in that hand. And the higher it goes, the lighter it feels. The lighter it feels, the higher it goes. Just floating up all by itself. Drifting higher and lighter and higher and lighter. Now imagine a soft breeze. That hand may float over toward your lap, or it may float even higher, or it may just stay where it is now. Very comfortable, very relaxed all over. You can just let that hand [or arm] float or, if you choose, you can let the string loosen and the balloons float away and let that hand slowly drift back

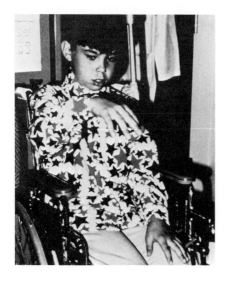

Figure 5-2. *Hand levitation technique.*

down to a comfortable resting place. So easy. Just effortless." If the child seems to be having difficulty, the therapist can first induce a hand or arm catalepsy and then suggest further movement.

Arm lowering. "Stretch one arm out straight in front of you with the palm of your hand facing up." Assist child if necessary. "Good. Now imagine that I am putting a dictionary on that hand." For young children a rock might be preferable. "You may notice that it begins to feel heavy. Now imagine a second dictionary on top of the first one. That arm can feel even heavier. Soon it will want to drift down. When it feels heavy, just let it drift down. Heavier and heavier, down and down. I can see it moving down now. Good. Just let that happen." As with most inductions, timing is essential. The therapist can add dictionaries or rocks as needed, but should be careful to comment on actual movement. For the few children who resist this technique, the therapist can shift to arm rigidity or arm catalepsy.

Finger lowering. This method appeals to young children and may also be used with older children for whom arm lowering is difficult, perhaps because of physical debilitation. The therapist helps the child rest the little finger on the bed or arm of the chair, leaving the other fingers extended in the air. "Pretend that this little finger is having a nice rest on the arm of the chair. The other fingers would like to rest too. Watch them. Soon they will want to drift down and down until they are resting too. I wonder which finger will drift down first. Look, that one is resting now. When they are all resting, you can feel very comfortable all over. You can close your eyes if you like. More and more comfortable."

Arm rigidity. "Stretch one arm straight out to the side and make a tight first. Imagine that the arm is very strong just like the straight strong branch on a tree. Stronger and stronger. So strong that I cannot push it down. I cannot bend it. That arm is very powerful. It can be as strong and powerful as it wants" (Fig. 5-3). Note how easily this method can lead into ego-strengthening suggestions.

Mighty oak tree. This method is especially useful in groups, but also appealing to young children who do not naturally sit still. "Stand up, tall and straight as a strong oak tree. That's good. Let your arms be branches and stretch toward the sky. Your feet are roots which go

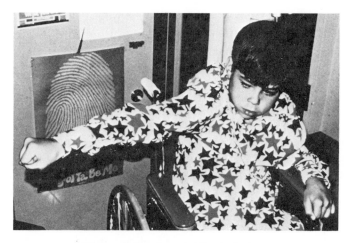

Figure 5-3. *Arm rigidity technique.*

down through the floor. Feel how strong you are. Very strong. You can't be moved. Feel the sun and air and rain come in through your branches to make you even stronger. Feel those strong tough roots. When you're ready, when you really feel like a powerful oak tree, I'll try to lift you."

Arm catalepsy. "Is it okay with you if I pick up this hand? Good. Just let it relax. Let me do the work." If the child cooperates by raising the hand and arm, indicate that such conscious cooperation is not necessary and repeat until there is no conscious cooperation. "Good. Just let the hand rest. Let me do the work of lifting it. Fine. Now look at that hand as though it were part of a sculpture, just floating there by itself. Just imagine it floating there all by itself." The therapist gradually loosens hold of the hand, sensing when the catalepsy has been achieved. "Good. That hand is floating by itself now. Just consciously raise the other hand and notice the difference. Now you can begin to understand how your strong unconscious mind can help you do what you want."

Progressive Relaxation Techniques

These methods are essentially the same for children as for adults. They are often used as inductions with adolescents and sometimes with younger children who have medical problems that can benefit by deliberate programming of physiological relaxation (e.g., the child with quadriceps spasm associated with a fractured femur). The main difference in response between children and adults is that children often respond very quickly with total body relaxation. The therapist must observe the rate of response and be ready to terminate the induction with a simple suggestion of complete relaxation. Lengthy details about specific muscle groups may be necessary for some children; others will experience boredom that can then interfere with response to further suggestions.

Following breathing. "Focus your eyes easily on some point on your lap or anywhere you like and pay attention to each time you breathe out. That feeling is relaxation. When you breathe out you loosen your chest muscles. Each of us does that 10 or 12 times a minute. Pay attention to breathing out and each time extend your own relaxation a little further. Relax your tummy muscles. Next time you breathe out, extend the comfortable feeling into your upper leg muscles. Relax your lower leg muscles and feel a flow of comfort, loosening, relaxation from your chest muscles down to your toes. Go at your own pace and your own speed. When you're ready, focus on your lower back muscles. Let them feel very comfortable. Loosen your upper back muscles. Let a flow of relaxation spread through your shoulders down your upper arms, gradually into your lower arm muscles, into the small muscles of your hands . . . your fingers. When you're ready, allow your neck muscles to become comfortable. Loosen them but just enough to keep your head very comfortable. Let the flow of relaxation move into your cheek muscles, your forehead, around your eyes, even to the tiny muscles of the scalp. When you're nice and comfortable all over please give me a signal by nodding your head or raising a finger. You can tell me if there is any part of your body that doesn't seem ready to be comfortable yet, and we can do some other things so that you can be comfortable all over."

Teddy bear. This method may be especially useful for young children for whom sleep is desirable—as in pre- or postoperative situations—but for whom direct suggestion of sleep might produce resistance. A doll or stuffed animal may be substituted, according to the child's preference. "What does your teddy bear do when he is sleepy? Hold him the way he likes to be held. Let his head get very comfortable. Maybe you should pat him gently, so gently. That's good. Is he getting sleepy? Let his arms get cozy and comfortable. Don't forget his tummy, comfortable, sleepy. Let his feet get comfortable. Pretty soon the whole teddy bear is sleepy. Comfortable, drowsy, dozy. You can rock him if you like. So comfortable. So nice. Such a good feeling. So easy. So quiet."

Balancing muscles. "Sit forward, drop hands to your sides, and move your feet out and spread them a little apart from each other on the floor. Move your body forward until you feel your abdominal muscles pull, then move back until your back pulls. Do this until you find a balanced, neutral position for your trunk. Do the same with your head. Move a little forward, a little back until it feels right. Imagine a thread from the ceiling to your head. Think of your head stretched up a little, hold the position easily for as long as you wish, then think of the thread being cut and your head bending forward, very relaxed and comfortable throughout."

Floppy Raggedy Ann or Andy. "Pretend that you are Raggedy Ann, floppy all over, so loose and comfortable. Let's be like Raggedy Ann and feel floppy. Let me check this arm. Good. See how it flops down when I pick it up. Just like Raggedy Ann. Now let me check the other arm. Good. That's floppy too. Now let yourself feel floppy all over, loose all over, and very comfortable all over."

Eye Fixation Techniques

Coin technique. Present a coin and ask the child to hold it between the thumb and first finger (Fig. 5-4). For some children, attention is heightened by first drawing a smiling face with a colored marking pen on the thumbnail. Younger children often prefer to have their favorite stuffed animal hold the coin, sometimes in a paw, sometimes under a nose. Whether they fix their eyes on the coin held by them-

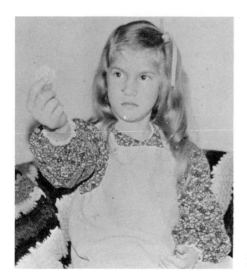

Figure 5-4. *Coin technique.*

selves or by the stuffed animal seems immaterial. "Just look at that smiling face on the thumb that's holding the coin [or just look at that coin, real easy]. That's good. After awhile the fingers [or paws] begin to get a little tired of holding it and after awhile the coin can slip down to the floor [or sofa or bed]. It will be safe there. You can get it later. When it falls, just close your eyes."

Looking at point on hand. "Move around until you have a comfortable position and let your eyes look down, easily, at a point on your hands or fingers, on your ring or on a painted nail or some other spot. Just hold your eyes there easily while you take five long, deep, comfortable breaths. After the fifth breath let your eyes close easily and comfortably."

Stereoscopic viewer. The photo chosen must be of something which the patient is known to enjoy. "Hold this viewer easily in front of your eyes. I'll turn the light on. Can you see the kitty walking in the leaves? Maybe she's looking for someone to play with. See the colors. What else do you see?"

Biofeedback. Children as young as 3 or 4 are intrigued by watching changing numbers on a thermal monitor and have a remarkably long attention span for the machine (Fig. 5-5). Some children may be asked just to watch the numbers change. Others may be encouraged to change finger temperature by thinking hot or cold. The latter

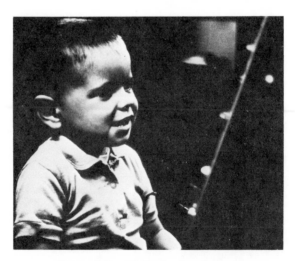

Figure 5-5. *Biofeedback technique.*

method emphasizes bodily control and may be a good introduction to related therapeutic suggestions. "This machine tells you how warm or cool your fingers are. Look at the numbers. When they go up, that means your fingers are warmer. When they go down, that means your fingers are cooler. Sometimes you can make the numbers change by just thinking about your fingers being warm or cool. I wonder which way the numbers will go for you. Good. The number went up. Your fingers are warm and comfortable. Look. The number has changed again. Just watch the numbers and feel more and more comfortable."

Distraction and Utilization Techniques

These methods, based on techniques developed by Erickson (1959), are especially helpful with children who are frightened or in severe pain. They attract attention often by a seeming lack of logic, shifting focus from a negative to a positive aspect of the situation. Once the therapist can get the child's attention, trance may occur spontaneously and therapeutic suggestions may be easily accepted. The success of these techniques is chiefly a function of the therapist's creativity. We give only a few examples.

"It hurts and it's going to hurt a while longer. I wonder if it will stop hurting in 5 minutes or 7 minutes or 30 seconds or right now."

"Your right hand is hurt. Let's be sure the left hand is not also injured. Does it hurt here . . . or here . . . or here?"

"Those are pretty sparkling tears. Can you cry some more of them? I wonder which eye will have more tears."

"What's that dog in the corner doing?"

"What color is the air today?"

"Listen to that scream. You certainly have strong lungs. Now scream a few more times and then we'll count in a whisper. One, two, three. . . . You're good at whispering. We'll count when you scream and we'll count when you whisper. Four, five. . . ."

Machine-Aided Induction Techniques

Videotape.   Young children who are shy or hesitant may benefit by watching a videotape of a child of similar age responding to hypnotic induction.

Audiotape.   For some children who have difficulty learning to go into hypnosis without the therapist present, inductions may be recorded on cassette tapes for use at home or in a hospital room. We prefer, however, that children achieve full independence in using hypnosis for their own benefit; tape recorders may not always be available or may not function properly. When a tape is requested by a child or family, the therapist should ask for recommendations from the child regarding what should be placed on the tape. Each tape should be tailored to the child's particular needs. Some children like to dictate their own induction onto the tape, thus taking a step toward mastery. The child should be told that this tape is for his or her use only, and is not to be played for other children. We have not seen children abuse taped inductions when the therapist explains that the tape would probably not be helpful to other children.

Telephone. We have both found that children respond easily to hypnotic induction by telephone so long as patient and therapist are well known to one another. Sometimes distance precludes a face-to-face visit or the therapist is not immediately available when some unexpected special circumstance arises in which immediate reinforcement of hypnotic suggestions is advisable. For instance, a burned child may suddenly be faced with an unexpected procedure or may otherwise experience intense pain and be unable to use techniques of self-hypnosis. Although privacy and quiet are desirable, we have used telephone inductions in a busy intensive care unit where as many as a dozen adults were working with our patient and others. In long-term follow-up of children with habit problems, Olness (1976) has children telephone the office on a regular basis. During these conversations, the patient verbally reviews self-hypnosis exercises and the therapist reinforces suggestions. Obviously, it is important that the patient be able to use inductions which do not require the therapist's actual presence. After the patient has told the therapist about the current situation, the therapist can begin the induction. In a few cases, it may be necessary for some other person to hold the telephone receiver near the child's ear and mouth.

Group Inductions

Simultaneous induction of several children in a group has been reported to be successful, particularly with children who have chronic illnesses such as hemophilia (LaBaw, 1975). This method may be especially useful with very young children, who often feel more comfortable in groups and can capitalize on their natural tendencies to imitate their peers. Sometimes parents also enjoy desired relaxation and confidence when they are given the opportunity to participate with their children in group exercises. They may also enjoy sharing the benefits of learning self-hypnosis to reinforce these general goals.

The therapist may choose to have all participants use the same induction, such as favorite place imagery or the coin technique. At other times, and especially if the children differ widely in age, the therapist may use a patient's-choice induction in which each patient uses a self-hypnotic technique most beneficial in the past. During this time the therapist may remain silent, may address general comments to the group or may make particular statements to individual group members. Likewise, when the therapist makes hypnotherapeutic suggestions, these may be addressed to the group as a whole or to individual members; in the latter case, rivalry will be minimized if all members receive a brief individual comment or suggestion.

In group inductions, some children—especially the younger ones—may choose to have their eyes open, at least at the beginning, so that they can observe and imitate their peers. For most children, the therapist may comment that distraction will be lessened and concentration heightened if they close their eyes at the outset, perhaps opening them briefly from time to time as needed.

Dehypnotization or Arousal

When choosing a method of terminating a trance, the therapist takes into account the patient's need for structure and tendency to resist dehypnotization. As compared with adults, children usually need less formality and ritual. If structure seems helpful the therapist may count—or ask patients to count—to a certain number. Or children may count silently using suggestions that they will open their eyes at some point in the counting and feel fully alert, aware, and refreshed by the end of the count. If a less structured approach seems best, the therapist might say, "Enjoy that experience [or scene or place] a little while longer and then, when you're ready, slowly, comfortably, easily, open your eyes and return to your usual state of awareness." For a younger child, "Do that a little longer and, when you're ready, go back [or return] to what you were doing before we began this practice." If the child was in pain or distress before the induction, the therapist needs to add some clarification such as "lying in your bed with your teddy bear, and you can keep all the comfortable, nice feelings you have now." Some children may be told to enjoy the hypnotic state "for as long as you like," but this phrase should be avoided with children who might use it to extend the session beyond appropriate limits or otherwise manipulate the therapist. Occasionally a child in a group hypnotherapy session may compete with peers by resisting dehypnotization. The therapist can usually solve the problem with a casual remark such as "I wonder who will be the first one to be able to get fully alert again." Rarely, a direct comment to the child may be in order.

Consistent with our usual avoidance of the terms "asleep, sleepy, tired, drowsy," we avoid the term "wake up." However, when doing an induction with a child for whom it would be appropriate to drift from the state of hypnosis to the state of sleep without intermediate arousal, we would say, "Now, if you wish, you can just drift off to sleep. When you wake up, you can feel fully refreshed and alert. When you wake up, you will no longer be in hypnosis; you will be in your usual state of awareness and will enjoy the rest of the day."

INDUCTION TECHNIQUES FOR DIFFERENT AGES

Children of different ages often prefer different induction techniques. Although we can group techniques roughly according to the age groups for which they are most often appropriate, there are no hard and fast rules, especially in cases where levels of cognitive or social-emotional development are at variance with expectations based on chronological age. Immature adolescents may do well with techniques that normally would appeal to younger children. Likewise, some young children succeed best with methods which appeal to older age groups, especially techniques they know are used by older siblings or parents. As usual, we remain flexible and let the patient be the guide.

In Table 5-1, we have included methods that need no description and therefore have not been discussed previously.

MODIFICATIONS FOR CHILDREN WITH SPECIAL PROBLEMS

It is especially important that the therapist working with children who have various handicaps be familiar with a variety of induction techniques and be capable of creative modification to suit special needs.

Physical Disabilities

Hypnotherapeutic induction can be successful with children who are at bedrest or who have motor limitations, verbal dysfluencies, blindness, or deafness. Even delirious or comatose children may respond (Markowitz, 1980). In general, the therapist chooses a method

Table 5-1
Induction Techniques by Age

Preverbal (0–2 years)
Tactile stimulation: stroking,
  patting
Kinesthetic stimulation: rocking,
  moving an arm back and forth
Auditory stimulation: music or
  any whirring sound such as a
  hairdryer, electric shaver, or
  vacuum cleaner placed out of
  reach of the child
Visual stimulation: mobiles or
  other objects that change shape,
  color, or position
Holding a doll or stuffed animal

Early verbal (2–4 years)
Story telling
Stereoscopic viewer
Favorite activity
Speaking to the child through a
  doll or stuffed animal
Raggedy Ann or Andy
Teddy bear
Watching induction on videotape

Preschool and early school (4–6 years)
Favorite place
Multiple animals
Flower garden
Story telling
Mighty oak tree
Coin watching
Letter watching
Television fantasy
Stereoscopic viewer
Videotape
Bouncing ball
Thermal biofeedback
Finger lowering
Playground activity

Middle childhood (7–11 years)
Favorite place
Favorite activity
Cloud gazing
Flying blanket
Riding a bike
Arm lowering
Favorite music
Listening to self on tape
Coin watching
Fixation at point on hand
Hands moving together
Arm rigidity

Adolescence (12–18 years)
Favorite place
Sports activity
Arm catalepsy
Following breathing
Eye fixation on hand
Driving a car
Playing or hearing music
Hand levitation
Balancing muscles
Virtually any adult induction
  method

in which the handicap is not involved or modifies a method to take account of the problem. For example, in the case of a deaf patient, it may be necessary to agree on written suggestions or to enlist the aid of someone who knows sign language.

Korn and Johnson (1978) reported using hypnotherapy to facilitate rehabilitation of a 16-year-old girl with significant brain damage. The patient was comatose when the therapists first began making suggestions for induction of hypnosis. She responded to specific imagery designed to help her recapture her ability to swallow, to move extremities, to dress herself ("Imagine yourself dressing a life-size doll"), and to speak. Over a period of weeks, this patient became alert and regained autonomic reflex responses, motor skills, and speech.

Mental Retardation

Hypnotic induction in retarded children and adolescents must take into account the mental age of the patient. The therapist can then proceed to some extent as if the child's chronological age were the same as his or her mental age. Development in retarded children may be very uneven, with social skills sometimes far more advanced than cognitive skills. We have had successful experiences with relatively mildly retarded children (IQ 50 to 70). Children with more severe retardation usually respond poorly or not at all to hypnotic induction. Such patients do not seem capable of necessary levels of ability to relate to the therapist, focusing attention selectively and following instructions. Even if they do respond to induction, they usually do not benefit from hypnotherapeutic suggestions, probably because of limited conceptualization, memory, and language skills.

Learning Disabilities

As much as possible, the therapist must understand the specific areas of disability in order to modify induction accordingly. Often these patients are hyperactive and have very short attention spans. Induction methods that involve movement (either ideomotor or movement imagery techniques) are often most successful.

Autistic and Severely Disturbed Children

There is one case report (Gardner & Tarnow, 1980) of the use of hypnotic induction with a mildly autistic adolescent. Efforts to use traditional approaches to induction were met with minimal responses. Listening to a favorite piece of music proved a successful induction, during which this patient responded with spontaneous eye closure, neck and jaw relaxation, and hand catalepsy. Severely autistic children who have little capacity for interpersonal relationships are not likely to respond to hypnotic induction.

Olness has found use of eye fixation on a thermal biofeedback monitor to be a successful induction method for severely disturbed children. As they watch the numbers change, appropriate suggestions are made regarding their ability to concentrate, to control their body, and to do positive things for themselves.

It seems reasonable that children with severe ego deficits might respond best to induction techniques that are adaptations of soothing, comforting, nonverbal methods similar to those recommended for use with young children.

Terminally Ill Children

It is very important that induction of hypnosis in terminally ill children enhance their sense of mastery. It should be clear to such patients that they are involved in treatment planning from the beginning and that the methods chosen are their own. Unfortunately, many of these patients are weak and sometimes affected by sedatives and pain medications. If possible, the time of initial hypnotic induction should be the maximum possible number of hours after the last sedative or pain medication. Sometimes, however, a heavily sedated child will respond. For these patients reinforcement via cassette tapes may be helpful. Parental assistance and telephone reinforcement from the therapist are necessary more often than in patients with self-limited or non-life-threatening problems.

TEACHING SELF-HYPNOSIS

It is often useful to teach children self-hypnosis, particularly when problems relate to recurrent discomfort or to undesirable habits. This subject has been discussed as a separate entity only once in the published literature (Gardner, 1981). A few writers have discussed self-hypnosis in the context of treatment of specific pediatric problems such as hemophilia (LaBaw, 1975) or functional megacolon (Olness, 1976). For children who practice self-hypnosis, the advantages are (1) their sense of control and mastery is acknowledged and (2) desired behavior is more frequently reinforced by repetition of appropriate imagery exercises.

Gardner (1981) noted that brief didactic teaching concerning abuse of self-hypnosis is usually sufficient to prevent children from giving demonstrations to their friends or acting as well-meaning but untrained hypnotherapists. The risk of abuse is higher in children with poor judgment or poor impulse control or children with socio-pathic tendencies; teaching self-hypnosis is usually contraindicated in such cases. Using these guidelines, we have not known any of our patients to abuse their self-hypnotic skills.

We find that the major problem with teaching children self-hypnosis is ensuring that they actually do practice the exercises on a prescribed daily basis. In one study (Kohen, Olness, Colwell, & Heimel, 1980), children often got bored with the prescribed practice or "forgot" to do it. Even with cooperative parents, an excellent response to hypnotherapy, and office or telephone reinforcement from the therapist, relatively few children will continue self-hypnosis practice beyond a few months.

Some children resist the recommendation of using self-hypnosis. Factors producing resistance include inadequate motivation to solve the problem, age and developmental level of the child, transference to the therapist, fear that therapy visits will cease if the child uses hypnosis independently, and parental interference.

It is usually possible to deal successfully with resistance to using self-hypnosis. In the case of very young children, we prepare a cassette tape for the child or involve a parent in the practice. The latter often serves a dual purpose, for parents of children with chronic illness benefit from acknowledgment by health care providers that they are able to contribute in some way to the therapeutic process.

Children who resist self-hypnosis because of fear that therapy visits will cease can be specifically reassured on this point. The therapist can also make phone calls for a time in order to effect a smooth termination. We have also found that writing letters to the patient can have a positive effect in encouraging regular self-hypnosis practice.

Some children resist self-hypnosis as a reaction against parental interference, sometimes well intentioned and sometimes not. The problem is especially likely to arise in the case of enuretic children (Kohen, Olness, Colwell, & Heimel, 1980), probably because wet beds can be especially vexing to parents and can trigger their anger more easily than other problems such as pain or anxiety.

Jacobs (1962) reported a case history of a 6-year-old girl suffering from enuresis. The child believed that her parents didn't love her. When the child was in trance suggestions were given that she would learn a "signal" when her bladder was full and also that her parents loved her whether or not she wet. At first, she did very well. Each night the mother was instructed to put the child to bed, to hold her and kiss her, tell her what a good girl she was, how much the family loved her, and how easy it would be to remember the signal, thus reinforcing the therapist's suggestions. After family financial setbacks the mother subsequently became distraught, shouted at the patient, spanked her, and the patient relapsed. After discussion with the therapist, the previous suggestions were reinforced and the patient had no further problems. It is important to remember that unpleasant habits in children induce unpleasant habit reaction patterns in family members, and therapists must consider those in prescribing treatment.

Olness (1976) specifically requests that parents not remind children who have habit problems to practice self-hypnosis, often suggesting more positive ways for them to give attention. She informs children in the presence of the parent that their parents are not to remind them. Then she goes into detail with the child concerning how best to remember to practice. Possibilities include putting a sign on the door, tying a string around the toothbrush, having a placecard beside the dinner plate, and tying a sign around the neck of a favorite stuffed animal. The parent acknowledges the child's decision. Following this, the parent is asked to leave, and the therapist works with the child alone.

It also seems useful to agree on the place where the child will practice and to allow for trips out of town or overnight visits to friends. In general, we ask that the child practice, in a sitting position, in his or her room. Occasionally, in consultation with the parent, the therapist and child might decide on a particular chair in the study. The chosen place should be quiet. The child should usually practice alone, although we know of children who successfully practice during rest periods at school.

When desired therapeutic objectives are being accomplished and frequent office visits are not necessary, we recommend that the child call the therapist on a regularly scheduled basis. The child is then asked to verbalize the self-hypnosis exercise over the phone and the therapist reinforces where necessary. It is also essential to arrange for a time to terminate self-hypnosis exercises, for example, 1 month after all beds are dry. This implies that the therapist expects success, and the patient is motivated to continue. Occasionally a child will be bored or tired of a certain image in the induction, and suggestions can be made for change.

Gardner (1981) described a three-step method for teaching children self-hypnosis, easily accomplished in one session:

Step 1. The therapist uses various induction and deepening methods, usually emphasizing imagery and ideomotor techniques.

The latter are especially useful for children who want some outward and visible sign that hypnosis has been achieved. After allowing time for enjoyment of the imagery, the therapist asks the child to count silently up to five, eyes opening at three, fully alert at five. The therapist comments that the child now knows how to come out of hypnosis and return to the alert state without help. Rapid dehypnotization in emergencies may also be discussed.

Step 2. Therapist and patient discuss which of the induction techniques employed in step 1 were most helpful and agree to discard the rest. The child is then asked to describe to the therapist in detail the techniques chosen for induction, to feel the same good feelings, and to go into hypnosis easily and naturally as the description proceeds. The therapist may add details if the child's wording is too general. After another pause and a reassuring comment, the therapist asks the child to return to the normal alert state. Problems are discussed as necessary.

Step 3. This is the same as step 2 except that the child is asked to recall and to decide to experience the induction silently. Neither child nor therapist speaks. The child nods when trance is achieved. After another pause, the child returns again to the normal waking state. Any remaining problems or questions are discussed.

The child is then ready for fully independent use of self-hypnosis.

CONCLUSIONS

Hypnotic induction is usually a pleasant and creative experience both for child patients and for their therapists. Techniques can be modified to suit children of different ages or with special problems such as physical disability. Most children readily learn self-hypnosis and can benefit from this additional skill. The choice of specific induction techniques is based on the therapist's ingenuity as well as on the child's needs, preferences, and abilities. While such choices are now based on clinical judgment, future research may show that some problems or some children respond better to one technique than to another. To date, such studies have not been reported.

REFERENCES

Erickson, M. H. Pediatric hypnotherapy. *The American Journal of Clinical Hypnosis,* 1958, 1, 25–29.

Erickson, M. H. Further techniques of hypnosis: Utilization techniques. *The American Journal of Clinical Hypnosis,* 1959, 2, 3–21.

Gardner, G. G., & Tarnow, J. D. Adjunctive hypnotherapy with an autistic boy. *American Journal of Clinical Hypnosis,* 1980, *22,* 173–179.

Gardner, G. G. Teaching Self-hypnosis to children. *The International Journal of Clinical and Experimental Hypnosis,* 1981, *29,* 300–312.

Jacobs, L. Hypnosis in clinical pediatrics. *New York State Journal of Medicine,* 1962, *62,* 3781–3787.

Kohen, D., Olness, K., Colwell, S., & Heimel, A. Evaluation of hypnotherapy in 500 pediatric behavioral problems. Paper presented at the annual meeting of the American Society of Clinical Hypnosis, Minneapolis, November, 1980.

Korn, E. R., & Johnson, K. Hypnosis and imagery in rehabilitation of a brain damaged patient. Paper presented at the annual meeting of The American Society of Clinical Hypnosis, St. Louis, October, 1978.

LaBaw, W. L. Auto-hypnosis in hemophilia. *Haematologia,* 1975, *9,* 103–110.

Markowitz, D. M. Personal communication, August, 1980.

Olness, K. Auto-hypnosis in functional megacolon in children. *The American Journal of Clinical Hypnosis,* 1976, *19,* 23–32.

PART II
Hypnotherapy with Children

6

General Principles of Child Hypnotherapy

We will now review techniques and results of hypnotherapy for a wide range of childhood problems. Most published accounts of hypnotherapy for specific childhood problems include some general comments concerning principles, indications, contraindications, and pitfalls of this therapeutic modality. A few papers (Call, 1976; Kaffman, 1968; Williams & Singh, 1976; Wright, 1960) focus directly on basic issues.

In order to avoid excessive repetition in succeeding chapters, we devote this chapter to a discussion of general principles of child hypnotherapy. Some of our thoughts are shared by most people in the field, whereas others will provoke varying degrees of controversy.

DEFINITION AND BOUNDARIES OF HYPNOTHERAPY

Hypnosis and hypnotherapy are two different entities. *Hypnosis is an altered state of consciousness* that may have certain temporary beneficial effects, such as tension reduction, but is not in itself designed for that purpose. *Hypnotherapy is a treatment modality* with specific therapeutic goals and specific techniques utilized while the patient is in the state of hypnosis.

We also distinguish between a hypnotist and a hypnotherapist, for these terms are often confused in the context of clinical work.* A hypnotist—often found in the classified advertisements of newspapers or in the yellow pages of the telephone directory under "Hypnotists"—may be a person with limited education whose only skill is the use of hypnosis and who accepts virtually everyone for treatment. While such people often get good results—otherwise they could not stay in business—they may engage in indiscriminate use of their one skill, sometimes with unfortunate results.

A hypnotherapist is, first of all, a therapist. A child hypnotherapist has advanced training in one of the child health professions and uses hypnotherapeutic techniques as part of a comprehensive approach to the diagnosis and treatment of certain disorders. In this context, it is a good rule of thumb that one should not attempt to treat a problem with hypnotherapy unless one is also competent to assess the problem and recommend other therapies if appropriate. When parents ask us about hypnotists, we do our best to educate them with regard to these distinctions.

We believe that the practice of hypnotherapy with children should be limited to health professionals who typically assume primary responsibility for treating children's problems, for example, child psychologists and psychiatrists, dentists, pediatricians, and other physicians and surgeons who work with children. Furthermore, these professionals limit hypnotherapeutic work to their own areas of competence. This does not mean, for instance, that a psychologist should never treat organic pain with hypnotherapy. It does mean that the psychologist who does so is also competent to treat organic pain with other methods (e.g., supportive psychotherapy or biofeedback).

In selected cases, it is appropriate for nurses, physical therapists, speech pathologists, and other specialists to use hypnotherapy. If their specialized treatment of a child is performed under the supervision and/or responsibility of a physician, dentist, or psychologist, then their use of hypnotherapy should also be conducted under the direct supervision of a health professional who assumes responsibility for the patient and who is competent in the use of hypnotherapy.

To give an example—complex for the sake of clarity—a surgeon might have primary responsibility for the care of a burned child and may have ordered extensive physical therapy as part of the total treat-

---

*We do not mean to imply that the term "hypnotist" always has a negative connotation. For instance, in research on various hypnotic phenomena, the scientist who does a hypnotic induction and explores the subject's hypnotic behavior is a hypnotist, not a hypnotherapist.

ment regimen. The surgeon—if he or she is not trained in hypnotherapy and is not also a psychotherapist—might request that a psychologist, who is trained in hypnotherapy, assume primary responsibility for the child's emotional well-being and for helping to maximize the child's cooperation with treatment, including painful physical therapy sessions. The psychologist consults with the surgeon and the physical therapist and evaluates the child in order to design specific hypnotherapeutic strategies to maximize the child's opportunity for physical and emotional recovery. The psychologist might then train the physical therapist in some of these methods for the purpose of facilitating cooperation with necessary procedures in physical therapy, remaining available for continuing consultation and supervision.

GOAL OF HYPNOTHERAPY

People who come to us requesting hypnotherapy begin by saying, "I have a problem." Often they really mean to say, "A problem has me." That is, they perceive themselves as having been rendered passive and helpless, the victim of a situation over which they have virtually no control. Previous therapeutic efforts either have been of limited value or have contributed to the patient's passive-dependent stance by forcing continued reliance on external powers such as machines and medication.

The goal of hypnotherapy is always to teach the patient an attitude of hope in the context of mastery. The patient learns to be an active participant in his or her own behalf, to focus on creating a solution rather than on enduring a problem, and to discover and use resources for inner control as much as possible.

The goal of mastery does not mean that the patient turns away necessarily from external aid, although this may sometimes be possible. An anxious child may no longer need tranquilizers; an asthmatic child may no longer need a nebulizer. Often, however, the child successfully using hypnotherapy continues to require external help, albeit now in a different psychological context. Thus, a child in renal failure continues regular dialysis, but has less anxiety and depression, is more motivated to participate in treatment, more cooperative with necessary dietary restrictions. Such a child keeps the need for dialysis to a minimum and may perceive the machine as a useful aid rather than as an external imposition.

RECOGNIZING DEVELOPMENTAL ISSUES

That a child is not an adult seems obvious, but is sometimes over-looked in hypnotherapy. If a child patient is to achieve the goal of mastery through successful response to hypnotic induction and treatment techniques, language must be adapted to the level and interests of that child, being neither too complex nor too simple and patronizing. As in any therapy, the hypnotherapist must take into account the child's perceptual and conceptual skills with respect to problems and possible solutions. For this reason, it is often best to let the child select some of the details of imagery used in hypnotherapeutic suggestions. The therapist might say, "Think of a way you can feel safe" and then follow the child's lead instead of suggesting a particular plan.

If the child patient is seen at different points over a period of time, it is important to remember that techniques that were appealing and helpful at one age may have no value or even be aversive at a later age.

The degree to which children mix reality and fantasy is often a cause of fears and other problems. But this developmental tendency can become an advantage in hypnotherapy. For example, the child may respond particularly well to imagery techniques such as rehearsal in fantasy, experiencing a new behavior first in hypnotic imagery and then quickly becoming able to make the transition to incorporating that behavior in reality situations.

PARENTAL INVOLVEMENT

In some instances, particularly when the parent has been overprotective or when the child needs greater autonomy, it is best to minimize the parental role in hypnotherapy. The parents may be asked specifically to refrain from reminding the child to practice self-hypnosis and to allow the child privacy during practice sessions. The therapist gives the parent a general explanation of the treatment program. The following vignette is an example of this approach.

Hugh N., age 7, suffered from severe asthma. Finding self-hypnosis very helpful, he became able to participate more fully in school and in sports, and was especially proud of being able to help himself and not always having to rely on his parents for medication. Soon after hypnotherapy began, his mother said to the therapist, "When Hugh begins to wheeze, he goes to his room and closes the door. After about 5 minutes, he comes out and he's not wheezing, and I don't know what he does in there!" The therapist answered, "I know what I asked him to do, but I don't know what he really does in there either. What is important is that Hugh is better." The mother continued to allow her son the privacy and independence he needed.

In some cases, the child may need the parent's presence either in the therapist's office or during use of self-hypnosis, in order to help focus on hypnotic suggestions or to provide reassurance. For example, Ellen L., an adolescent girl, had difficulty sleeping because of chronic, progressive organic pain with associated anxiety. Although she learned self-hypnosis, the severity of her pain sometimes interfered with her ability to concentrate on hypnotic suggestions. Her mother willingly served as a surrogate therapist when needed, with the result that both mother and Ellen got more sleep and felt more hopeful about Ellen's condition.

Most parents abide by the therapist's recommendations concerning the degree of their involvement. A few parents consciously or unconsciously sabotage the therapy. In a particularly unfortunate case, Billy R., a 6-year-old, was brought for hypnotherapy to seek relief from the itching of severe eczema. He responded well in the first few sessions, easily controlling the itching as he sat in the therapist's lap. He learned self-hypnosis and was asked to practice twice daily for 5 to 10 minutes at home. He said he needed his mother to help him, and the therapist agreed that mother's presence would be useful. But the mother refused, saying she already spent too much of her time with his extensive skin care. She also refused to seek help for her own resentment and related problems. Billy's itching continued unabated.

Sometimes careful assessment points to the need for the parents or other family members to be involved, not just to support the child but as full participants in family therapy, with or without hypnotherapy. Just as in child psychotherapy, parents of children presenting for hypnotherapy may focus the pathology on the child when they also need help. If the parents absolutely refuse to participate in therapy, sometimes it is possible to make at least partial gains with the child alone. In such cases, the parents may be willing to be seen every few weeks for counseling or for a review of the current home situation. We usually prefer this "half-measure" approach to that of absolutely refusing therapy for the child alone. Sometimes the parents' trust will eventually increase to the point that they enter therapy. At the least, it may be possible to teach the child more effective ways of coping in the family situation. We realize, however, that this therapeutic strategy may reinforce the parents' conviction that the locus of the problem is in the child, making the parents even more resistant to treatment for themselves. There is the added risk, if hypnotherapy with the child is successful, that the parents may then find another target for the pathology, perhaps another child or even the marital relationship itself.

TYPES OF HYPNOTHERAPY

To say that a child is using hypnotherapy really tells us very little except that hypnosis is being employed somehow in the treatment program. Hypnotherapy refers to the use of a variety of hypnotic techniques in the context of some form of psychotherapy, using that term in its broadest sense. Thus, hypnotherapeutic methods may be employed in the context of relationship or supportive therapy, behavior modification, psychoanalysis and dynamic therapies, gestalt therapy, or rational-emotive therapy. Some hypnotherapeutic methods are common across several psychotherapeutic approaches, whereas others have more limited application. For example, hypnotic relaxation is used to facilitate progress both in analytically oriented therapy and in behavior modification. Hypnotically induced dreaming, on the other hand, might be employed in the analytic approach but probably not in a behavior modification program.

The specific hypnotherapeutic techniques used with a particular patient are derived from the nature of the presenting problem, the patient's goals, other patient characteristics, the therapist's theoretical orientation, and certain situational factors such as the amount of time available for treatment. There are a large number of possible hypnotherapeutic techniques, each with many variations. Specific examples will be described in Chapters 7 through 13. At this point, we simply divide hypnotherapeutic methods into three broad categories.

Supportive, Ego-Enhancing Methods

The chief goal here is to help the patient feel more worthy, more capable of dealing effectively with problems and challenges, more able to contribute to his or her own well-being and be in control of circumstances, both internal and external. Patients who fear necessary surgery, who experience pervasive anxiety, or who manifest borderline or psychotic behavior often derive special benefit from supportive techniques. Such patients might actually be harmed by approaches that deal more directly and intensively with psychopathology.

Symptom-Oriented Methods

Here the therapeutic effort is directed at removing, altering, or alleviating specific symptoms, either physical or emotional in nature. Difficulties associated with phobias, pain control, and habit control, among many others, often respond to symptom-oriented approaches, especially if the patient is highly motivated to be rid of the symptom. These symptom-oriented approaches are contraindicated if the symptom serves a major defensive purpose such as to protect the patient from severe underlying depression or the outbreak of psychosis.

Dynamic, Insight-Oriented Methods

Again the goals are symptom relief and ego strengthening, but now special methods are employed to help the patient understand issues that create and maintain problems, gain insight into and work through underlying conflicts, and achieve a more extensive shift toward personality maturation in broad cognitive, affective, and social spheres.

Generally speaking, supportive and symptom-oriented methods are most often used with children, and dynamic methods are used to a somewhat lesser extent. For many child patients, hypnotherapy includes a combination of all three methods.

INDICATIONS FOR HYPNOTHERAPY

Since the rest of this book is devoted to a detailed review of situations in which children can benefit from hypnotherapy, we limit this section to a few general comments. It is generally accepted that hypnotherapy is underutilized in the treatment of children. Moreover, hypnotherapy is too often considered as a last resort, despite the fact that it might have several advantages over other treatment modalities. These advantages include frequent appeal to and acceptance by the child patient, few risks and side effects, frequent rapid response to treatment, and the fact that hypnotherapy fosters attitudes of independence and mastery in coping with problems.

A child can be considered a suitable candidate for hypnotherapy if (1) the child is responsive to hypnotic induction methods, (2) the problem is treatable by hypnotherapy, (3) the child can relate positively to the therapist, (4) the child has at least minimal motivation to solve the problem, (5) the parents or other responsible adults agree to the treatment plan, and (6) the use of hypnotherapy for the problem at hand would not harm the patient.

CONTRAINDICATIONS

As child hypnotherapy achieves greater acceptance by health professionals and the general public, the problem of underutilization gives way to excessive enthusiasm and inappropriate utilization. Parents and other well-meaning adults sometimes put great pressure on us to use hypnotherapy as rapidly and forcefully as possible with child patients so as to eliminate troublesome symptoms. Children, too, sometimes make inappropriate demands for hypnotherapy. It is encumbent on us to resist this pressure. A few parents and children will then threaten to seek the help of a "hypnotist." At this juncture, sometimes we are successful in offering guidance and sometimes not.

We also see excessive enthusiasm about hypnotherapy in some health professionals who have just begun training in this subspecialty and have been exposed to accounts of dramatic cures such as those one often hears about in hypnosis workshops or reads about in hypnosis journals. Sometimes these professionals think of their most difficult patients and conclude that hypnotherapy is bound to be the answer to their unsolved problems. Occasionally this is true; more often it is not. In detailed discussion of such cases, we tend to find either that the therapist has underestimated the patient's degree of pathology or that the therapist has problems with a countertransferential need "to be all things to all people." In such cases, we try to educate toward more rational use of hypnotherapy.

The situations in which we believe hypnotherapy is absolutely contraindicated may be subsumed in the following categories of patient requests: (1) granting the request could lead to physical endangerment for the patient, (2) granting the request could aggravate existing emotional problems or create new ones, (3) the request is simply to "have fun" experimenting with hypnosis, (4) the problem is more effectively treated by some method other than hypnotherapy, and (5) the diagnosis is incorrect, and the real problem should be treated some other way.

There are also some relative contraindications for hypnotherapy, usually based on inappropriate timing of the referral. In these situations, granting the request for immediate hypnotherapeutic treatment would involve overlooking a significant medical problem, overwhelming the patient's ego, or trying to impose change on an unmotivated child. In such situations, hypnotherapy may be appropriate if utilized at a later time or in a manner different from what the patient or parent demands.

Absolute Contraindication: Risking Physical Endangerment

Eddie Y., 15 years old, admitted with some embarrassment that although he enjoyed playing football he became frightened when he was rushed by larger players. Convinced that anxiety impaired his running and passing skills, he said, "Could you hypnotize me so that I couldn't see those big guys, and then I wouldn't be afraid?" Eddie was told that it might be possible for him to experience such a hypnotic negative hallucination, but that it was most inadvisable since he couldn't dodge players if he couldn't see them. He quickly understood that he would not only endanger himself by such use of hypnosis but would also quickly become a detriment to the team. He also agreed with the idea that a mild degree of anxiety can be appropriate and even beneficial to his performance. Reconsidering, he concluded that his anxiety was within normal limits. He felt assured that he could seek more appropriate kinds of treatment, with or without hypnotherapy, if ever his anxiety truly reached irrational and maladaptive proportions. He continued playing football without further difficulty.

Absolute Contraindication: Risking Aggravation of Emotional Problems

Cynthia N., an angry and depressed adolescent girl, telephoned the therapist to report a very unhappy experience with a boyfriend and requested one or two sessions of hypnotherapy for the sole purpose of developing amnesia for her entire relationship with him. The therapist explained that it was unlikely that she could achieve and maintain such an extensive amnesia; hypnotherapy could not produce such "magic cures." Even if she could accomplish this goal, it was inadvisable since she might then develop much more serious emotional difficulties. For example, instead of learning skills for coping with this circumscribed problem, she might achieve only partial repression and then develop a maladaptive reaction such as general depression or anxiety, perhaps leading to deeper problems in relating to men. The therapist suggested a longer course of psychotherapy which might include hypnotherapy, but not for the purpose of creating amnesia. Cynthia refused and insisted that she would continue her search until she found someone who would grant her request. We have no follow-up on this girl.

Absolute Contraindication: Hypnosis for Fun

Walter B., an adolescent boy who had recently met the therapist socially, asked to be hypnotized "just for fun." The therapist denied the request and explained why hypnosis should be limited to research and therapeutic situations. Walter agreed with the decision after he understood that hypnosis is an altered state of consciousness in which he might have unexpected emotional reactions that could not and should not be treated in a brief social encounter. He was impressed by a few vignettes of professionals participating in hypnotic inductions as part of hypnosis workshops. Although the hypnotic suggestion was simply to recall and enjoy a pleasant experience, two persons developed unexpected grief reactions and a third developed a mild paranoid reaction. Though such reactions are rare, they are unfortunate. Walter saw that one might choose to risk such a reaction as a participant in a hypnosis workshop or as a subject in a research study, but that there was no sense in taking such a risk when the only goal was to have fun.

Absolute Contraindication: Hypnotherapy Considered Not the Most Effective Treatment

Bobby A.'s mother sought hypnotherapy for her 5-year-old son to help him overcome an extreme fear of dogs. He refused to play outdoors for fear of meeting a dog, and his little sister was now beginning to share his fear. In an initial interview, Bobby demonstrated little fear when talking about dogs and cheerfully joined the therapist in playing with toy dogs. Further discussion with the mother soon revealed that it was really she who had a moderate fear of dogs and that Bobby was basically doing what she expected him to do, although he did have a mild degree of fear. The therapist counseled with the mother, who achieved rapid fear reduction. As a further means of helping her family move from inappropriate fear to adaptive enjoyment of dogs, she agreed to buy a puppy. A week later, the dog joined with the therapist, the mother, and her two children in a playful visit on the lawn outside the therapist's office. Bobby and his little sister easily resolved their fear, and the boy proudly took charge of feeding his new pet.

Absolute Contraindication: Request for Hypnotherapy Based on Misdiagnosis

Tim R., 6 years old, had trouble paying attention in school and failed to follow the teacher's instructions although he had at least average intelligence. When his mother requested that Tim have hypnotherapy for his "behavior problem," the therapist insisted on taking a careful history. It turned out that Tim had had recurring middle-ear infections and that his failure to pay attention was chiefly related to a previously undetected hearing loss. When Tim was treated for his medical problem, his behavior problem disappeared.

Relative Contraindication: Immediate Medical or Surgical Treatment Takes Precedence Over Hypnotherapy

Anne C., 10 years old, had a long history of complaints of vague abdominal pain associated with reluctance to go to school. One day, when the complaints became particularly severe, the mother requested hypnotherapy for Anne. The therapist insisted on a physical examination that resulted in a diagnosis of acute appendicitis and immediate surgery. Following Anne's recovery from surgery, the therapist reevaluated her, and she successfully used hypnotherapy to resolve a relatively mild school phobia.

Relative Contraindication: Another Form of Psychotherapeutic Management Takes Precedence

Larry W., age 14, was hospitalized because of total body weakness and rapidly developing inability to walk. Finding no organic basis for the problem, the physician made a diagnosis of conversion reaction and requested hypnotherapy. In psychodiagnostic interviews, it became clear that Larry's symptoms served as a defense against psychosis. After consulting with the physician, the therapist refused hypnotherapy for symptom relief and urged the parents to admit their son to an inpatient psychiatric program for intensive treatment. The parents denied that their son could have such a serious psychological problem, and they took him home. Follow-up about 1 year later revealed that he had indeed developed a frank psychosis. It is possible that, at some point in the course of intensive inpatient psychotherapy, hypnotherapy might have been a useful adjunct, but its use for abrupt symptom removal was clearly contraindicated.

Relative Contraindication: The Symptom Provides Significant Secondary Gain for the Child

Roy E.'s parents requested hypnotherapy for their 13-year-old son to help him control enuresis. Physical examination had revealed no organic basis for the problem. At first, Roy seemed motivated, but after a few sessions of hypnotherapy it became obvious that he used enuresis to express hostility toward his over-controlling parents, and he really had no intention of giving up the symptom. The therapist recommended that hypnotherapy be terminated and that the parents consider family therapy. The therapist added that hypnotherapy might be profitably utilized after Roy had achieved some resolution of his underlying conflicts, if he still continued to be enuretic. We have no follow-up on this case.

CONCLUSIONS

This brief review of general principles is intended to provide a framework in which to consider the disparate problems presented in succeeding chapters.

The following clinical material includes techniques that were utilized and why, what suggestions were given, and how the results were interpreted. We have done this in spite of the fact that there is little conclusive evidence bearing on the efficacy of any of the hypnotherapeutic programs. We take the position that as long as a given hypnotherapeutic endeavor has not been shown clearly not to be effective there may be at least some features of it useful to child hypnotherapists and their patients. We maintain this position even when we are critical of the claims made for positive results, departing from it only when it appears obvious that the use of hypnotherapy had no relationship to the results obtained.

Given the scope and complexity of problems to be discussed, we have sometimes had to be arbitrary about including a particular problem in one chapter rather than another.

REFERENCES

Call, J. D. Children, parents, and hypnosis: A discussion. *The International Journal of Clinical and Experimental Hypnosis*, 1976, 24, 149–155.

Kaffman, M. Hypnosis as an adjunct to psychotherapy in child psychiatry. *Archives of General Psychiatry*, 1968, 18, 725–738.

Williams, D. T., & Singh, M. Hypnosis as a facilitating therapeutic adjunct in child psychiatry. *Journal of the American Academy of Child Psychiatry*, 1976, 15, 326–342.

Wright, M. E. Hypnosis and child therapy. *American Journal of Clinical Hypnosis*, 1960, 2, 197–205.

7

Hypnotherapy for Psychological Disorders

Hypnosis is not a therapy in itself. When it is combined with various forms of medical and psychological treatment, it becomes hypnotherapy. Some authors express this clarification by avoiding the term "hypnotherapy" and utilizing the phrase "hypnosis as a therapeutic adjunct," but these efforts often result in a return to semantic confusion with the use of such phrases as "the patient was treated with hypnosis" or "hypnosis produced no substitute symptoms." Therefore we maintain the distinction between "hypnosis" as an altered state of consciousness and "hypnotherapy" as a treatment modality in which the patient is in hypnosis at least part of the time. Our only departure from this distinction is in our use of the term "self-hypnosis." Technically we refer to "self-hypnotherapy," but we will avoid that term since it is not yet in general use.

In this chapter, our discussion of hypnotherapy refers to the use of hypnosis in the context of psychotherapy, omitting treatment of habit disorders and learning problems. There are fewer reports of child hypnotherapy for primary psychological problems than for medical and surgical problems. The difference may be related to the greater frequency of positive attitudes toward hypnotherapy expressed by pediatricians and pediatric nurses as compared with child psychologists and psychiatrists (Gardner, 1976). Yet interest and acceptance of hypnosis in psychotherapy is growing, as evidenced by an entire chapter devoted to this subject in the recently published *Basic Handbook of Child*

99

Psychiatry (Williams, 1979). We hope that our review of this area will stimulate further use of psychological hypnotherapy by pointing out some of its advantages and applications. Cautions and contraindications have already been discussed and will therefore receive less emphasis.

ADVANTAGES OF PSYCHOLOGICAL HYPNOTHERAPY

Williams (1979) commented on the essential value of psychological hypnotherapy: "Hypnosis can accelerate and augment the impact of psychotherapeutic intervention. . . . The increased therapeutic leverage afforded by hypnosis can often facilitate both the conversion of insight into action and the more rapid relief of disabling symptoms" (p. 108).

We believe that children in hypnotherapy are more able to accept the therapist's interpretations and to utilize their own capacities for achieving insight into conflicts and other dynamic issues. Increased readiness for insight follows from the combination of heightened ego receptivity and ego activity, intensified transference, and focused attention that characterize the hypnotic state. Moreover, the emphasis on mastery that underlies contemporary permissive hypnotherapy further enhances children's motivation to solve their problems, for they are taught that the solution truly belongs to them and not to anyone else (Fromm & Gardner, 1979).

The chief difference between hypnotherapy for children and for adults is that child therapists are less likely to use hypnotic techniques for the purpose of eliciting intense emotional abreactions (Williams, 1979). This difference is most pronounced in work with young children, where play therapy serves the therapeutic purpose as well or better.

Specific hypnotherapeutic techniques vary with the age of the child, the nature of the problem, and the therapist's theoretical orientation. The techniques described below are not an exhaustive inventory, but rather a sample based on available clinical material.

In presenting clinical data, we are aware of the problem of diagnostic nomenclature, an area in which the very nature of child development makes for greater disagreement among child therapists than among those working with adults. Changing trends in the meaning and use of diagnostic labels further complicate the issue. In general, we have retained diagnostic labels contained in published reports or as they were used when we treated those patients described. In grouping cases, we have usually followed the guidelines of the American Psychiatric Association's *Diagnostic and Statistical Manual of Mental Disorders (DSM-III)* (1980).

BEHAVIOR DISORDERS

The problems in this group are manifested by children of all ages and are essentially characterized by impulsive and/or aggressive infringement on the basic rights of others or violation of major societal rules. Examples include delinquent behavior, rebellion at home or at school, poor self-control, and tantrum behavior. Hypnotherapy is rarely utilized early in the treatment of such problems. Psychotherapists often use behavior modification as a first approach, although insight therapy may also be employed. Once the courts become involved, "treatment" approaches more often involve punitive measures, although behavior modification including positive reinforcement for good behavior is increasingly popular in juvenile centers.

Although hypnotherapy is often a last resort in treating primary behavior disorders, reports describing its value tend to be positive provided both that the patient experiences distress and therefore is motivated for change and that the parents are willing to cooperate in the treatment program. Younger children often respond better than older ones. By the time the behavior problem has crystallized into character pathology, manifested by ego syntonicity and minimal anxiety, then treatment by any method becomes exceedingly difficult if not impossible (Crasilneck & Hall, 1975; Mellor, 1960; Solovey de Milechnin, 1955).

Behavior Disorders in Young Children

Behavior problems in preadolescent children are sometimes described as tension discharge disorders, usually a reaction against inconsistent parenting, family strife, or inability to adjust at school. Occasionally a physical problem leads to disruptive behavior. In virtually all these cases the behavior disorder represents an immature and maladaptive defense against anxiety and low self-esteem. The therapeutic task, then, is to provide a context in which the child can cope more adaptively. Hypnotic relaxation and the intensity of the transference to a benign therapist may provide such a context when other methods fail.

Williams and Singh (1976) reported briefly upon the case of a 10-

year-old boy who presented a 3-year history of temper tantrums. Psychiatric diagnosis was minimal brain damage; tension discharge disorder with depressive features. He had not responded to previous therapeutic efforts including medication, psychotherapy, and behavior modification. After three sessions of weekly hypnotherapy, there was marked abatement of temper tantrums. Specific hypnotherapeutic techniques with this patient were not described. Over the next 19 months, he maintained his gains in individual and family therapy, together with medication and special class placement. He also used self-hypnosis successfully at times of stress. We can assume that the parents willingly involved themselves in the treatment and that negative reactions to the tantrums from peers and family enhanced the child's motivation. This case is an example of the way in which hypnotherapy seems to provide the added impetus necessary for change to occur.

Crasilneck and Hall (1975) described in more detail their treatment of a 3-year-old boy whose problems included extreme overactivity, throwing food, beating other children, and soiling himself. Previous trials of medication and conventional psychotherapy had been of no avail. In hypnotherapy,

> it was possible to use a TV screen technique with him only with the modification of holding his hand, which seemed to bring some calmness and reassurance. His responses to suggestions were indicated by squeezing the therapist's hand rather than by verbal response. In hypnosis, he was told that he would be helped with his problem so that he would be able to learn to have people like him for being a good boy, that it would not be necessary to get attention by upsetting people. After ten sessions of hypnotherapy he began to respond. Counseling with the parents produced a different expectation for him in the home, rewarding each positive change that he made and reinforcing the image of a "good boy" whenever appropriate. He soon became a normal, adjusted child, still full of life and energy but not disruptive. [pp. 180–181]*

The authors' final comment on this case underscores the therapeutic value of helping the child rechannel energy constructively, in line with temperamental and physiological needs. By contrast, some methods of behavior change, for example, sedation or heavy punishment, often exacerbate the problem or lead to equally maladaptive behavior in the direction of withdrawal and timidity.

Two single case reports (Erickson, 1962; Lazar & Jedliczka, 1979) describe hypnotherapeutic treatment without any formal hypnotic in-

---

*From *Clinical Hypnosis: Principles and Applications* by H. B. Crasilneck and J. A. Hall, New York: Grune & Stratton, 1975. With permission.

duction, emphasizing utilization techniques, especially "prescribing the symptom." Both cases concerned "uncontrollable" children who in fact did control their environments, albeit maladaptively, and who then learned ways of more adaptive control.

Erickson's (1962) patient was an 8-year-old boy who became progressively defiant and destructive following his mother's divorce. Her scoldings, spankings, and deprivations served mainly to further the power struggle in which the child invariably proved himself the stronger. At the same time, he unconsciously communicated his need to know that he was not all-powerful and that there was a secure reality in which he could thrive. Erickson worked first with the mother, using double-bind techniques to enlist her cooperation to prove absolutely to her son that she was more powerful than he. Several months later, when symptoms recurred, Erickson worked directly with the boy, establishing his own authority by challenging the child to live up to his boast that he could stomp the floor or stand still for extremely long periods. This maneuver shifted the child's focus of attention so as to permit him to benefit from reality confrontation, with resultant positive behavior change. Follow-up after 2 years indicated that the gains were maintained.

Lazar and Jedliczka (1979) described a single session of hypnotherapy with a moderately mentally retarded, cerebral-palsied boy whose behavior problems included ignoring his mother, making himself late for school, using unacceptable language, and deliberately waking his parents by coughing at night. The child and his mother agreed that he was "a cripple." As a result, she never disciplined him, and he used disruptive behavior as a means of gaining some sense of control and probably also as a way of asking for appropriate external control.

The therapist used several techniques including prescribing the symptom, confusion, and double bind in order to help the boy alter his perception of the value of his behavior. For example, she asked him to spend a certain time each day saying bad words, and she asked him to choose which nights he would cough. In this way, she neutralized the pleasure of the bad language and subtly suggested that he would also choose nights when he would not cough. Similarly, she devalued his misbehavior in her office, either by ignoring it or by asking him to increase it until he stopped from fatigue and boredom. At the same time, she gave the mother very specific suggestions as to how to demonstrate parental control to the boy. Both mother and therapist deemphasized the identification of the boy as a helpless cripple and focused instead on the fact that he could experience mastery in his own development and enjoy more positive experiences with others. The child's behavior problems virtually disappeared in 1 week, and follow-up 20 months later revealed no recurrence.

While some might argue that neither of these cases really involved the use of hypnosis, we consider them both examples of the breadth of hypnotherapeutic approaches to which children can respond, especially in light of the fact that hypnosis can occur without any formal induction.

The following case is an example of our work with young children who have behavior disorders. Ray Y., a 10-year-old adopted boy, was seen for hypnotherapy regarding frequent temper outbursts that occurred both at home and at school. These were triggered by seemingly minor frustrations, for example, being unable to accomplish a task, being denied a privilege, being asked to go to bed (at normal bedtime). His mother perceived him as being easily frustrated and having a short attention span, although he did well academically in school. The patient was adopted in infancy. When he was 4½ years, his parents adopted two biologic sisters, ages 3 and 6 years. The patient had subsequently manifested frequent jealousy of his adopted sisters. He had been examined by his pediatrician and a neurologist, and had been receiving psychotherapy for several months without noticeable improvement.

At the time of the first visit for hypnotherapy, Ray appeared angry and embarrassed. The therapist first demonstrated peripheral temperature biofeedback and gave him the opportunity to raise his fingertip temperature, which he did very successfully on the first attempt. The therapist explained that he had accomplished this because of his own control, just as he had developed controls in many performance areas, such as body control when he performed on athletic teams. He was then taught a simple breathing relaxation hypnotic induction and was asked to practice daily. He was also asked to organize practice sessions for the entire family during which they would review relaxation imagery exercises from *The Centering Book* (Hendricks & Wills, 1975).

Because of illness in the patient, the second visit did not occur for 3 weeks. However, telephone follow-up revealed that Ray seemed much more confident and happy, reported that the family was practicing relaxation exercises, and, in addition, he was practicing self-hypnosis at home. He said he had had no tantrums in school and only a few at home. During the second visit, after induction of hypnosis, he was taught a jettison technique for ridding himself of things that bothered him without the need for tantrums.

In the third visit, the parents reported a marked reduction in Ray's tantrums. The session was audiotaped and Ray took the tape home for review three times weekly. Telephone follow-up 1 month later confirmed that he "has pretty much quit temper tantrums." The mother said that, other than fidgeting in church services, he was doing well and feeling much better about himself.

In the case of young children with behavior disorders, some therapists prefer to work primarily with the parents. Petty (1976) used this approach with the mothers of two children, a 4-year-old girl and a 5-year-old boy, both with severe tantrum behavior. Both mothers were initially instructed to ignore the tantrums but simply could not do so. Petty then utilized hypnotic relaxation and desensitization techniques. The mothers developed hypnotic images of past tantrums without feeling anxious or disturbed, then repeated the procedure with an imaginary future tantrum. In the first case, the tantrums abated after 3 months; improvement continued during the following year. In the second case, follow-up after 1 month also revealed marked decrease in tantrum behavior. Petty concluded that, as a result of the mothers' changed attitudes and responses, the children's tantrums lost their reinforcing value and extinguished.

Behavior Disorders in Older Children

Kaffman (1968) described a 14-year-old kibbutz boy who displayed a 4-year history of poor self-control and marked antisocial behavior including lying, stealing, property damage, and physical attacks on other children. Both the referring therapist and the boy's teacher had recommended residential treatment. Although the boy had refused to cooperate with earlier psychotherapy lasting 2 years, he now quickly accepted the suggestion of a 10-session trial of hypnotherapy, with the knowledge that the decision for residential treatment would be temporarily postponed. According to Kaffman, "hypnotic suggestions included the strengthening of his will to be and behave like other children, emphasis on his own responsibility and capacity to achieve this aim in the area of school, work, and social interaction, together with increased motivation to cooperate in treatment" (p. 733). From that day forward the boy's behavior problems ceased. He completed the 10 hypnotic sessions, and continued in psychotherapy every 2 to 4 weeks. At the end of 2½ years, he had maintained his gains, described by the author as "remarkable." While the behavior change may have been due to the introduction of hypnotherapy, we wonder about the effect of the serious threat of residential treatment. This is a case in which a 5- to 10-year follow-up would be particularly helpful in determining whether the boy really wanted to change his behavior or merely wanted to avoid the "punishment" of residential treatment. In the latter instance, we would expect eventual return of antisocial behavior.

The question of patient motivation arises for similar reasons in Mellor's (1960) series of 14 cases of juvenile delinquents, all of whom had been in a juvenile hall. Their acceptance of hypnotherapy was part of the requirement for probation. The patients, age 13 to 17 years, included 2 girls and 12 boys. The average total treatment lasted 6 hours, with successful results in 13 of the 14 cases. Follow-up ranged from 7 to 17 months, with 4-year follow-up in one case. The one treatment failure was a narcotic addict who showed no motivation for behavior change after five sessions.

Mellor's technique consisted of using ideomotor finger signaling to help the patients get at underlying emotional tensions and to elicit confidence that they could acquire more appropriate behavior patterns. Mellor believed that this technique facilitated regression, recall, and reorientation of thoughts and feelings. Since the patients were maintained in a light to medium trance, they experienced rapid integration and soon developed insight and took responsibility for overcoming their problems. They moved from the ego passivity that often accompanies impulsive behavior to ego activity and true self-control. These results are certainly impressive and the relatively short-term follow-up encouraging. But, given the children's histories, one would need a 5- to 10-year follow-up in order to be able to judge more clearly the value of the treatment. As with Kaffman's (1968) patient, we have to wonder whether the motivation for treatment was based chiefly on desire for change or on a wish to avoid the punishment of incarceration. Based on developmental issues raised at the beginning of this section, we are more confident of the validity of the positive reports of young children with behavior disorders than of those concerning adolescents.

ANXIETY DISORDERS

This category includes children consciously aware of and distressed by excessive anxiety, as manifested by phobic reactions, sleep disorders, posttraumatic stress disorders, or social anxiety.

Phobic Reactions

In general, the longer a child has had a phobia, the more difficult it is to resolve. Parents and other well-meaning adults often insist that a child will soon "outgrow" his or her fears. Sometimes this is true.

Often, however, the child develops a series of avoidance strategies so as not to have to confront the feared situation. Parents may reinforce and even encourage such avoidance behavior, thereby unwittingly communicating to the child that the fear is valid and depriving the child of opportunities for corrective experiences and mastery. As the avoidance strategies become more complex, with increasing involvement of parents and siblings, the problem may eventuate in a folie à famille. Given the ease of resolving recently developed phobias, early intervention makes much more sense than the approach of hoping the child will outgrow them (Gardner, 1978).

In the hypnotherapeutic treatment of phobias, our most common approach is based on desensitization, similar to the method used in behavior modification. In a state of hypnotic relaxation, the children develop images in which they experience safety and mastery. Then they develop a series of images related to the feared event, maintaining the feeling of mastery as they visualize each image. The therapist then gives posthypnotic suggestions that they can increasingly experience the same feelings of mastery in related reality situations. Sometimes the hypnotherapy sessions include in vivo desensitization. Research has suggested that these active participation techniques are as good as the use of imagery alone and may, in some instances, be more effective (Hatzenbuehler & Schroeder, 1978). Symptom substitution is rare.

Ambrose (1968) described another method for helping children cope effectively with anxiety. In hypnosis, the child is asked to make a fist and then "is told that he has all his fears and problems clasped in his fist. On the count of three he will open his fist and all his anxieties will disappear into thin air and he will feel happy, confident, etc." (p. 3). As in the desensitization method, the emphasis here is on mastery. Ambrose further stated that, especially in the case of deep-seated phobias, dynamically oriented therapy—with or without hypnosis—is necessary for lasting results. We have a notion that anlaytic work may be necessary more often with Ambrose's brief, almost magical, method than with the desensitization techniques in which the child can easily see the connection between therapeutic method and problem resolution. However, there are no data comparing the relative efficacy of the two methods.

School Phobia

As in all therapeutic approaches to school phobia, the hypnotherapist must first understand the underlying dynamics, a task often accomplished quite rapidly. Although the problem is usually related to fear of separation from mother, there may be other precipitating factors. Crasilneck and Hall (1975) described a 7-year-old boy whose mother had impressed on him that he should "do what he was told" in school. When older children on the school playground threatened to pull his pants down, his fantasized participation and its attendant anxiety led to refusal to go to school. In another case, a young child's "fear of school" turned out really to be fear of the school stationwagon that reminded him of an ambulance and associated fear of sickness. In both cases, assurance and clarification in the waking state and in hypnosis produced rapid symptom relief and return to school. Crasilneck and Hall further noted the importance of parent counseling in such cases in order to avoid parental behavior that either reinforces the fear by excessive comfort or is overly critical.

Lawlor (1976) described three cases of school phobia, two of which included hypnotherapeutic intervention as well as parent counseling and environmental manipulation. In both cases—a 5-year-old boy and a 4-year-old girl—the purpose of hypnotherapy was to interview the child in a relaxed state in order to gain information about the dynamics of the problem. The first child readily verbalized feelings of hostility and destructive wishes toward parents and siblings, with concurrent fears of abandonment. After reassurance from the therapist and the mother, the boy soon made a satisfactory school adjustment. In the second case, the situation was more complicated, including the mother's suicide shortly before the onset of phobic symptoms. Hypnotic interview revealed that the child blamed herself for her mother's death, feared her own death, and hoped to reunite with mother by staying home. She was placed with an aunt and uncle. The security of her new home combined with therapeutic reassurance to facilitate a good adjustment in her new school.

In both these cases, it is not clear whether the clarification of dynamics and therapeutic reassurance might have been equally successful without hypnotherapy. There were no previous attempts at psychotherapeutic intervention. In our own practice we find rapid success with young school-phobic children using play therapy, nonhypnotic interviews, and parent counseling. It is probably reasonable to conclude that hypnotherapy is at least as useful as more traditional methods of treating school phobia in young children.

We have little data concerning hypnotherapy with older school-phobic children, a group usually much more refractory to treatment. We used hypnotic desensitization with one school-phobic adolescent girl whose problems were complicated by poorly controlled diabetes for which she was hospitalized at the time she was seen. After two sessions of hypnotherapy, she willingly attended a school near the hospital. When she returned to her home in another state, she initially made a good school adjustment, but she later resumed school avoidant behavior. We were unable to maintain follow-up.

Needle Phobia

Because we both work in pediatric settings where many patients require repeated injections, we are asked to treat children of all ages whose fear of being stuck with a needle produces violent reactions such as tantrums, vomiting, struggling enough to require being restrained, and physical assaults on the person doing the procedure. Since the injection usually cannot be postponed, requests for help are often urgent, and we must work as rapidly as possible. Techniques depend on the age of the patients and the approaches to which they seem most likely to respond.

We reported treatment of a 7-year-old boy who required repeated intravenous infusions of plasma in the treatment of Bruton's agammaglobulinemia (Olness & Gardner, 1978). He responded with hysterical outbursts and had to be restrained by six people. The treatment was as follows:

> It was explained to the patient that his unique imaginative ability, better than that of many adults, could help him learn a method to "turn off his pain switches." When he learned the method, he could then turn off these switches prior to his injections and it would no longer be necessary for him to feel uncomfortable or upset. The patient was taught a standard method of relaxation, visual imagery exercises, and the switch-off technique [see Chapter 10]. During the first visit he demonstrated immediate ability to tolerate pin pricks in his self-anesthetized hands and arms. Subsequently, he joined a group of hemophiliacs who met regularly for review sessions. The next visit for gammaglobulin, which occurred three weeks after his initial visit to our hospital, was calm. He proudly turned off his switches and held out his arm for the injection. He has been followed up for one year with no further difficulties, and one nurse now starts the intravenous infusion. [pp. 230–231]*

Another of our patients was a husky 17-year-old boy, with a needle phobia of many years duration, who was being treated for meningitis with a 6-week course of continuous intravenous antibiotics. Each time the IV had to be restarted, he became hysterical and had to be restrained by several people. When offered hypnotherapy to overcome his phobic response, he responded enthusiastically. The treatment consisted mainly of imagery and in vivo desensitization, beginning with a very small tuberculin needle in his forearm, then increasing the size of the needle, and later injecting him with normal

---

*From "Some Guidelines for Uses of Hypnotherapy in Pediatrics" by K. Olness and G. G. Gardner, *Pediatrics*, 1978, *62*, 228–233. Copyright American Academy of Pediatrics 1978. With permission.

saline and sterile water. Instead of suggesting anesthesia, he was told in hypnosis to recall feelings of comfort in his arm and to fill his arm completely with comfort until there was simply no room for any other feeling. He rapidly developed a strong positive transference to the therapist and began to share her confidence that he could conquer his problem. His enjoyment of adolescent bravado further contributed to his motivation for success. After three hypnotherapy sessions, he tolerated restarting his IV without having to be restrained. A few days later, with the therapist present, he tolerated a lumbar puncture with only moderate anxiety. By the end of his hospital stay, his anxiety was minimal and his cooperation excellent. He called the therapist some months later to report that he had had no difficulty when he required a tetanus shot after a minor injury.

Not all cases of needle phobia respond as well to hypnotherapy. In the case of one adolescent boy, the phobic behavior remained unchanged after several sessions, despite good response to hypnotic induction. The boy was generally passive and fearful, afraid to go out alone at night, and rather isolated. The therapist wondered if, in this case, the reaction to needle sticks might be a symbolic expression of latent homosexual conflict. Unfortunately, the patient was lost to follow-up. Had he remained available, he might have required psychotherapeutic treatment of deep-seated problems concurrent with or even prior to direct treatment of the needle phobia (Hinton, 1980). This case brings up the question of whether all phobias are really symbolic expressions of deeper conflicts. While certainly true in some instances, we think many phobias result from conditioned anxiety responses or simple misunderstandings. Frequent accounts of rapid cure without symptom substitution support our hypothesis.

Animal Phobia

Crasilneck and Hall (1975) reported a case of animal phobia in which hypnotherapy was used both to understand the dynamics and to help the child master the problem.

A grade-school girl was brought to treatment because of a persistent fear of cats and other furry animals, for which no conscious explanation could be found in her past experiences. Under hypnosis, using an age-regression technique, we found that the fear had begun at a time when she had been in the outhouse privy on the farm where she was living as a child. She had been masturbating, feeling mixed excitement and guilt, when the door began to slowly open. Frightened and fearing discovery, she had run from the outhouse, only to trip over the family cat that had apparently pushed the door open. She was bruised in the fall, skinning her knees, and had gone crying to the house, ashamed to tell what had happened. At first her aversion had been to cats, though later it had generalized to other small animals. As time passed, she remembered only the fear of animals, seeming to forget the onset.

Under hypnosis, after the original traumatic situation had been uncovered, she was asked to imagine that she was the only spectator in a darkened theater. A red light came on, a buzzer sounded, and she saw a large red curtain rise, revealing a stage. It was suggested that on the stage she would see the original situation—the outhouse, herself, the cat. She was told, "Now you will see what really went on, and you will compare and contrast it to what you remember." From the point of view of her present, older ego, she watched the childhood scene unfold with a detached, more objective eye. After hypnosis was terminated, the events were discussed with her in the waking state, emphasis being placed on the way that her guilt and fear at the forbidden masturbation had been transferred to the cat, then to other similar animals. Her "phobic" symptoms rapidly improved. [pp. 182–183]*

Posttraumatic Psychogenic Amnesia

Crasilneck and Hall (1975) described their work with an adolescent girl suffering psychogenic amnesia.

A 17-year-old girl, angry after an argument with her mother and stepfather, had walked away from her home at night, intending to walk to the house of an aunt some miles away. While crossing a long bridge, she was offered a ride by an older man whom she did not know. The man drove to a secluded area, where he repeatedly raped her. Hours after leaving home she was found by a policeman wandering aimlessly in a deserted area. Brought to the emergency room, she denied any memory after the man had picked her up. She was vague and obviously disturbed.

Following an arm-levitation induction, the patient entered a state of somnambulism. She was told the following: "Recall of feeling and emotions often helps us get well even if such events are frightening. Your recent experience was so frightening that you have forgotten many facts about yourself, but under a state of hypnosis you can recall . . . everything that you have forgotten . . . every fact . . . every emotion . . . every detail . . . and so you are going to go back in terms of time and space . . . back in terms of space and time . . . to that experience that caused you to lose your memory . . . you are going back to the exact time and you can recall, relive . . . revive . . . feel . . . and experience everything that happened."

As the patient began to talk, cry, and abreact the traumatic scene that led to her amnesia, her memory abruptly returned and she dramatically abreacted the rape scene, struggling frantically against an imagined attacker and crying out in fear and pain. As the reenactment subsided, she regained her composure, had an intact memory for the entire event, and was reunited with her family.

*From *Clinical Hypnosis: Principles and Applications* by H. B. Crasilneck and J. A. Hall, New York: Grune & Stratton, 1975. With permission.

She was followed in the psychiatric clinic afterward and given an opportunity to understand not only her repressed feelings about the assault, but also the difficulties with her family that had led to the situation. [pp. 234–235]*

In our hypnotherapeutic work with amnesic patients, we give an additional permissive suggestion for reinstatement of the amnesia: "When you come out of hypnosis, you can remember as much as you are now ready to cope with, now ready to face. Whatever you need to forget, you will be able to forget until a later time when you are ready to deal with it." This wording does not authoritatively impose reinstatement of amnesia, a maneuver which we think often has more to do with the narcissism or anxiety of the therapist than with the needs of the patient. Instead, it communicates respect for the patient's defenses while also implying that the patient may—either now or in the future—be strong enough to face and integrate the traumatic material.

Sometimes a child has good recall of a traumatic event and wants to talk about it, but is unwilling to do so for any of several reasons. Here again, the combination of hypnotic relaxation and heightened positive transference often provides a setting in which the child feels free enough to communicate.

Recent developments in forensic psychiatry have led to increased utilization of hypnosis both to assist children in recalling details of crimes in which they were victims or witnesses and to assist in comprehensive psychological and psychiatric evaluation of juvenile defendants (Kline, 1979; Kroger & Doucé, 1979; Orne, 1979). Although hypnotic interrogation is sometimes extremely valuable in criminal investigation, the process is fraught with pitfalls that sometimes lead to serious miscarriages of justice. In an effort to clarify the complex issues involved in forensic hypnosis, *The International Journal of Clinical and Experimental Hypnosis* has published a special monograph issue devoted entirely to this topic (October, 1979). The issue contains an especially valuable paper by Orne (1979) describing uses and abuses of forensic hypnosis and offering guidelines for using hypnosis in the judicial process. Child hypnotherapists must realize that techniques suitable for helping a child recall and master an emotional trauma differ in significant ways from appropriate techniques for working with the same child in the context of criminal investigation. The most competent child hypnotherapist should obtain additional special training before engaging in forensic hypnosis.

---

*From *Clinical Hypnosis: Principles and Applications* by H. B. Crasilneck and J. A. Hall, New York: Grune & Stratton, 1975. With permission.

Sleep Disorders

Fear of Going to Sleep

Jacobs (1962, 1964) described three children, age 6, 8, and 9, who suffered anxiety associated with going to sleep. He emphasized the importance of understanding the dynamics that, in these cases, included equating sleep with death, associating sleep with anesthesia and postoperative pain, and psychic trauma resulting in generalized feelings of insecurity. Jacobs directed his treatment at the underlying anxiety, reminding the children in hypnosis of their parents' love for them, and assuring them that they could feel increasingly safe and confident. In all three cases, normal sleep patterns returned within several weeks.

Nightmares

While all children occasionally have nightmares, some children have them so frequently that they become truly disruptive, making the child afraid to go to sleep and causing the parents to be roused at night. In contrast to night terrors, the child usually is able to recall at least some details of the nightmare. If there is a known precipitating event, the child can be encouraged to recall that event in hypnosis and then be reminded that he or she is now older or safer or in some way able to deal with the problem. Whether or not there is a known precipitant, the child can be asked to experience hypnotic safety and then to redream the nightmare in hypnosis, but this time changing the ending so as to emerge the master rather than the victim of the situation. The child is then told that it is possible to do the same thing when actually sleeping, if the nightmare should recur. Children enjoy this challenge, and their nightmares usually cease after one or two sessions of hypnotherapy (Gardner, 1978).

Occasionally parent counseling is also necessary, especially if the parents are unwittingly reinforcing the child for having nightmares. For instance, some parents employ a whole series of comforting measures which may include a snack, a backrub, a story, getting up to watch television, and even sleeping in bed with the parents. No wonder the nightmares continue!

Night Terrors

Since children do not recall night terrors, one cannot use the hypnotic dream alteration method employed for nightmares. One can, however, try to clarify the precipitating event and then use hypnotic imagery to increase the child's sense of confidence and safety. Taboada (1975) used this method with a 7-year-old boy who had had night terrors for 15 consecutive nights after a frightening incident at camp. The night terrors ceased after one hypnotherapeutic session, with no recurrence at a follow-up 18 months later.

Social Anxiety

For both temperamental and psychodynamic reasons, some small children feel especially insecure in social situations outside the immediate family. Many of these youngsters learn adaptive social skills as a result of participation in preschool groups, with the support of parents, teachers, and other helping adults. Some, however, continue to be generally shy and withdrawn, and their difficulties may become pronounced when there is additional social stress such as occurs with a move to a new neighborhood or a change of schools. While long-term psychotherapy may be indicated, sometimes brief supportive hypnotherapy can help these children use their strengths to overcome the problem. The following case example illustrates the possible value of short-term hypnotherapy.

Diana C., age 15, came into the office with her mother to request help in overcoming shyness that had become incapacitating in school and in social situations. The patient described herself as always being introverted, especially when compared to three older siblings, but this became more of a problem at age 13 when she entered junior high school. Previously she had attended parochial school and had known the same classmates for 6 years. In the new junior high school, she found herself unable to stand up in class and recite or raise her hand to answer questions. She preferred accepting failing grades rather than giving oral presentations. In the therapist's office, she also expressed her reluctance to initiate friendships except with her siblings and said that she engaged in social activities only when with her older sister and two older brothers.

The patient was a strikingly beautiful, well-groomed adolescent. According to her mother, she had been a good student until entering junior high school. She got along well with parents, siblings, and other relatives and a few girlfriends. Her mother volunteered that, although she accompanied her daughter for the first visit, she would encourage her daughter to come alone on subsequent visits. This and other comments suggested that the mother truly wanted her child to achieve greater independence and social participation. There was no evidence of severe family pathology.

Diana was seen three times for hypnotherapy. In the first interview, it became apparent that she was interested in becoming a model, perhaps a counterphobic reaction but still one that could be used to her advantage. Hypnosis was induced with eye fixation and progressive relaxation. Diana was asked to visualize herself feeling comfortable as a model. She was asked to practice self-hypnosis twice daily, using ego-strengthening imagery. When seen 2 weeks later, she said she was feeling more comfortable in social situations and had been able to recite in class. During this visit she was asked to regress to a past experience that was pleasant and that represented success to her. She was asked to squeeze her right fist to make the recollection of positive, happy feelings more vivid. When she did this, the therapist asked her to let herself be aware of something that might be bothering her, to consider whether or not she could let go of this, and then to imagine sending it off on a plane or freight train. She was told that she could repeat this imagery in her self-hypnosis exercises at home, if she wished.

On the third visit, 6 weeks later, Diana reported proudly that she had had her first date, that she was comfortable in the classroom, and was now practicing self-hypnosis once daily. In hypnosis, the therapist asked her to image herself on a stage, performing in front of people whom she liked and feeling good about herself. She was followed by telephone and continued to do well during 6 months' follow-up.

SOMATOFORM DISORDERS

The problems discussed here have in common a presenting complaint of a physical problem for which the basis is primarily psychogenic. We include conversion reactions, psychogenic pain, psychogenic seizures, and anorexia nervosa. In some cases, the psychological disorder is precipitated by a bona fide physical problem; in other cases the origins are purely psychogenic. In all cases, however, psychological factors play a major role in maintaining or aggravating a somatic complaint.

Conversion Reactions

Historically, conversion reaction has been conceptualized as an expression of neurotic—often sexual—conflict, usually occurring in young women. More recently, it has become clear that the conflict may center around other issues such as expression of hostility or independence and that the conversion may be expressed in borderline and psychotic individuals as well as in neurotics (Jones, 1980). The likelihood of the problem occurring in children is still largely ignored. For example, Jones did not mention children in her extensive review of the problem, and the *DSM-III* lists conversion reaction only under adult disorders.

Williams and Singh (1976) reported a case of conversion reaction, manifested by hysterical amblyopia, in an 8-year-old girl. We quote their report in full, since it is an excellent example of careful diagnostic assessment, detailed description of hypnotherapeutic treatment, and appropriate follow-up.

Maria, an 8-year-old Puerto Rican girl, was admitted from the emergency room to the pediatric service after an urgent referral from school, which reported a progression of visual difficulties over a 3-week period. These difficulties involved markedly diminished acuity in distance and peripheral vision, culminating in total inability to function in school. Neurological, ophthalmological, and psychiatric evaluations upon admission all concurred in the diagnosis of a conversion reaction.

Precipitating environmental stresses included: (1) a 10-year-old female cousin of Maria had an enucleation of her right eye after a traumatic injury 2 months prior to Maria's admission; (2) the arrival of a new infant in Maria's household (already rife with sibling rivalry) 1 month prior to admission; (3) a television program Maria saw, 3 weeks prior to admission, portraying an episode of hysterical blindness; (4) Maria's class was changed without appropriate explanation 2 weeks prior to admission; and (5) a man approached Maria on the street 1 week prior to admission and pulled her hair before he ran off.

Maria was found to be in the midrange of hypnotizability (grade 2–3). A hypnotic exercise was developed and utilized, together with supportive explanation and a family session to achieve several related goals. These included helping Maria to recognize and accept the connection between cumulated anxiety and loss of vision; to develop a retrospective emotional–cognitive mastery of previous traumatic experiences; and to relinquish the regressed symptom complex in favor of a more healthy (premorbid) mode of dealing with ongoing life situations and stresses. The implementation of these goals yielded marked symptom attenuation and essentially restored full visual function in two sessions over a 3-day period.

The exercise itself, first with Maria alone and then in joint session with Maria and her mother, involved Maria's repeating out loud the following three statements while in a trance state:

1. When people are very scared and upset, they may stop being able to see.
2. By relaxing (with this exercise), I can overcome my scared and upset feelings.
3. As soon as I am able to see better, I can go home and do all the things I like to do.

Maria was discharged after the second session, with only a mild subjective report of "blurriness," taken as a call for continued psychotherapeutic support. She was seen in follow-up 10 days later, by which time her visual symptoms had fully cleared. During further outpatient sessions, the therapist placed emphasis on significant issues of ongoing concern within the family as well as upon Maria's school performance. He gave positive reinforcement to Maria for having overcome her visual difficulties, and this mastery was used as a paradigm for her capacity similarly to struggle with and overcome other problems.

Although there was no recurrence of visual symptoms over a 3-month period following discharge, the therapist recommended continued supportive psychotherapy at monthly intervals because of the somewhat turbulent family interaction. The family declined to follow this recommendation, but we have nevertheless received no reports from them or from the school of any recurrent visual problems during the subsequent 14 months. Follow-up contact with the school guidance counselor 17 months after discharge confirmed that there had been no recurrent visual or behavioral problems and disclosed that school adjustment had actually improved. [pp. 331–332]*

The authors hypothesized that the rapid symptom relief following hypnotherapy was chiefly due to helping the patient focus on the twin issues of postulating causes of the presenting symptom and realizing her capacity to reorient autonomously to her contribution to the symptom by directing thoughts and efforts along new, more adaptive lines.

Williams and Singh briefly reported other cases of childhood conversion reaction: (1) A 12-year-old boy presented with a 9-month history of abdominal pain with flexion of the trunk and inability to walk. After two sessions of hypnotherapy over 1 week, the patient began walking during the following week. (2) A 12-year-old girl with a seizure disorder presented with inability to walk and blindness of one day's duration. Ability to see and walk were restored after one hypnotherapy session. (3) A 13-year-old girl complained of a 6-month history of polyarthralgia of hips, knees, and ankles, with gait impairment. Her joint pains resolved completely after three weekly hypnotherapy sessions. In all these cases, continued individual and family therapy were recommended. Follow-up ranged from 7 to 16 months. There were no cases of symptom substitution, although some symptoms transiently recurred, usually associated with situational stress or premature termination of outpatient psychotherapy.

Williams (1979) reported hypnotherapeutic treatment of a 13-year-old boy with lower back pain, eventually diagnosed as conversion. His method was essentially the same as that used by Williams and Singh (1976). The pain disappeared after one hypnotherapeutic ses-

---

*From "Hypnosis as a Facilitating Therapeutic Adjunct in Child Psychiatry" by D. T. Williams and M. Singh, *Journal of the American Academy of Child Psychiatry*, 1976, *15*, 326–342. With permission.

sion. At the time of Williams' report, the boy had remained symptom-free for 2 years.

Sarles (1975) briefly described a 16-year-old girl who was hospitalized after sudden onset of total paralysis from her neck down. Physical examination revealed no organic disease. Psychiatric evaluation disclosed hysterical features and a precipitating event in which the girl was berated for kissing a boyfriend and warned that he would "watch every step she took." During an 8-week course of family counseling and hypnotherapy that used regressive techniques to explore the dynamics of the paralysis, the girl made a complete recovery. No follow-up data were given in this report.

In a paper on pediatric hypnotherapy, Olness and Gardner (1978) included a short case report of a conversion reaction. We now present the case in more detail, with special emphasis on the use of hypnotherapy and its role in the larger treatment context.

Kit T., was a bright, active 8-year-old boy, the youngest of eight children in a middle-class, intact, Catholic family. He developed a documented streptococcal pharyngitis and, soon thereafter, experienced pain and weakness in his extremities, progressing over 2 weeks to the point that he could not walk or use his arms and required total care. Admitted to the neurological service of a large hospital, diagnostic work-up revealed no organic basis for his complaints. Psychological evaluation pointed to conflict in the area of independence–dependence of which the boy was partially aware. He said he enjoyed the role of baby in the family, including special attention from mother; at the same time, he wished he was old enough to have more of the privileges enjoyed by his older siblings. Kit's mother acknowledged that she had always loved babies and derived gratification from continuing to think of Kit as her baby. Kit was aware of his mother's feelings, and his wish to please her contributed to his conflict. It seemed that the strep throat tipped the balance, providing Kit with even more maternal attention. He unconsciously attempted to resolve the conflict by becoming a baby, thereby gratifying both himself and his mother. At the same time, the conversion reaction allowed unconscious expression of hostility toward the mother who seemed to interfere with his developmental needs.

The therapist explained the dynamics to the boy and his mother, assuring them that Kit was not malingering. The mother was shocked that her conscious wishes could have such a profound effect on her son, and she imediately asked for help with her problems. Both Kit and his mother were relieved that there was no permanent physical disability, and readily accepted the recommendation of brief hypnotherapy for Kit to alleviate his symptoms, followed by individual and family therapy to work through the underlying conflicts.

That afternoon, in the first of two hypnotherapy sessions, the therapist talked further with Kit about mind–body relationships, the dynamics of his conversion reaction, and the way hypnotherapy could help him get conscious and unconscious wishes in better alignment. He was fascinated with the idea that, while consciously he could not move his arms, he probably could do so in the altered state of hypnosis. As an initial demonstration, the therapist used an arm levitation hypnotic induction with eyes open, to which Kit readily responded.

Then the therapist employed the method of combined age regression and age progression to facilitate the recovery of a lost skill. First, Kit was asked in hypnosis to recall a specific time when he walked or ran with confidence and enjoyment and to relive that past experience. Having accomplished this, he was then asked to let go of the situational details of the memory but to hold on to the good, strong feelings in his legs, now experiencing them in the present. He said, "My legs feel very strong; I don't think they could feel any stronger." It was then suggested that he could imagine using his strong legs in the future. He did so. Then he was told that, if he was ready, he could remain in hypnosis and walk across the room. Having followed this suggestion with obvious pleasure, he was given a posthypnotic suggestion that he could, if he wished, choose to retain the use of his legs when he came out of hypnosis. He did so, generally happy, but disappointed that we had not yet "cured his arms." The therapist said he could work on that the next day, planning to use the interim to observe his response to the partial recovery.

By the following morning, Kit had maintained his gains with no evidence of new problems. The second hypnotherapy session proceeded along the lines of the first, now focusing on his arms. He achieved hypnotic arm rigidity and experienced normal strength and sensation first in hypnosis and then in the waking state. He was discharged from the hospital later that day. The symptoms briefly recurred the next day but then disappeared totally.

Kit and his family were followed in outpatient therapy over several months, and the basic conflicts were satisfactorily resolved. Annual cards from Kit's mother have indicated that he has been symptom-free for more than 3 years and once more leads an active, happy life.

Sometimes cultural factors suggest that nontraditional methods in the general domain of hypnotherapy will be most useful. Carla S. was a 10-year-old Mexican-American girl with nonorganic total body paralysis and a diagnosis of conversion reaction. The child was hesitant to relate to Anglo-American doctors and responded only minimally to one session of traditional hypnotherapy. Although adequate history was difficult to obtain, it eventually came out that the child had been hexed. We then contacted a curandera (faith healer) who saw the child for three sessions. She produced a necklace and suggested that the power of the necklace could be transferred to the child. By touching the necklace, Carla regained movement of her arms and upper torso in two sessions. She also regained her ability to walk, though at a slower rate, since she had been confined to a wheelchair for 4 months. She was given the necklace to wear as a continuing reminder of her own power and as a symbol to the community that she could no longer be hexed.

One must not conclude from these reports that it is always the treatment of choice to use hypnotherapy to achieve rapid symptom relief in conversion reactions. As noted in the case of Larry W., conversion reaction may occur in the context of a borderline psychotic state, serving a major defensive purpose. In such cases, hypnotherapy should be employed—if it is used at all—first for ego strengthening and only later and very gradually to aid in symptom removal or amelioration.

Psychogenic Seizures

In cases of psychogenic seizures, psychological problems play a major role in precipitating seizure activity. The patient may or may not also have an organically based seizure disorder. Although not conscious during a true seizure, the patient often has heard descriptions of the details of the seizure activity. Sometimes the child has witnessed true seizures in relatives or close friends. Although it is difficult for casual observers to differentiate between true and psychogenic seizures, there are distinguishing characteristics. For example, if the patient exhibits dramatic movements that look like a grand mal seizure but does not lose consciousness, has no incontinence, and experiences no stupor immediately afterwards, one should suspect that the seizure has a psychogenic origin (Glenn & Simonds, 1977).

Gardner (1973) described her treatment of Tracy N., an 8-year-old girl with familial epilepsy, whose first generalized convulsion occurred at age 9 months. From age 3, her EEG showed a petit mal variant disturbance, with seizure activity manifested chiefly by eye-fluttering spells. Seizure frequency increased markedly when the child was in kindergarten, and the problem worsened over the next 2 years despite several medication changes and a trial ketogenic diet. At age

8, Tracy was diagnosed as having both true and psychogenic seizures. No longer able to function either at home or at school, she was highly motivated to improve seizure control. Treatment lasted for 18 sessions, consisting of a combination of hypnotherapy, play therapy, and parent counseling.

The therapist avoided suggesting any sensations associated with the seizures, such as eye closure, drowsiness, amnesia, or time distortion. The hypnotic induction consisted of relaxation with eyes open, followed by hand levitation as a demonstration that the child could learn new ways to control her body. In hypnosis, she was given repeated suggestions that it could be fun to keep her eyes open and see what was going on. Ego-strengthening suggestions were also utilized, praising her for cooperation and improvement and reminding her of the happy consequences of positive change. She learned self-hypnosis and enjoyed home practice sessions focused on "being able to keep her eyes open more and more."

By the fifth session, Tracy showed clear improvement. She then developed a new problem, namely difficulty getting to sleep at night. This problem quickly resolved when the therapist reminded her that there were times when it was appropriate to close her eyes. Play therapy emphasized carry-over of the hypnotic behavior to the waking state and modification of low self-esteem. The parents were counseled to reinforce behavioral improvement and to ignore periods of eye fluttering. We did not deal with other complex family issues that would have required long-term therapy. At the time of termination, the seizure frequency was markedly reduced, and the child was enjoying success both at home and at school. Ten months after initiation of hypnotherapy she continued to make good progress in all areas.

About 8 months later, Tracy's symptoms returned. In a second course of hypnotherapy she made marked gains initially but then deteriorated again. Therapy was terminated after about 6 months. The parents sought help for the child elsewhere, and we have no further follow-up.

Glenn and Simonds (1977) treated a 13-year-old girl who had been having psychogenic seizures for about 2 weeks. There was no underlying organic seizure disorder. The child did have a 4-year history of emotional problems, apparently precipitated by the death of her father. Early in hypnoanalytic treatment she experienced a seizure concurrent with describing a vivid rape fantasy, probably related to conflicts over emerging sexual desires. The treatment included hypnotically induced seizures and training the patient to prevent the seizures by pressing her right thumb and forefinger together. She was also taught to verbalize her fantasies. She participated in an inpatient behavior modification program with emphasis on improving self-esteem. Her mother and stepfather were seen twice monthly for counseling. There were no seizures after the first week of a 4-month hospitalization, and follow-up revealed that the patient remained seizure-free for 2 years after discharge. It is not clear in this report whether hypnotherapy continued during the 2 years after discharge or was limited to the period of inpatient treatment.

Williams and Singh (1976) briefly described two cases of psychogenic seizures. In the first case, a 15-year-old girl presented with a 4-year history of both true and psychogenic psychomotor seizures, markedly exacerbated in the last month. She was seizure-free after a 10-day hospitalization that included both hypnotherapy and family therapy. During 14 months of continued outpatient therapy, both individual and family, she had only occasional seizures, associated with situational stress. In the second case, a 12-year-old girl presented with a 4-year history of mixed-type seizures, both organic and psychogenic, unresponsive to medications. After initial improvement in a hospital program including hypnotherapy, behavior modification, and family therapy, the girl's condition worsened after discharge. She improved again after readmission and maintained her gains over the next 12 months at home where she continued in supportive psychotherapy.

Psychogenic Pain

Williams and Singh (1976) described an 11-year-old boy with a long history of recurring psychogenic abdominal pain, complicated by many factors including serious organic illness that had been misdiagnosed as psychogenic. The child was seen for brief hypnotherapy aimed at understanding sources of tension and using relaxation to reduce and eliminate pain. He was symptom-free in 48 hours. He was followed in outpatient psychotherapy for 20 months during which there was only one transient recurrence of abdominal pain, possibly attributable to gastroenteritis.

Sarles (1975) treated a 14-year-old girl with a 12-week history of severe hip pain determined to be of psychogenic origin, probably related to family discord. Her pain was relieved after one session of hypnotherapy and she ambulated 3 days later. She successfully used self-hypnosis whenever the pain recurred. Follow-up revealed that she had returned to school and that the family was involved in family therapy.

When psychogenic pain serves major defensive functions or provides significant secondary gain, it is much less likely to respond to hypnotherapy. Kelly C. was a 14-year-old girl referred to us because of knee pain that began when she dislocated her knee 12 months earlier. Corrective surgery had been deemed successful, but the pain continued. Nerve blocks and various medications had been of little help.

In the first hypnotherapeutic session, Kelly was constricted and markedly depressed, expressing doubt that hypnotherapy would be of any value. Despite the fact that she responded well to hypnotic induction, she derived no benefit from several hypnotherapeutic approaches designed to alleviate her pain. Diagnostic interviews and psychological testing suggested that the pain might be binding severe anxiety and might also be providing significant secondary gain including passively expressing hostility and dependency needs, neither of which she could admit into consciousness. The girl vigorously denied any sort of emotional distress and responded negatively to the suggestion of extended psychotherapy. She terminated hypnotherapy after four sessions, her condition unchanged. Though her parents were hesitant to accept the idea of a psychological basis for her pain, 1 month later they did take her to a psychotherapist nearer her home. We have no follow-up on the outcome of this case.

Anorexia Nervosa

Crasilneck and Hall (1975) emphasize the importance of recognizing the debilitating and sometimes life-threatening consequences of continued voluntary starvation. Therefore, they begin hypnotherapeutic treatment with direct suggestions for increased food intake. When the patient begins to gain weight and the medical situation is stabilized, they then begin psychodynamic exploration, both with and without hypnoanalytic techniques. They note that the underlying dynamics often center around sexual conflicts, but may stem primarily from other issues such as need for control, aggressive impulses, and frank death wishes. Their technique is illustrated in the following case report:

One rather mild case began in a high school girl after a girl friend became pregnant. She noticed people watching the girl friend's abdomen as the pregnancy became more and more apparent. The patient became concerned that she, too, would mistakenly be thought pregnant since she was slightly overweight. To counter this fear, she began to eat less and less, losing to a point that caused anemia and fatigue.

In spite of advice from her family physician that she must increase her food intake, the patient continued to lose weight. When it was obvious that her weight was dangerously low, we were called to see the patient with the hope that hypnotherapy might counter the negative attitude towards food intake.

After we established rapport, hypnosis was accepted by the patient and she was able to enter a deep trance. She was then told, "You will be hungry. Food will taste good, and your body weight will be necessary for your own good health and welfare." The patient began increasing her caloric intake, starting with her next meal. Her body weight, although on the slim side, came into the normal range for her height. She was encouraged continually to verbalize her many feelings of shame, sorrow, and hostility concerning her girl friend's pregnancy. She was also quite aware of strong libidinous drives within herself, which had caused much guilt. When she was able to express the affect concerning her conflicts, the obsessive thoughts concerning food intake resolved themselves. One year later, although no longer in treatment, she was a slim attractive young lady who could accept the actions of others without introjecting their feelings. She understood that libidinous drives are normal in adults and that they should not lead to feelings of guilt, shame, and masochistic acts. [p. 162]*

Davis (1961) used hypnotherapy in the treatment of a 12-year-old girl with anorexia nervosa whose underlying problems included severe depression eventually treated with electroconvulsive therapy (ECT). This child seemed much more disturbed than the patient described by Crasilneck and Hall (1975). Hypnotic trances were utilized both for direct suggestions regarding increased food intake and for dynamic exploration. The patient gained weight and was discharged from the hospital after about 3 months. Follow-up 5 months after discharge revealed that she had maintained her weight gain and was adjusting well.

Most of the anorexic patients we see in a tertiary care setting are dangerously ill, often having lost 50 percent of their normal body weight. The threat of death demands immediate increase in food intake. We therefore begin with a strictly controlled behavior modification program in which the patient either eats and retains frequent small meals or is tube fed an equivalent amount. Either hypnotherapy or conventional psychotherapy is used for anxiety reduction and for dynamic exploration and conflict resolution.

AUTISM

Gardner and Tarnow (1980) published a case report describing the use of hypnotherapy with Tom A., a 16-year-old boy diagnosed as mildly autistic at age 3½ years. The child had made gains in traditional psychotherapy and in special education programs, though he remained socially isolated and unable to integrate new experiences.

*From *Clinical Hypnosis: Principles and Applications* by H. B. Crasilneck and J. A. Hall, New York: Grune & Stratton, 1975. With permission.

He had a long-standing habit of biting his finger in response to frustrating situations, and he had developed a large callous, with intermittent bleeding and infection.

At age 16, it seemed that Tom might be able to transfer to a regular high school, but his continued finger-biting behavior—refractory to previous treatment—seemed certain to elicit peer rejection and interfere with school adjustment. He was therefore referred for hypnotherapy in an attempt to eliminate this problem.

Unresponsive to traditional hypnotic induction methods, Tom mentioned that Aria no. 47 from the Bach *Saint Matthew Passion* helped him feel calm. Thereafter, when the therapist played him a tape recording of this aria, he easily entered hypnotic trance. Skilled in music, he wrote two short musical compositions for use in hypnotherapeutic treatment. He listened to the first, entitled "Frustration in C Minor," after recalling a frustrating experience, with the suggestion that recall of the music could replace the finger-biting behavior. Then he listened to the second composition, "Happiness in C Major," with the suggestion that recall could strengthen feelings of confidence and increased self-control. The therapist also discussed the construction of the Bach aria, focusing on the way it implied different possible responses to particular events. The finger biting, which occurred two to three times weekly prior to hypnotherapy, extinguished entirely after 4 weeks, with the exception of one episode when both Tom's parents and his primary therapist were out of town. He maintained his gains over a follow-up period of 18 months.

Interestingly, Tom was able to describe frustrating events with greater detail and understanding when he was in hypnosis. At first, there was a marked difference between hypnotic and waking state verbalizations. Later, the hypnotic communication skills generalized to the waking state. Improvement also generalized to other areas of behavior at home and at school where he continued a satisfactory adjustment in regular classes and became a member of the school jazz band. Throughout the treatment, the therapists emphasized competence and mastery in several ways:

(1) involving the patient in treatment planning from the very beginning, (2) communicating to the patient that *he* was acceptable, while agreeing that aspects of his *behavior* were unacceptable, (3) focusing immediately on developing a *solution* rather than getting bogged down in discussing the *problem,* (4) praising the patient for cooperation and responding quickly to his efforts, e.g., using his compositions before he had achieved a hypnotic trance, (5) utilizing the patient's obsession with music as a strength on which to base therapeutic strategy rather than perceiving it negatively as resistance or as an obstacle in the way of progress, and (6) helping the patient observe his own

progress, thus further enhancing his confidence in his ability to master problems in living. [p. 178]*

The authors concluded that hypnotherapy may be a suitable technique for youngsters with severe ego deficits, provided induction techniques are modified to suit special needs and interests and therapeutic suggestions focus on patient skills and ego strengthening rather than on stressful uncovering of repressed material.

CONCLUSIONS

Hypnotherapy can be useful for a great variety of emotional problems, both recent and of long duration, with children of all ages. Poor results are usually associated with lack of motivation, deep-seated conflicts which the patient refuses or is unable to acknowledge, severe underlying pathology for which the symptom serves as a major defense, significant secondary gain from the symptom, and premature termination of treatment. Parental attitudes also play an important role, especially in cases where parents deny that physical symptoms are chiefly the result of psychological problems. When the child's problems are the most obvious manifestation of complex family pathology, hypnotherapy is likely to fail unless family therapy is also accepted as a treatment modality.

REFERENCES

Ambrose, G. Hypnosis in the treatment of children. *The American Journal of Clinical Hypnosis,* 1968, *11,* 1–5.

Crasilneck, H. B., & Hall, J. A. *Clinical hypnosis: Principles and applications.* New York: Grune & Stratton, 1975.

Davis, H. K. Anorexia nervosa: Treatment with hypnosis and ECT. *Diseases of the Nervous System,* 1961, *22,* 627–631.

Diagnostic and Statistical Manual of Mental Disorders (DSM-III) (3rd ed.). Washington, D.C.: American Psychiatric Association, 1980.

Erickson, M. H. The identification of a secure reality. *Family Process,* 1962, *1,* 294–303.

Fromm, E., & Gardner, G. G. Ego psychology and hypnoanalysis: An integration of theory and technique. *Bulletin of the Menninger Clinic,* 1979, *43,* 413–423.

Gardner, G. G. Use of hypnosis for psychogenic epilepsy in a child. *The American Journal of Clinical Hypnosis,* 1973, *15,* 166–169.

Gardner, G. G. Attitudes of child health professionals toward hypnosis: Implications for

*From "Adjunctive Hypnotherapy with an Autistic Boy" by G. G. Gardner and J. D. Tarnow, *The American Journal of Clinical Hypnosis,* 1980, *22,* 173–179. With permission.

training. *The International Journal of Clinical and Experimental Hypnosis*, 1976, *24*, 63–73.

Gardner, G. G. The use of hypnotherapy in a pediatric setting. In E. Gellert (Ed.), *Psychosocial aspects of pediatric care*. New York: Grune & Stratton, 1978.

Gardner, G. G. & Tarnow, J. D. Adjunctive hypnotherapy with an autistic boy. *The American Journal of Clinical Hypnosis*, 1980, *22*, 173–179.

Glenn, T. J. & Simonds, J. F. Hypnotherapy of a psychogenic seizure disorder in an adolescent. *The American Journal of Clinical Hypnosis*, 1977, *19*, 245–250.

Hatzenbuehler, L. C., & Schroeder, H. E. Desensitization procedures in the treatment of childhood disorders. *Psychological Bulletin*, 1978, *85*, 831–844.

Hendricks, C. G., & Wills, R. *The centering book*. New York: Transpersonal Books, 1975.

Hinton, R. M. Personal communication, June, 1980.

Jacobs, L. Hypnosis in clinical pediatrics. *New York State Journal of Medicine*, 1962, *62*, 3781–3787.

Jacobs, L. Sleep problems of children: Treatment by hypnosis. *New York State Journal of Medicine*, 1964, *64*, 629–634.

Jones, M. M. Conversion reaction: Anachronism or evolutionary form? A review of the neurologic, behavior, and psychoanalytic literature. *Psychological Bulletin*, 1980, *87*, 427–441.

Kaffman, M. Hypnosis as an adjunct to psychotherapy in child psychiatry. *Archives of General Psychiatry*, 1968, *18*, 725–738.

Kline, M. V. Defending the mentally ill: The insanity defense and the role of forensic hypnosis. *The International Journal of Clinical and Experimental Hypnosis*, 1979, *27*, 375–401.

Kroger, W. S., & Doucé, R. G. Hypnosis in criminal investigation. *The International Journal of Clinical and Experimental Hypnosis*, 1979, *27*, 358–374.

Lawlor, E. D. Hypnotic intervention with "school phobic" children. *The International Journal of Clinical and Experimental Hypnosis*, 1976, *24*, 74–86.

Lazar, B. S., & Jedliczka, Z. T. Utilization of manipulative behavior in a retarded asthmatic child. *The American Journal of Clinical Hypnosis*, 1979, *21*, 287–292.

Mellor, N. H. Hypnosis in juvenile delinquency. *G.P.*, 1960, *22*, 83–87.

Olness, K., & Gardner, G. G. Some guidelines for uses of hypnotherapy in pediatrics. *Pediatrics*, 1978, *62*, 228–233.

Orne, M. T. The use and misuse of hypnosis in court. *The International Journal of Clinical and Experimental Hypnosis*, 1979, *27*, 311–341.

Petty, G. L. Desensitization of parents to tantrum behavior. *The American Journal of Clinical Hypnosis*, 1976, *19*, 95–97.

Sarles, R. M. The use of hypnosis with hospitalized children. *Journal of Clinical Child Psychology*, 1975, *4*, 36–38.

Solovey de Milechnin, G. Conduct problems in children and hypnosis. *Diseases of the Nervous System*, 1955, *16*, 249–253.

Taboada, E. L. Night terrors in a child treated with hypnosis. *The American Journal of Clinical Hypnosis*, 1975, *17*, 270–271.

Williams, D. T. Hypnosis as a therapeutic adjunct. In J. D. Noshpitz (Ed.), *Basic handbook of child psychiatry* (Vol. 3). New York: Basic Books, 1979.

Williams, D. T., & Singh, M. Hypnosis as a facilitating therapeutic adjunct in child psychiatry. *Journal of the American Academy of Child Psychiatry*, 1976, *15*, 326–342.

8

Hypnotherapy for Habit Disorders

Childhood habit problems potentially responsive to hypnotherapy include enuresis, fecal soiling, verbal dysfluencies, habitual coughs and other tics, nail biting, hair pulling, thumb sucking, sleep walking, certain eating disorders, and drug abuse. Although many habits may have once had emotional significance for the child, often the habit has lost its meaning and become functionally autonomous by the time the child is referred for treatment. Sometimes habits seem to develop without any underlying emotional significance and are perpetuated simply by repetition in association with certain situations.

In all cases, before beginning hypnotherapy, it is important to try to determine whether the habit still serves any important psychological function, whether there is any secondary gain. Does the child achieve a position of control by making his or her habit the center of family concern? Is there pleasure in making the parents angry in a passive way which avoids punishment? If there is significant secondary gain, it may be best to postpone symptom-oriented hypnotherapy. The child and/or the family may first need dynamically oriented psychotherapy to work through the underlying problems. Occasionally, however, the child can resolve dynamic issues concurrently with a symptom-oriented approach.

Even if there is no apparent secondary gain, the therapist must assess the child's motivation for overcoming the habit. Assessment can be made either directly by verbal questioning or indirectly by ideomotor signaling in hypnosis. The latter method is more likely to reveal unconscious conflict, as, for example, when the child raises both "yes" and "no" fingers simultaneously. It is valuable to determine how the child thinks life will be different if the problem is resolved. If a child still obtains much pleasure from the habit, has little desire to give it up, and has come for therapy chiefly as a result of parental pressure, there will probably be little benefit from hypnotherapy. In this case, the therapist might suggest that the parents postpone treatment. Sometimes parents expect too much of a small child who is not developmentally ready to change certain behavior. Again, treatment should be postponed.

In hypnotherapy for habit disorders, we have not found symptom substitution to be a problem, although we sometimes hear dire warnings in this regard. Our experience suggests that children either gladly give up habits or indicate a continuing need for them, sometimes despite an earnest desire to the contrary. In general, a trial of 4 to 6 sessions of hypnotherapy suffices to determine whether the child is really ready for habit change. In the case of some habits, successful treatment depends on removal of misconceptions about the problem. Sometimes such misconceptions can be resolved by verbal explanations. In other cases, the therapist may choose to use diagrams to explain anatomical or physiological relationships, and these may enable a child to develop suitable images for success while in a hypnotic state. Many parents have also benefitted from such explanations. In order to detect persisting confusion, it is helpful to request that the child bring his or her own drawing or diagram to the therapist on the next visit.

Whenever a habit may be a symptom of an underlying physical disorder, it is crucial that the child be appropriately evaluated from a medical standpoint prior to the initiation of hypnotherapy. Since this possibility is most likely in cases of enuresis and soiling, we will include issues of differential diagnosis in our discussion of these problems. These habits may have both psychological and medical components, and too often the former are emphasized while the latter are ignored. A psychotherapist must not yield to parental pressure for hypnotherapy without proper diagnostic evaluation.

Finally, hypnotherapeutic approaches to habit problems should focus on the patient's competence and ability for mastery, emphasizing that it is ultimately the child, not the therapist, who makes the change. Hypnotic suggestions should include images of future recognition that the problem is solved. Parents should be asked to focus on family life without the problem and thereby affirm confidence in their child's ability to overcome it.

ENURESIS

Through the ages, nocturnal enuresis has been the most common chronic behavioral problem faced by the pediatrician (Olness, 1977b). Glicklich (1951) reported that this problem was discussed in a 16th century pediatrics text, in a section entitled, "Of Pyssying in the Bedde." One study has estimated that enuresis has occurred in approximately 20 million Americans over the age of 5 (Cohen, 1975). It is generally agreed that the symptom does not warrant extensive investigation or treatment under age 5 unless information from history and physical examination suggests organic causes. The majority of bedwetting beyond age 5 is associated with no discernible organic or psychological causes.

Evaluation

The approach to evaluation of enuresis varies depending on whether or not the symptom is *primary* (i.e., the child has never had a prolonged period of consecutive dry beds) or *onset* (i.e., the child had several months of dry beds followed by a relapse) (Olness, 1977b). It is also important to ascertain whether or not the enuresis is at night only, or a combination of day and nighttime. The presence of concurrent day and night enuresis indicates that more intensive investigation is needed to rule out organic causes which might include diabetes mellitus, occult spinal dysraphism, urinary tract infections, congenital urinary tract anomalies, or seizures (Anderson, 1975; Kolvin, 1973; Olness, 1977b). Rarely, the presence of nocturnal enuresis is caused by hyperthyroidism, diuretic medications such as theophylline given for asthma, chronic constipation, or a child's habit of taking large amounts of caffeine drinks such as coffee or colas. There is also a likely association between documented allergies and the presence of nocturnal enuresis. The mechanism is unknown (Gerrard, et al., 1971; Olness & Immershein, 1976).

Initial evaluation of enuresis must include questions regarding the meaning of the symptom for the family. Although there may have been no original emotional trigger, emotional problems often develop as bedwetting persists. It is important to ascertain the expectations of parents regarding achievement of dry beds. If, for example, the parents believe that "All children should be dry by age 3," it is possible that unreasonable parental pressure has made the child lose confidence even when neurophysiological maturity has developed somewhat later than 3 years. In the case of onset bedwetting, it is helpful to know about stresses which may have triggered the symptom (Doleys, 1977). These may be events such as an emergency appendectomy for the child, emergency surgery for a parent, death of a pet, death of a grandparent, or a move to a new home resulting in increased distance from bed to bathroom. A model questionnaire for assessment of enuresis is presented in Appendix C.

Physical examination should endeavor to rule out the rare neurological etiologies of enuresis. Therefore, it is important to undertake a careful neurological assessment with emphasis on lower extremity muscle tone and strength, sensation, gait, and deep tendon reflexes. Examination of the spine and back, abdomen, external genitalia, and perineum is important. If concomitant soiling is present, it is crucial to do a rectal examination. Impacted stool present in the rectal ampulla might suggest constipation that is causally associated with enuresis. Poor anal sphincter tone or an abnormal anal wink response might suggest a neurological impairment. The physician should also observe the urine stream of the child.

Each child presenting with the complaint of enuresis should have a urinalysis done. If there are symptoms or physical findings suggestive of a urinary tract infection, a urine culture should also be done. X-ray studies are not indicated unless physical findings suggest physical abnormalities.

General Management

Given the high incidence of enuresis and of its spontaneous remission, it seems logical that, in general, bedwetting should not be regarded as a major problem. Unfortunately, the perceptions of physicians, parents, and children often differ in defining when it is a problem. If the youngster is less than 5 years old and has no historical or physical findings that suggest an underlying medical problem, the possibility of developmental delay should be explained to the parents who may then accept patience as the best approach. For children, bedwetting is usually regarded as a problem when the possibility of camp-outs or sleep-overs develops. At this time the symptom may engender a sense of incompetence and a feeling of being different from siblings and peers.

If the parents and child wish treatment, it is important to agree on a plan acceptable to all parties involved, especially the child. Studies indicate that the most successful treatment methods are those reinforcing the child's own responsibility for success (Marshall et al., 1973). One such method is hypnotherapy.

A Hypnotherapeutic Approach

Initially we meet with child and parents together. Statistics about the incidence of enuresis are presented as well as a brief review of ideas concerning cause. We routinely ask for the child's perception about the cause of the problem. Occasionally a child, particularly in the case of onset enuresis, will recall some trigger event which the parents have not considered significant.

We determine the child's words for urination and defecation. Anatomy is discussed with the aid of diagrams. We ask the child to bring a similar drawing for us at the time of the next visit. We then explain that success will depend on the child's involvement and commitment to practice self-hypnosis. We ask parents not to remind the child to practice, again emphasizing the child's responsibility in the treatment process. We give the parents a printed summary concerning enuresis and their part in the self-hypnosis treatment (Appendix D) and ask them to leave.

In hypnotherapeutic sessions with enuretic patients, we discuss in detail the best time for practice of suggested exercises. It is usually not a good idea to practice just before bedtime if the child is very tired. We recommend practice just after dinner or an hour before bedtime. We review the path from bed to bathroom and sometimes have the child draw us a map of this path. We encourage the child to decide on a specific reminder for practice (e.g., string around the toothbrush handle, ribbon around the neck of a favorite stuffed toy, sign on the door). We emphasize that the bladder is a muscle and that the patient has previously learned control of many muscles. We also use the analogy of the therapist being the coach asking the patient to practice muscle control, thereby further placing ultimate responsibility on the child.

We proceed to ask the child to explain likes and dislikes, such as hobbies, interests, favorite colors, and favorite dreams. We then choose an induction method which seems appropriate. Following the induction, we often ask the child to show us a "yes" finger and a "no" finger and then ask a series of questions, most irrelevant, such as "Do you like the color purple?" or "Do you like to eat chocolate ice cream?" and, without changing pace, insert the question "Would you like to have all dry beds?" or "Are you ready to work on solving the problem of wet beds today?" If the answer is no, as it is occasionally, this suggests that the child may be receiving significant secondary gain from the problem (e.g., being allowed to get into bed with parents when bed is wet) or simply that there is not sufficient motivation to work on the problem at this time.

Following a yes response, we ask the child to imagine being in a favorite place and to signal a yes when ready to give instructions to his or her bladder. At this point, we might say, "Tell yourself that you will sleep well tonight. Tell your bladder to send a message to your brain to awaken you when it is full of urine [or pee]. When you awaken, tell yourself to get out of your dry bed, walk across the room, through the door, down the hall to the bathroom, turn on the light, urinate in the toilet, turn the light off, return to your dry bed, and go back to sleep. Then think of yourself, awakening in a dry bed, knowing you will have a good day. Enjoy knowing your bed is dry because of your efforts, because you're the boss of your bladder muscle. Enjoy the good feeling of waking up in a dry bed as long as you like. Then, when you're ready, you can open your eyes and enjoy the rest of the day." The child is to practice this exercise daily.

In general the initial visit takes from 30 to 40 minutes; we have the child come for a 15- to 20-minute review 1 week later. Subsequent visits are tailored to the particular child. Many older children do very well after one or two visits and are followed by letter and phone. Younger children seem to require more professional reinforcement and may have return visits every 2 weeks for several months. We ask younger children to keep calendars or cumulative graphs of their successes. After termination of office visits, these are mailed to us monthly for several months.

Observations about Special Cases

- Occasionally, children do better with a cassette tape made during the office visit. They play this at home each evening. We do not know any way of predicting which children can benefit most from the cassette tape.
- Occasionally, 4-year-olds do very well in spite of our concern that many are not physiologically capable of night time bladder control. In one case, a therapist refused to work with a 4-year-old, saying he was "too young," but she did work with his 6-year-old brother. A week later they returned. The 6-year-old had taught the 4-year-old, and both were dry.
- We have worked with siblings concurrently up to a maximum of five in a single family. The siblings seem to reinforce each other in these situations although most siblings prefer to be seen separately.
- A mother who is also a nurse adapted what she called the "quarter trick" (coin induction) from an article on treatment of enuresis with self-hypnosis. Her son, age 6½, had never had a dry bed. After 5 days of practice, he had no further wet beds. Generally, the process goes less well if parents teach or reinforce. Several

physician parents have reported total failures in working with their own children who then do well when referred to a nonrelative for hypnotherapy.

- Occasionally children relapse after more than 1 year of dry beds. When they review self-hypnosis, they usually recapture control quickly.
- Occasionally children who fail with self-hypnosis exercises will move on to use a bell and pad system with rapid success. At present, we have no way to predict which children will benefit most from hypnotherapy and which from some other form of treatment.

Results of Hypnotherapy

There are several published accounts of successful use of hypnotherapy with enuretic children. Some are single case reports (Jacobs, 1962; Olness & Gardner, 1978; Tilton, 1980). Solovey and Milechnin (1959) described their hypnotherapeutic approach to the problem but presented no data concerning results.

Collison (1970) employed hypnotherapy with nine children, age 9 to 16, with onset enuresis. Treatment lasted 6 to 20 weeks and included direct suggestion, ego-strengthening methods, and insight therapy. All nine children achieved dry beds and remained dry during follow-up lasting 1 to 5 years.

Baumann and Hinman (1974) reported improvement in 64 of 73 enuretic boys, age 7 to 13, treated with hypnotherapy in combination with imipramine and other medical management, parental instruction, and monetary rewards for dry beds. Duration of treatment and of follow-up were not reported.

While at George Washington University, Olness (1975) taught self-hypnosis to 40 enuretic children, age 4 to 16 years. Treatment focused on direct suggestions that the children were asked to review daily. Parental involvement was minimal. Of the 40 children, 31 were cured of bedwetting, most within the first month of treatment. Six others improved. Of three children who did not improve, one said he did not want dry beds and was receiving significant secondary gain from his symptom. A second child refused to practice at home. The third child had significant urologic anomalies that had required surgery. The successful children required no more than two visits before improvement was apparent. Follow-up lasted 6 to 28 months. No concurrent medications were employed.

Stanton (1979) included background music along with a variety of hypnotic techniques in his treatment of 28 enuretic children, age 7 to 18 years. After one to three sessions, 20 children stopped wetting. Of these, 15 remained dry after 1-year follow-up. The five who relapsed were among the younger children. Characteristics of the eight who did not improve were not described.

Kohen and associates (1980) reviewed data for 257 enuretic children treated with hypnotherapy at Minneapolis Children's Health Center. In all, 44 percent achieved complete dryness, defined as 30 consecutive dry beds and requiring a 12-month follow-up without relapse. Another 31 percent showed significant improvement. Most children referred had tried two or three other treatment methods first, including bell and pad, imipramine, and other drugs. Failures related primarily to lack of motivation on the part of the child and excessive involvement by parents. For example, if parents said, "We had two dry beds last week," preempting the child's own report, failure was likely. If parents reminded children to practice their self-hypnosis exercises, progress was much slower. Many parents would say, "I know I shouldn't, but I can't help it." In these cases, further exploration of the parent–child relationship was sometimes useful.

Two recent studies (Kohen et al., 1980; Stanton, 1979) concluded that hypnotherapy is not likely to help enuretic children if there is not marked improvement over the first two or three sessions. Prolonging treatment rarely produces gains commensurate with the investment of time and money involved.

SOILING

Evaluation and Medical Management

The symptom of soiling in a child past usual toilet-training age represents constipation until proved otherwise. Pure encopresis, (soiling without stool retention) is rare, although parents will often insist that their child's symptoms do not represent constipation (Fleisher, 1976; Levine, 1975). The presence of primary fecal incontinence in association with urine incontinence should lead the examiner to suspect a neurological problem. Occasionally, a congenital defect (e.g., spinal dysraphism) will not manifest itself by symptoms of fecal and/or urinary incontinence until the child is 5 or 6 years of age (Anderson, 1975).

Much emphasis has been placed on the psychological concomitants of fecal incontinence (Claydon & Lawson, 1976; Halpern, 1977). There is no doubt that many secondary emotional problems develop in a child with this symptom, but the original cause is more often physical than psychological. It is important to note that psychotherapy, while often indicated for the ego damage caused by soiling, cannot unblock a stuffed colon! Practitioners may reflexly send a child with fecal incontinence to a mental health professional before undertaking a complete evaluation. The following information is essential before undertaking treatment:

- *How often and when does the child soil?* Children with underlying constipation are likely to soil multiple times a day, whereas the pure encopretic child may have a normal bowel movement once a day into a place other than the toilet.
- *Does anyone else in the family have bowel problems?* This question is important with respect to the vaguely defined entity of familial constipation, which may reflect family eating habits. The question may aid in assessment of the family focus on bowel function and expectancies with respect to outcome.
- *What was the child's stool pattern in early infancy?* Constipation in early infancy may be present in the case of congenital aganglionoses (Nixon, 1964) or in the irritable colon syndrome described by Davidson and Wasserman (1966).
- *How was the child fed in early infancy?* Feeding habits established in infancy may potentiate later constipation, for example, continuation of large amounts of cow's milk into the second year of life.
- *Was there any change in diet, family constellation, caretaker, or bathroom options around the onset of constipation?* Frequently one finds that, just prior to onset of bowel problems, the family moved and the bathroom changed or the family went camping and the child didn't like outdoor toilets or the child had a febrile illness and was dehydrated, following which he or she had a hard, painful stool, or the child suddenly began drinking an extra quart of milk a day.
- *Ask the parents to describe the child's accidents.* Information concerning size and appearance of stool aids in determining whether or not there is constipation with overflow soiling or pure encopresis. Overflow stools tend to be runny and small in amount. Occasionally, particularly after an enema or suppository, the stool of a chronically constipated child will plug the toilet.
- *Is the child taking any medicines?* Certain medications such as imipramine, codeine, and Ritalin are constipating, and their use must be considered in any management plan (Fleisher, 1976). Occasionally, parents or physicians misinterpret the problem as diarrhea and inadvertently prescribe kaopectate, which will increase the problem.

- *Has the child complained of tingling, numbness, or funny feelings in his or her legs? Is there poor coordination?* It is important to look into the possibility of lower extremity paresthesias that might suggest the presence of spinal dysraphism.

With respect to planning management, it is important to know how the child handles the problem, how siblings and schoolmates respond, what interventions have been tried, and what the family believes to be the cause of soiling.

A thorough evaluation requires that a physical examination be done and that this include a careful neurological examination as well as abdominal palpation. A rectal examination is reasonable after careful preparation of the child for this procedure. If the examination does not confirm constipation, it may be necessary to obtain x-rays of the abdomen in order to determine whether or not stool is present. A diagnostic anal manometry may be indicated if there is a question of rectal aganglionoses. Thyroid function tests should be done if there are any signs of hypothyroidism. If history and physical examination uncover occult spinal dysraphism or aganglionoses or hypothyroidism or other conditions requiring specific treatment, these conditions must be treated.

If the diagnosis is constipation with overflow soiling, appropriate intervention is as follows:

1. Anatomy should be explained carefully, with the aid of drawings.
2. Mechanical problems associated with prolonged retention should be carefully explained.
3. If the patient currently has significant retention, a series of enemas for thorough evacuation should be prescribed.
4. Concurrently, the diet should be regulated. Dietary changes should be explained in detail to the child with emphasis on gradual reentry of proscribed foods (e.g., milk, apples, bananas, rice, jello, carrots) after a period of 4 to 6 weeks.
5. The child should choose to sit on the toilet either after breakfast for 10 minutes or after dinner for 10 minutes. This decision should be communicated to the parents.
6. In the initial period some enemas may need to be given. It is recommended that an enema be given every 48 hours if the child has not voluntarily defecated. If this rule is broken, the ultimate curative process is only delayed by the continued excessive stretching of the lower colon.

Hypnotherapy

Fleisher (1976) has stressed the need for children to be given responsibility in treatment of soiling. Conventional medical and surgical management does not do this. Hypnotherapy, alone, in patients who have had the problem for many years is unlikely to affect the mechanical components. But it does give the child personal responsibility and the opportunity to remain in control of his or her bowels while eliminating an undesirable habit. We ask parents to refrain from reminding the child to practice self-hypnosis exercises and to indicate in their praise of the child's successes that the child was responsible for the happy outcome.

Some children with long-standing soiling will continue to have some residual soiling, although they learn to defecate regularly. This problem may be due to long-term stretching of the anorectal sphincters.

The Minnesota Children's Health Center has offered biofeedback training of the anorectal sphincters to some of these children (Olness, 1977a). In one unpublished study from this center, 10 children from a self-hypnosis therapy group were matched with 10 children from a biofeedback group. The 20 children had each had previous medical evaluation and treatment for soiling. Children in the self-hypnosis group were taught to practice suggestions that they could keep anal muscles closed except when in the bathroom for defecation, that they could be physically and mentally comfortable and relaxed during defecation, and that they could enjoy future anticipated events without worrying about soiling. Of the children in the self-hypnosis group, there were two failures of which one was a relapse some months after doing well with self-hypnosis. This child was moved into biofeedback training and did well. In the biofeedback group there was one failure, a 4-year-old boy who seemed not to focus on the machine or his muscle control and showed no improvement after three visits. It was elected to discontinue further efforts until he was older, while maintaining diet and enemas as necessary. He was matched to a 4-year-old who did extremely well using self-hypnosis. In this retrospective analysis of 20 patients, the median time from onset of biofeedback or self-hypnosis practice to dramatic improvement was 1 week in the biofeedback group and 1 month in the self-hypnosis group.

Prospective studies need to be done. These findings may be the tip of an enormous iceberg. Encouragement and positive reinforcement are part of both self-hypnosis and biofeedback. Some of the biofeedback subjects volunteered feelings of relaxation while practicing.

These results suggest several questions: Does the direct visual feedback in biofeedback sessions make it easier for children to comprehend what they must do for themselves as they sit on the toilet? Does the oscilloscope serve as a better induction of hypnosis than verbal communication? Do both procedures stimulate imagery which becomes the reality of bowel control? Clearly, we have much to learn about the relationship between biofeedback and hypnotherapy as they relate to habit disorders.

In some clinical reports, hypnotherapy has been directed at dynamic issues with little or no attention paid to the need for medical management. In such cases there may be improvement, but the problem is rarely fully resolved.

Goldsmith (1962) described hypnotherapy with a 9-year-old girl with constipation who soiled herself several times each day. The poor bowel control was interpreted as an unconscious expression of aggression toward the mother, and hypnotherapy was directed at understanding these underlying issues as well as including direct suggestions for symptom relief. The child was told in hypnosis that she would not be able to eliminate until she was actually sitting on the toilet. In the next week the child had no major "accidents," but experienced continuous seepage. Medical aspects of the problem were still not addressed, and the seepage was again interpreted as an expression of hostility toward the mother. Further dynamic hypnotherapy resulted in some improvement, but the child continued to have "an occasional lapse," again thought to represent hostility.

Silber (1968) did distinguish between soiling based on mechanical problems and encopresis, which he defined as psychologically motivated soiling. He employed hypnotherapy in combination with enemas with nine encopretic children, age 5 to 9 years. Treatment, which lasted approximately three sessions, helped the child focus on anthropomorphic images related to defecation, for example, the anal sphincter as an intelligent watchman. Dynamic issues were dealt with only indirectly through these images. All nine children were reported as cured.

Olness (1976) reported successful hypnotherapeutic treatment of four children with functional megacolon, of whom three were in the 3- to 5-year age range. All were taught self-hypnosis and gave themselves daily suggestions regarding their ability to control their bowels in appropriate ways. Olness concluded that success was chiefly due to the children's being given responsibility for their own solution. Parents were involved only to the extent that they praised the child for improvement and reinforced feelings of mastery.

SPEECH AND VOICE PROBLEMS

Stuttering

The problem of stuttering has been described from many points of view, with treatment approaches derived from presumed neurological, educational, and psychological causes. Hypnotherapy has been found a helpful adjunct in the context of differing treatment approaches. A key factor in success may be the children's feelings of mastery and confidence in the hypnotherapeutic relationship. Published accounts consist of technical considerations, with isolated case reports (Moore, 1946; Falck, 1964; Silber, 1973). Silber (1973) utilized fairy tales, folklore, and symbols to help children who stutter get in touch with potential verbal fluency and self-esteem and to strengthen their ability to cope effectively with environmental stress. He used his own imaginative skills to engage the child's creative abilities in working toward a solution to the problem.

Defects of Articulation

Silber's (1973) hypnotherapeutic approach to children with significant articulation problems again focused on imaginative use of fairy tales, folklore, and symbols. He described his successful work with a 10-year-old boy, seen for 26 sessions over a period of 18 weeks. The child continued to speak clearly 2 years later. Silber concluded that success was related to the fact that the "patient is committed by co-operation and participation in a creative endeavor of the imagination" (p. 281).

Voice Problems

Laguaite (1976) reported her hypnotherapeutic treatment of 18 children, age 4 to 10 years, with deviant voices, usually associated with excessive shouting. In some cases, the problem was related to vocal nodules or hypertrophy of the vocal bands. Five children had normal larynges, and two could not be visualized adequately. Three children did not complete the course of treatment. For the remaining 15, hypnotherapy focused on encouraging the patients not to yell so much, ego strengthening, and insight-oriented techniques. Of these 15, all but 2 showed improvement in the appearance of the larynx or the complete disappearance of the nodules. Laguaite noted that another group of children, treated for nodules without hypnotherapy, also showed improvement but required an average of 14 sessions of treatment as opposed to only 10 sessions for the hypnotherapy group.

One of our patients was an 11-year-old boy who swallowed lye at age 21 months and subsequently underwent numerous surgical procedures. He had not spoken normally since esophageal surgery at age 9. When asked questions in the therapist's office, the patient whispered answers. In the preliminary conversation, he said that fishing was one of his favorite pastimes, and that he looked forward to being able to sing when he recaptured his voice. He was told that there may have been a temporary organic cause for his loss of voice, such as swelling around the vocal cords associated with surgery, and perhaps he had continued to whisper as a habit. His mother said she believed this because she had heard him speak aloud in his sleep. At the first visit, the boy learned progressive relaxation, synchronized with breathing. He then imagined himself in a favorite place. He later reported that while imagining himself in a favorite place, he went fishing and caught three walleyed pike. Following the therapist's request, he then recalled a time in the past when he was enjoying singing a particular favorite song and carried this forward to a time in the future when he could imagine himself singing the same song aloud. He appeared very relaxed throughout the 15-minute exercise. He was asked to review it at home twice daily.

The patient returned 1 week later. After review of progressive relaxation and favorite place imagery, he visualized a calendar going backwards week by week. He used previously arranged ideomotor signals to indicate that the problem leading to his loss of voice occurred in September 1977. As the therapist described moving from week 3 to 2 in September, he coughed, had a choking expression, and tensed his left hand. Asked to return to his favorite place, he reviewed the suggestions of the first visit. In checking records of his outpatient visits to the surgeon's office, it was noted that he was seen by the surgeon on September 15, 1977, with a chart notation "surgery to follow."

The third visit occurred 2 weeks later. The parents reported they now heard the boy speak in a normal voice interspersed with whispering. At this visit he reviewed the progressive relaxation and favorite place imagery. He was taught the clenched fist technique (Stein, 1963) as a device for letting go of something which might be bothering him and related to the vocal loss. Following this he was asked to describe his favorite place and he said "fishing" in a normal voice. He was encouraged to speak immediately following relaxation exercises at home and was asked to call the therapist when his voice returned.

He called 2 weeks later to say he could speak again, but he would like to come for an additional visit. He explained that he heard himself singing loudly as he completed one of his relaxation exercises. His mother confirmed, "He's talking and doesn't need to come back, but he wants to come back once more." His mother said he was very happy after school on the day following the return of his voice. He said, "School is more fun when you can talk." However, on the second day he returned home saying, "Talking can get you into trouble." In follow-up 4 months later he continued to speak normally.

INTRACTABLE COUGH

Many children develop cough habits that are annoying to parents, teachers, and peers. They may represent prolongation of a response to an infectious or allergic disease. The following demonstrates an approach to this problem. A 13-year-old patient was referred to us by a pediatrician for a trial of self-hypnosis in treatment of a cough that had been present for 6 months. Three months after onset of the cough, the patient was hospitalized for a bronchoscopy, the results of which were normal. He also had normal pediatric and psychological evaluations and negative allergy tests. The patient and his mother associated the onset of the cough with the time when he helped his father with a soybean harvest. He and the therapist discussed the possibility that the cough may have begun as a response to inhaled irritants from the harvest dust and had later become an annoying habit. The therapist drew diagrams of anatomy, the bronchial tree, and the cough reflex. She also explored, at length, the patient's interests, hobbies, likes, and dislikes. He especially enjoyed bicycle riding.

The patient was approached from the perspective of symptom relief to be achieved through daily practice of a self-hypnosis exercise. Self-induction used backward counting followed by imagining a favorite place and then increasing relaxation by imagining a long bicycle ride. When he felt relaxed, he was asked to focus on the image of his bronchial tree and cough reflex and to suggest cessation of the cough to himself. He also focused on future anticipated happy events which he could enjoy without the cough. During the exercise he did not cough. The patient practiced the exercise twice daily for 1 week and returned for a follow-up visit. He reported having no severe coughing episodes since the last visit and said he was sleeping without coughing interruptions. He continued practice for an additional month. Subsequently, the mother sent a letter which said the patient was doing fine and she thought his symptoms had been "like those of a virus."

GIGGLE MICTURITION

Although rare, this entity is seen occasionally by physicians and may represent a conditioned reflex as demonstrated in the following case history.

A 14-year-old boy was referred for the problem of giggle micturition. Although he was popular among his peers and a good student, he was embarrassed by the problem of urinating whenever he laughed. His mother believed the problem had its origins in toilet training when she discovered that he would urinate if she tickled him. The patient had been evaluated by several urologists and pediatricians without improvement.

During the first visit, the boy used diagrams to understand urinary tract anatomy and bladder reflexes. After he had agreed to practice twice daily, he was taught a relaxation-imagery exercise. He relaxed by focusing on a favorite place of his choosing and also used imagery of stair descent to increase the depth of relaxation. He was asked to give himself suggestions for bladder control and to imagine himself in a laugh-provoking situation in which he could laugh freely without concurrent urination.

At the second visit 1 week later, he stated he was much improved and very pleased with his progress. He stated that he had "lost a few drops of urine" only three times while laughing. At the third visit, 2 weeks after the second, he reported only one accident.

Subsequent follow-up was by phone over the next 4 months. He was completely dry. Five months after his last call, his mother called saying he had no accidents in school but occasionally wet during group outings. He was no longer practicing the relaxation-imagery exercise. The mother was told that since he had solved the primary problem of control during school, perhaps he did not regard the residual problem as serious enough to warrant further practice. The mother was asked not to encourage him to return for therapy unless he made the request.

He returned for an additional visit 3 months later with the report that he laughed frequently and had no accidents of any kind during the preceding 4 weeks. He spoke of his plans to become a lawyer or psychiatrist, his plans to go to summer camp, and of his recent honor grades in geometry. Follow-up over the subsequent year indicated no recurrence of giggle micturition.

HAIR PULLING, NAIL BITING, THUMB SUCKING

These habits may have their origins in anxiety, emulation of a peer or an adult role model, or unsatisfied oral needs. They are non-lethal, of little physical medical significance (unless a child should ingest parasites, bacteria, or viruses in the course of biting or sucking), but they are exceedingly annoying to observers and often to the patients themselves. Frequent reminding from parents and resistance in the child may lead to significant family problems. The use of hypnotherapy for these problems may provide an acceptable way out.

As is true in management of all habit problems, it is useful to structure intervention in such a way that the child's confidence, sense of personal responsibility, and mastery are reinforced. The initial interview should be structured in similar fashion to those related to problems such as enuresis and soiling. We emphasize that the original cause for the problem may no longer be important because the child is older and sees things in a different perspective.

After discussion about the child's interests, likes, and dislikes, we plan an appropriate self-hypnosis exercise. Following induction of hypnosis, the child is taught use of ideomotor signals and asked questions related to desire to be rid of the habit, desired rate of progress, and other details. If it is evident that the child wishes to proceed, we ask the child to devise an appropriate suggestion.

These may be variations of the following:

"Whenever your hand begins to lift toward your hair or your mouth, move it instead to the other hand and give yourself a little pat for not pulling, sucking, or biting."

"Whenever your hand begins to lift, tell yourself that you can feel as comfortable as you do in your favorite place—as you do now—without any need to bite or suck or pull."

"At the close of your exercise, tell yourself to sit down with a clock and suck each finger for 5 minutes in order to treat them fairly." This often results in rapid extinguishing of the symptom.

"You will bite all fingers but your thumb nails. When they grow out you will let your pointer finger nails grow out."

"And the final suggestion is to see yourself without the symptom: buying nail polish and putting it on your lovely nails; hearing your friends admire your nails and color of nail polish; seeing a baby sucking his thumb and wishing you could help him the way you helped yourself; going on a trip and thinking, 'I'm not a thumbsucker anymore'; buying barrettes for your lovely hair; or going for a hair cut and styling."

In general, it is not a good idea to reinforce these suggestions with the image of parental praise, for that may encourage the child to resist.

Mohlman (1973) recommends that, after the patient is in trance, suggestions to eliminate thumb sucking should be as follows: "Instead of putting your thumb in your mouth, would it be all right to put your thumb in your fist?" After receiving a yes, the therapist says, "This will be even more pleasant to you than putting it in your mouth, and also it will be easier because your fist is nearer your thumb."

Erickson (1958) recommended prescribing the symptom of thumb sucking to a rebellious 16-year-old girl who rapidly lost interest in the habit after 10 evenings of deliberately irritating her parents with loud thumb sucking. Staples (1973) reported successful use of hypnotherapy in the case of a 4-year-old girl who sucked her thumb. Hypnosis was induced by having her imagine she was holding her sleeping teddy bear. Following induction of hypnosis, suggestions were made that the patient was growing bigger every day, that soon she would get so big that she would not suck her thumb anymore, that she might be big enough next week or next month. Secter (1973) has recommended a similar approach to thumb suckers.

Although these approaches, stressing maturation and elimination of the symptom, are often successful, they may embarrass older children who are clearly beyond the age of thumb sucking, bed wetting, and other preschool behaviors. In the case of older children, it seems more appropriate to provide a substitute comfortable feeling for the symptom and to enhance mastery by focusing on the patient's previous successes and future anticipated events without the symptom.

Gardner (1978) reported successful use of hypnotherapy with an 8-year-old girl who twisted and pulled out her hair, leaving obvious bald patches. As is true of many children with habit problems, she claimed to be unaware of the behavior and was highly motivated to change it. The symptom and resulting attention were interpreted as a manifestation of the child's need for power and control in her family. In hypnosis, she was told that she could find a way truly to be in control of her hair. She was given suggestions for awareness of hair-pulling behavior as soon as she lifted her hand for this purpose, and she was told that she could recall the phrase "Stop, please do not hurt" from the part of her that wanted pretty hair. In the first of three hypnotic sessions, the child added her own creative details to these ideas. When she lifted her hand to begin hair pulling, it trembled as it got near her head, then returned to her lap. She reported the sensation of a "force-field," an impenetrable barrier similar to the one in the television program "Star Trek." When not thinking of hair pulling, she could touch her head easily and enjoy new habits of good hair grooming. Although this child refused to practice self-hypnosis, she responded well to posthypnotic suggestions. After 2 weeks, the scalp lesions were healed, and there was new hair growth. After another 2 weeks, there was further hair growth, and the child was no longer wearing a bandanna. Follow-up 2 months later revealed no further hair pulling and improvement in other behavior patterns.

SLEEP WALKING

This problem has not been adequately studied to determine precise etiologic factors. Although the symptom may reflect anxiety, it also seems to be associated with certain developmental periods and to be more frequent in certain families. Although usually a benign symptom, sleep walkers occasionally fall down stairs and injure themselves. This is frightening to other family members who are likely to request investigation and treatment, while the sleep walker is unconcerned. The following case history describes our use of hypnotherapy in one such instance.

The patient was an 11-year-old boy whose sleep-walking problem had been present since he was approximately 4 and had increased to walking around the multilevel house at least once every night. Parents were concerned about possible injury, and the patient was afraid to stay at homes of friends or relatives. He was taught the coin induction method of relaxation with addition of favorite place imagery and a nice long walk down a hill during which time he became more and more comfortable. Prior to this, sleep levels had been discussed with him and, since sleep walking is thought to occur in the transition between REM and non-REM sleep, he was asked to program himself to remain in bed during this transition period. He practiced this every night prior to sleeping. There was an immediate decrease in sleep-walking incidents to two or three a week and, within 2 months, the sleep walking had ceased. His mother stated that she felt he was using his newly found possibilities for self-control in other areas such as school and personal relationships.

CHRONIC OVEREATING

Haber, Nitkin, and Shenker (1979) reported uniformly unsuccessful results of hypnotherapy with eight obese adolescents. Suggestions included maintenance of an appropriate diet, aversive response to fattening foods, increased exercise, and positive self-esteem. Four patients were not responsive to hypnotic induction. Of the other four, three experienced negative sequelae of hypnosis, including feelings of depersonalization, increased anxiety, and dissociative behavior. We have not found such a large incidence of untoward effects of hypnosis. The problems might have been due to peculiar patient characteristics.

In a previously unpublished study at George Washington University (Olness et al., 1974), group hypnotherapy was offered to 60 obese postmenarche adolescent females. Prestudy evaluations included many laboratory studies, psychological testing, and physical examinations. Criteria for inclusion into the study included weight greater than 140 pounds, weight 20 percent above the weight norm for the subject's age and height, and obesity by skin-fold measurements.

Patients were divided into three groups. Group A patients were taught self-hypnosis, and Group B patients spent equal time with a control physician who gave them support and counseling. Group C patients had no treatment. All patients were seen regularly by a nutritionist and nurse clinician. After undergoing the prestudy evaluations, patients were weighed on a monthly basis for 1 year. At the end of 1 year, the subjects in Groups A and B had lost an average of 5.8 pounds and the nonintervention Group C had gained an average of 5.0 pounds per person. However, within the group there were some significant differences which correlated with the ability of the girls to visualize themselves as thinner in the future, for example, buying clothing of a smaller size. Those girls had an average weight loss of 9.7 pounds, compared with an average loss of 0.6 pounds for the others in the group. Although this study officially ended after 1 year of follow-up, the girls in Groups A and B were weighed again after a second year. Those in Group A had maintained weight loss or continued weight loss, including those who had not lost appreciably during the first year. Those in Group B had gained weight in similar fashion to the control group.

A report (Kohen et al., 1980) of 500 children with behavior problems treated with hypnotherapy mentions five children with obesity who lost weight during periods when they practiced self-hypnosis. However, only one child maintained significant weight reduction. Treatment approaches followed those of other habit problems.

Specific suggestions included the following: enjoying eating the appropriate amount of food for health and correct weight; feeling comfortable between meals without eating snacks; and visualizing looking thinner, buying smaller sizes, being complimented for appearance, and seeing one's height and weight as compatible on a growth chart.

Our clinical impression is that it is important that obese children review the self-hypnosis exercises several times daily for several weeks and that frequent visits in the first months of treatment are more necessary than in management of other habit disorders.

TICS AND TREMORS

We find that children with tics and tremors are frequently referred for a trial of hypnotherapy and that these referrals often come from pediatricians or neurologists. These symptoms, perhaps more than many habit problems, seem to be the symbolic expression of unresolved intrapsychic conflicts. For this reason, we recommend psychological evaluation with emphasis on family interaction. Although it may not be necessary or appropriate to mention the hypothesis of psychogenic determinants of the child, it is essential to have a reasonable working hypothesis before beginning hypnotherapy.

Approaches are similar to those for all habit problems with the addition of the jettison technique in which the child releases tension and problems from his or her clenched fist. Suggested imagery should emphasize mastery and the child's own control, and should include a focus on future happy events in which the patient no longer has a tic or tremor. The following case demonstrates a jettison technique.

Alison D. was a well-developed, pretty 14-year-old girl who was referred by her pediatrician for "hypnosis to control a hand tremor." She described a series of psychophysiological complaints including headaches, epigastric pain, and lower abdominal pain; she had had extensive medical evaluations for each complaint. She was a good student who mentioned a desire to finish school and study medicine. As she described her previous symptoms and evaluations through grade school, she said, "I always knew there wouldn't be anything really wrong. I was just nervous."

When asked why she thought she was nervous, Alison hesitated and said, "Well, I'm nervous about my mother's boyfriend who attacked me many times when I was around 8 or 9." She stated that she had never discussed these episodes of sexual abuse with her mother, that her mother continued to see the boyfriend, and that she could not stand him. She said she was angry at her mother who "knew what was going on and did nothing." She stated that she had been asked out by a boy for the first time a few weeks ago and that the hand tremor began at the same time. She did not wish to discuss the problem with her mother or the boyfriend. Alison was taught progressive relaxation and favorite place imagery and was then taught the clenched fist technique for releasing what bothered her. During the first session she opened and closed her fist several times. On return visit, 2 weeks later, she said she had no recurrence of the tremor and was coping much better.

The therapist hypothesized that the hand tremor represented aggressive and/or sexual impulses but did not share this idea with Alison, since such insight might produce unnecessary conflict about discussing the problem with her family.

Heimel (1978) reported a case which required a longer course of hypnotherapy for a tic disorder. Erik P., a 10-year-old boy, had a tic consisting of shaking movements of the head and shoulders that occurred repeatedly each day for a 9-month period prior to presentation in the pediatrician's office. He was seen on 15 occasions over 16 months.

Since Erik found it very difficult to discuss his problems with the therapist, the dynamic meaning of the tic remained unclear for quite some time. Eventually, some information became available through the use of ideomotor signaling in hypnosis. The patient had a very poor self-image and feelings of nonacceptance by his parents, grandparents, and peers. He believed that his sister was much more accepted by family members. His father seemed to be very passive and played no active role in the patient's life. As these feelings were shared with his parents, they made efforts to improve the family relationships. The dynamics of Erik's tic were never entirely clear; the head shaking might have served as unconscious expressions of hostility while at the same time assuring increased attention and concern from the family. The relatively long duration of the symptom, together with the ongoing emotional difficulties, made rapid resolution unlikely.

Initially in hypnotherapy, Erik was taught progressive relaxation and given ego-strengthening suggestions. When there seemed to be no response after a few weeks, the hypnotherapist offered Erik the jettison technique—"wrapping or packing up what was bugging him, and sending it far away on a freight train or plane." During these sessions, the patient was noted to smile several times as he clenched his fist in the process of eliminating troublesome thoughts or ideas.

After addition of this technique, Erik's parents and teachers noted a 90 percent reduction in frequency of the tic. However, when the tics disappeared the patient developed a chronic cough. Consultation with an otolaryngologist was obtained and no pathology was found. Erik was again offered hypnotherapy, which he accepted. He was confronted with the possibility that he had used the cough as a substitute for the tic. The coughing disappeared within a few weeks after two hypnotherapy sessions.

In follow-up, 3 years later, the family stated that Erik was adjusting well as a sophomore in high school, that he had no tics, coughs, or other habit symptoms, and that he seemed happy and relaxed.

HABITUAL DRUG ABUSE

Baumann (1970) reviewed his experience with adolescents, from grades 6 to 12 in school, who abused a variety of drugs. With most of these patients, the hypnotherapeutic approach focused on asking the youngsters to develop a "hypnotic high" in which they used their own imaginative abilities to experience feelings even better than the similar feelings they had had following actual drug ingestion. Other forms of psychotherapy were also employed with many patients. Initially pleased with the finding that 50 percent of 80 marijuana users were no longer doing so 1 year after hypnotherapy, Baumann reviewed data for 80 more marijuana users who had not been treated for this problem. Again, about half had stopped drug use after 1 year. Neither group considered the drug physically harmful, and those who stopped did so from boredom, lack of satisfaction, or fear of the law. Baumann concluded that hypnotherapy could not be considered an effective therapeutic modality for this group.

Among adolescents who used drugs that they thought to be physically dangerous, Baumann (1970) found his methods more successful. Of 30 teenagers who had had only "good trips" with LSD, 26 stopped taking the drug completely and 4 reduced the frequency of usage. There was little change, however, for 12 other patients who had experienced "bad trips" with LSD; it was difficult to adapt the technique in these cases. Of 17 adolescents who were "shooting speed" (amphetamines), all stopped injecting the drug although 4 turned to oral amphetamines. Of 28 users of oral amphetamines, 6 stopped altogether, 20 decreased usage, and 2 remained unchanged. Of 10 patients who frequently used overdoses of barbiturates, 9 showed significant improvement following hypnotherapy. Since this group had no "high" experiences, imagery was directed more toward helping the youngsters satisfy other needs more appropriately. The treatment was not considered effective for two patients who used heroin or for two others who used multiple drugs.

Baumann (1970) concluded that hypnotherapy can be a useful adjunct in the management of adolescent drug abusers, provided they are well motivated for habit change. The greatest motivating factor seemed to be fear of physical damage to the patients themselves or to their children.

We have had little experience with adolescent drug abusers. However, we have sometimes adapted Baumann's imagery technique to help patients get rapid and maximal effect from prescribed sedatives and analgesics. Some of our patients have used hypnotic sedation and comfort to obviate the need for preoperative sedation or postoperative chemical analgesia. The technique might also be adapted in the hypnotherapeutic treatment of other habit disorders, providing the child with emotional gratifications and obviating the need to engage in the habit. Gardner's (1978) emphasis on giving the hair-pulling child a sense of controlling her hair is one example in which the basic need, i.e., control, was not changed but rather rechannelled in more appropriate directions.

CONCLUSIONS

Hypnotherapy appears to be valuable in the treatment of a wide variety of habit disorders, provided (1) there is no underlying organic problem, (2) the child is well motivated, and (3) the child is willing to assume primary responsibility for change. As compared with many other approaches, hypnotherapy is less expensive, less time-consuming, and less dangerous. Therefore, it would be advantageous to consider a hypnotherapeutic approach early rather than as a last resort, as is often the case. On the other hand, some of the better controlled studies have found that patients who resolve a habit problem after hypnotherapy may not do it because of hypnotherapy, but rather for other reasons. We need better controlled, prospective studies in order to determine which children with which habit problems are most likely to benefit from hypnotherapy.

REFERENCES

Anderson, F. M. Occult spinal dysraphism: A series of 73 cases. *Pediatrics*, 1975, *55*, 826–835.

Baumann, F. Hypnosis and the adolescent drug abuser. *The American Journal of Clinical Hypnosis*, 1970, *13*, 17–21.

Baumann, F. W., & Hinman, F. Treatment of incontinent boys with non-obstructive disease. *The Journal of Urology*, 1974, *111*, 114–116.

Claydon, G. S., & Lawson, J. Investigation and management of long-standing chronic constipation in childhood. *Archives of Diseases of Childhood*, 1976, *51*, 918–923.

Cohen, M. W. Enuresis. *The Pediatric Clinics of North America*, 1975, *22*, 545–560.

Collison, D. R. Hypnotherapy in the management of nocturnal enuresis. *The Medical Journal of Australia*, 1970, *1*, 52–54.

Davidson, M., & Wasserman, R. The irritable colon of childhood. *The Journal of Pediatrics*, 1966, *69*, 1027–1038.

Doleys, D. M. Behavioral treatments for nocturnal enuresis in children: A review of the literature. *Psychological Bulletin*, 1977, *84*, 30–54.

Erickson, M. H. Naturalistic techniques of hypnosis. *The American Journal of Clinical Hypnosis*, 1958, *1*, 3–8.

Falck, F. J. Stuttering and hypnosis. *The International Journal of Clinical and Experimental Hypnosis*, 1964, *12*, 67–74.

Fleisher, D. R. The diagnosis and treatment of disorders of defecation in children. *Pediatrics Annals*, 1976, *5*, 700–722.

Gardner, G. G. Hypnotherapy in the management of childhood habit disorders. *The Journal of Pediatrics*, 1978, *92*, 838–840.

Gerrard, J. W., Jones, B., Shokier, M. K., & Zaleski, A. Allergy and urinary infections: Is there an association? *Pediatrics*, 1971, *48*, 994–995.

Glicklich, L. B. An historical account of enuresis. *Pediatrics*, 1951, *8*, 859–876.

Goldsmith, H. Chronic loss of bowel control in a nine-year-old child. *The American Journal of Clinical Hypnosis*, 1962, *4*, 191–193.

Haber, C. H., Nitkin, R., & Shenker, L. R. Adverse reactions to hypnotherapy in obese adolescents: A developmental viewpoint. *Psychiatric Quarterly*, 1979, *51*, 55–63.

Halpern, W. I. The treatment of encopretic children. *Journal of the American Academy of Child Psychiatry*, 1977, *16*, 478–499.

Heimel, A. Use of hypnosis in pediatric clinical practice: A report of 68 patients. In *Proceedings of Northwestern Pediatric Society*, September 28, 1978. (Abstract)

Jacobs, L. Hypnosis in clinical pediatrics. *New York State Journal of Medicine*, 1962, *62*, 3781–3787.

Kohen, D., Olness, K., Colwell, S., & Heimel, A. 500 pediatric behavioral problems treated with hypnotherapy. Paper presented at the annual meeting of the American Society of Clinical Hypnosis, Minneapolis, November, 1980.

Kolvin, I. (Ed.). *Bladder control and enuresis*. Philadelphia: Lippincott, 1973.

Laguaite, J. K. The use of hypnosis with children with deviant voices. *The International Journal of Clinical and Experimental Hypnosis*, 1976, *24*, 98–104.

Levine, M. Children with encopresis: A descriptive analysis. *Pediatrics*, 1975, *56*, 412–416.

Marshall, S., Marshall, H. H., & Richards, P. L. Enuresis: An analysis of various therapeutic approaches. *Pediatrics*, 1973, *52*, 813–817.

Mohlman, H. J. Thumbsucking. In *A syllabus on hypnosis and a handbook of therapeutic suggestions*. Des Plaines, Ill.: The American Society of Clinical Hypnosis Education and Research Foundation, 1973.

Moore, W. E. Hypnosis in a system of therapy for stutterers. *Journal of Speech Disorders*, 1946, *11*, 117–122.

Nixon, H. H. Review: Hirschsprung's disease. *Archives of Disease in Childhood*, 1964, *39*, 109–115.

Olness, K. The use of self-hypnosis in the treatment of childhood nocturnal enuresis: A report on forty patients. *Clinical Pediatrics*, 1975, *14*, 273–279.

Olness, K. Autohypnosis in functional megacolon in children. *The American Journal of Clinical Hypnosis*, 1976, *19*, 28–32.

Olness, K. Comparison of hypnotherapy and biofeedback in management of fecal soiling in children. Paper presented at the annual meeting of the Society for Clinical and Experimental Hypnosis, Los Angeles, 1977. (a)

Olness, K. How to help the wet child and the frustrated parents. *Modern Medicine*, 1977, *45*, 42–46. (b)

Olness, K., & Immershein, R. Association of nocturnal enuresis and allergy. In *Proceedings of the Ambulatory Pediatric Association*, 1976. (Abstract)

Olness, K., Fallon, J., Coit, A., Fry, G., & Bassford, M. Group hypnotherapy in management of obesity in teenage girls. Paper presented at the annual meeting of the American Society of Clinical Hypnosis, New Orleans, 1974.

Olness, K., & Gardner, G. G. Some guidelines for uses of hypnotherapy in pediatrics. *Pediatrics*, 1978, *62*, 228–233.

Sector, I. I. Thumbsucking. In *A syllabus on hypnosis and a handbook of therapeutic suggestions*. Des Plaines, Ill.: The American Society of Clinical Hypnosis Education and Research Foundation, 1973.

Silber, S. Encopresis: Rectal rebellion and anal anarchy? *Journal of the American Society of Psychosomatic Dentistry and Medicine*, 1968, *15*, 97–106.

Silber, S. Fairy tales and symbols in hypnotherapy of children with certain speech disorders. *The International Journal of Clinical and Experimental Hypnosis*, 1973, *21*, 272–283.

Solovey, G., & Milechnin, A. Concerning the treatment of enuresis. *The American Journal of Clinical Hypnosis*, 1959, *3*, 22–30.

Stanton, H. E. Short-term treatment of enuresis. *The American Journal of Clinical Hypnosis*, 1979, *22*, 103–107.

Staples, L. M. Thumbsucking. In *A syllabus on hypnosis and a handbook of therapeutic suggestions*. Des Plaines, Ill.: The American Society of Clinical Hypnosis Education and Research Foundation, 1973.

Stein, C. The clenched fist technique as a hypnotic procedure in clinical psychotherapy. *The American Journal of Clinical Hypnosis*, 1963, *6*, 113–119.

Tilton, P. Hypnotic treatment of a child with thumbsucking, enuresis and encopresis. *The American Journal of Clinical Hypnosis*, 1980, *22*, 238–240.

9

Hypnotherapy for Problems in Learning and Performance

Many children experience problems both in learning certain material and in performing or demonstrating that they have mastered the material. Increasingly, children and their teachers and parents turn to hypnotherapy for help, spurred on by encouraging reports in the press and in professional journals.

Many reports of hypnotherapy for learning problems contain a measure of optimism that is not really warranted by the data. Hypnotherapy can sometimes be beneficial in treating emotional problems, such as low self-esteem or anxiety, that impede learning. But a hypnotherapist must take care to distinguish these emotional problems from true learning disabilities. Diagnostic work-up should include psychological and educational evaluation and, in some cases, the child should also be seen by a speech pathologist, a neurologist, and an ophthalmologist.

When clinical evaluation suggests that hypnotherapy might be helpful for patients with learning difficulties, we think it important that they understand that the process is under their own control and that they are, in large part, responsible for the outcome. Daily practice of self-hypnosis with appropriate suggestions is recommended. This approach helps to identify children not really motivated for change or who derive secondary gain from their problems.

Prior to embarking on hypnotherapy, specific goals should be discussed with the child, for example, to pass third-grade requirements, to increase reading level by 6 months, to complete arithmetic homework, to increase classroom participation, or to pass a particular test. Generally, the emphasis should first be on small goals and there should be clear feedback to the child. Often the hypnotherapist will need frequent consultation with the child's teachers.

When it seems clear that hypnotherapy will not be helpful, the patient and/or parents should be counseled as to more appropriate avenues of help. Parental pressure sometimes makes this referral process very difficult.

HYPNOTHERAPY WITH MENTALLY RETARDED CHILDREN

Parents of mentally retarded children sometimes turn to bizarre treatment methods that have no known efficacy and may actually do more harm than good. Hypnotherapy is no exception, probably because of its magical appeal and reports of dramatic cures in other areas. Clinical hypnosis researchers have also investigated this area, focusing on two issues: whether mentally retarded children are hypnotizable, and whether it is possible to increase their performance on intelligence tests and related learning tasks. All researchers do not agree on the definition of mental retardation. We define mental retardation as an intelligence quotient (IQ) below 70 on a standardized test, when the obtained IQ is interpreted as a valid reflection of the child's intellectual ability and not primarily the result of depression, anxiety, refusal to cooperate, or other behavioral or cultural variables.

It is important to remember that an intelligence test score measures a child's current intellectual functioning. In some instances, the response patterns on individual test items or subtests suggest that the child's potential may be higher. However, limited areas or "islands" of normal functioning in the midst of general performance at a mentally retarded level are not sufficient to conclude that a child's overall intelligence is really well above the obtained IQ score. In the past, this mistake was often made in evaluations of autistic children. Even when these children made significant gains in the emotional sphere, most of them did not achieve expected parallel gains in intellectual functioning.

Hypnotic Responsiveness

The normative studies of hypnotic responsiveness cited in Chapter 3 did not include retarded children and therefore contribute nothing to the question of whether such children can experience hypnosis.

Jacobs and Jacobs (1966) concluded that children with very low intelligence were generally not hypnotizable. However, there was no standardized measure of hypnotizability in that study.

Sternlicht and Wanderer (1963) addressed themselves specifically to the question of whether mentally retarded children are hypnotizable. Unfortunately, however, their study also had significant methodological limitations. The subjects were 20 "certified mentally defective" children who were institutionalized at the Willowbrook State School, near New York City. The children's chronological ages ranged from 7 to 15 years (mean age = 11). All children had been tested with the Revised Stanford-Binet Intelligence Scale, Form L, with IQs ranging from 37 to 68 (mean IQ = 52), and mental ages from 3 to 9 years.

The authors argued that use of a standardized hypnotizability scale, such as the Children's Hypnotic Susceptibility Scale (London, 1963), would be inappropriate because the emphasis on verbal instructions would put mentally retarded children, with their typically poor verbal skills, at a disadvantage as compared to subjects of normal intelligence. In place of a standardized scale, the authors used a "progressive anesthesia" induction technique (Watkins, 1962). The children were told that parts of their bodies would become more stiff and rigid and would be without any feeling. When this effect was achieved in the entire body, the children would then be "in a deep state of sleep" (p. 106). These verbal suggestions were enhanced with tactual stimulation on the children's fingers and hands. They were first asked to move a finger in which they felt altered sensation. They were then asked to report how deep a state of sleep had been achieved by giving a number on a scale in which 0 meant none at all and 10 meant deeper asleep than ever before.

Of the 20 children, 8 did not pass the initial finger-moving test and were declared nonhypnotizable. For the remaining 12 children, the scores were negatively skewed, with 10 reporting scores in the 7 to 10 range and the other 2 reporting a score of 1.

The authors concluded that 60 percent of their sample were hypnotizable. We cannot agree. The authors acknowledged the problems of using subjective reports of hypnotizability but defended their choice as the best available. We note the U-shaped curve of scores and come to a different conclusion. Institutionalized mentally retarded children tend to fall into two groups, those who demonstrate minimal cooperation and those who exert tremendous effort to cooperate and to please adults, apparently thriving on bits of social reinforcement so often lacking in large institutions. All 20 children in this study counted from 1 to 12 for the examiners, as part of the process of establishing rapport and in order to demonstrate ability to use the scoring system. We wonder whether they got verbal or nonverbal reinforcement for each higher number or for completing the task. If so, they may have concluded "the higher, the better." If they were given this sort of reinforcement, they might have simply been seeking further praise by giving a high number when later asked to estimate their depth of "sleep." We become even more suspicious of the high scores when we notice the emphasis on "sleep," in light of the repeated finding that children often respond negatively to hypnotic induction methods that suggest sleep.

In short, we think these data have more to do with social reinforcement and demand characteristics than with hypnosis, and we cannot conclude that retarded children are hypnotizable. Obviously the study suffers from other defects, including the lack of a control group of institutionalized children with normal IQ and lack of any evidence that the children really understood the anesthesia instructions. It may be notable that none of the 12 "hypnotizable" children responded to suggested age regression.

Before leaving the question of hypnotic responsiveness in mentally retarded children, we should mention the issue of pseudoretardation. That is, a child may test and function at a retarded level but may actually have normal intelligence. For instance, Gardner (1973) reported IQ data on an 8-year-old girl with psychogenic epilepsy. At the beginning of treatment, when she was virtually in petit mal status, her Binet IQ was 72, in the borderline retarded range. Eighteen months earlier, before exacerbation of her symptoms, her IQ on the Binet was 93 (average), and 3 months after initiation of psychotherapy, her Binet IQ was 103 (average). The fact that she was hypnotizable when her measured IQ was 72 obviously says nothing about the relationship between hypnotizability and intelligence, since the IQ score was not a true measure of her intellectual ability. In future research on hypnotic responsiveness of children with low intelligence, one must be careful not to include cases of pseudoretardation.

Can Hypnotherapy Increase IQ?

We know of no long-term studies that utilize hypnotherapy as an adjunct in the educational programs of mentally retarded children. The results were disappointing in one study (Woody & Billy, 1970) that included a single session of "clinical suggestion." Since the study was published in a hypnosis journal, we assume that the authors believed that they employed hypnosis but avoided that term—as did many authors cited in this chapter—because they feared it might not be acceptable in the school setting where the study was conducted.

Woody and Billy (1970) located 28 mentally retarded boys, age 9 to 13, in special-education classrooms. All had been given an individual intelligence test on which their IQs ranged from 50 to 75. The authors selected 32 nonretarded boys from regular classes in the same schools. Each of these groups was then divided into an experimental and a control group, equated for age and IQ. The retarded and nonretarded control groups were given the Peabody Picture Vocabulary Test (PPVT) on two occasions, 2 weeks apart. Apparently these groups received no intervening treatment or special attention. The two experimental groups received a "clinical suggestion session" immediately prior to the second PPVT administration. The suggestions focused on enhancing physical relaxation, minimizing anxiety over past test performance, and heightening motivation for and expectation of good performance. Neither of the nonretarded groups showed any change in PPVT scores. The mean IQ increase for the retarded "clinical suggestion" group was 4.79 points, while the mean gain for the retarded controls was 3.21 points. Although the authors indicated that the difference for retarded experimentals and controls is statistically significant, neither difference is greater than the standard error of measurement for individual IQ tests. The authors concluded that differences of such small magnitude are hardly likely to have any practical significance. Further statistical analysis led the authors to state that "it does not appear that clinical suggestions are any more effective for retarded boys than they are for non-retarded boys" (Woody & Billy, 1970, p. 270). They wondered whether several clinical suggestion sessions might have yielded different results.

Based on the data from this study, we find no evidence that hypnotic suggestions can increase IQ in children with primary mental retardation. Despite its several methodological weaknesses, it is probably the most carefully controlled study reported at this time.

The Utility of Hypnosis in Counseling

While we do not think it has been demonstrated that mentally retarded persons are hypnotizable, neither has it been shown clearly that they are not hypnotizable. Even if they do not seem to respond to hypnotherapeutic suggestions for enhanced intellectual performance, perhaps they can utilize hypnosis as an adjunct to counseling and psychotherapy.

Woody and Herr (1967) surveyed 102 psychologists in clinical and academic settings, all trained in the use of hypnosis, concerning their opinions as to the possible utility of hypnosis in counseling the mentally retarded. The 84 who responded tended to be uncertain rather than having clear positive or negative opinions; most had no experience using clinical hypnosis with this population.

Lazar (1977) reported successful hypnotherapy with a moderately retarded boy with behavior problems (see Chapter 7). Of course, in this and other single case reports, it is impossible to be sure whether the positive results should be ascribed to hypnosis or to some other aspect of the therapeutic interaction. Lazar (1977) did not measure her patient's hypnotic responsiveness by any standardized scale, and one could conceptualize her techniques for extinguishing undesirable behavior as belonging more in the realm of behavior modification than of hypnotherapy.

Based on available research and our own clinical experience with mentally retarded children, we conclude that their capacity to respond to hypnotic induction is, at best, quite limited. In cases of true mental retardation, we doubt that hypnotherapy can significantly enhance intellectual functioning. In treating such children for emotional and behavior problems, we think behavior modification and parent counseling are probably the most effective approaches. It should be possible to design methodologically sound research studies that would clarify these issues.

HYPNOTHERAPY FOR CHILDREN WITH LEARNING DISABILITIES

Minimal Brain Dysfunction

Among educators, psychologists, and others who work with learning-disabled children, there are varied opinions as to the cause of so-called minimal brain dysfunction (MBD), its precise nature, and the best treatment approach. However, most people agree (1) that these children have normal intelligence with specific learning deficits; (2) that they often manifest hyperactivity, short attention span, distractibility, emotional lability, and poor impulse control; (3) that they experience repeated failure in school because of their academic and behavior problems; and (4) that these difficulties result in low self-esteem, anxiety, depression, and poor attitudes toward learning. These children then may decrease effort to succeed in school, thus lowering grades further and creating a vicious cycle of ever-increasing problems. The use of MBD as a diagnostic label is often thought to be of doubtful value except that it establishes that the children are not mentally retarded and that, in general, the learning disabilities are primary and the emotional problems are secondary.

Special educational techniques have been developed to remediate the learning deficits associated with MBD, and these are available in many schools. Sometimes, however, the children's low self-esteem, negative attitudes toward learning, and related emotional problems combine to make it almost impossible for them to benefit from remedial training. We agree with Crasilneck and Hall (1975) that hypnotherapy is not a primary treatment for MBD. We also agree that hypnotherapy can often help the child with MBD lower anxiety, increase capacity to recognize lability, develop strategies for controlling emotional outbursts, and modify attitudes toward learning in general and school in particular.

Crasilneck and Hall (1975) described their treatment of an 8-year-old girl with MBD whose secondary emotional problems were manifested not only in school but also at home and with her peers. Diagnostic evaluation revealed no evidence of neurological damage or primary emotional disorder. Intelligence was average, with indications of higher potential. The child benefited from hypnotherapy designed to ameliorate the secondary problems. The chief contribution of this single case report consists of the inclusion of details of the hypnotic suggestions given and the results obtained.

Hypnosis was instituted on a trial basis to decrease anxiety and instill a sense of confidence in the child. She was told that she would find herself wanting to study more and would find pleasure and gratification in doing the very best job possible. She was told in the trance that some of the energy that was causing her trouble would be redirected into more useful work. She would find herself capable of making better grades in school. Such a suggestion for improved grades would *not* have been made had it not seemed, on balance, that the reality of her situation was such that she had not been using her full capabilities. She was next told that she would be able to concentrate much better and would begin to enjoy getting along in school and with her parents.

Following each hypnotic session, the child was encouraged to discuss her fears, her fantasies, her feelings about past failures, and any unusual problems or successes that she had experienced since the last visit.

At the end of nine weeks her report card had come up one letter grade, on average. Her attention span seemed improved, and her ability to concentrate seemed more stable. She was enjoying school more and showed marked improvement on her examinations. Her interpersonal relations with her parents, her schoolmates, and her teachers indicated good adjustment. Six months later her grades were above average, and she had become more happy. Her anxiety was rarely sufficient to cause any of her past difficulties.

Throughout her treatment great care was taken not to set goals that were unrealistically high for her apparent abilities, as this would have induced a further conflict of perhaps greater severity than her presenting complaints.

This precaution makes accurate clinical assessment of great importance in using hypnosis for such cases. [p. 193]*

Illovsky and Fredman (1976) utilized hypnotherapy with 48 children, age 6 to 8 years, selected from among 180 children referred to a
clinic because of behavior and learning problems in school. Excluding
children with major psychiatric disorders or perceptual difficulties, the
authors selected children manifesting short attention span, acting-out
behavior, and distractibility. All these children had a history of good
school attendance, an IQ above 85, and parental consent. Concurrently
with hypnotherapy, the students received remedial academic instruction, as they had before the hypnotic sessions were begun, albeit with
little success. On 55 occasions—no child was present for all sessions—
the children listened to tape-recorded hypnotic suggestions, under the
supervision of one of their reading teachers. The taped hypnotic induction included eye fixation, eye closure, general relaxation, counting
from 1 to 10, and imagining a pleasant outdoor scene. The suggestions
for improved learning and increased ability to cope with emotional
problems were as follows:

From now on, you are going to think of what to do for yourself. If you
think of something bad that happened to you before, think about whether
you could have done it better. If you could have done it better, then, think
that when the same thing happens again, you will do it better. . . . Go into
a deeper and deeper relaxation . . . deeper and deeper. . . . There is nothing
to disturb you and there is nothing to bother you. . . . You are feeling nice
and relaxed and you are sinking into a still deeper relaxation. . . .

If you think that someone wants to do something bad to you, imagine
that you are in his place and you want to do the same thing to him. Then
think about why you would be doing it in his place. Then think that he was
also not doing it to hurt you but for some other reason. Go into a deeper and
deeper. . . . etc.

You feel like talking to people, because you want to know what they think
and you want to learn something from them and also you want people to like
you. For this reason, you feel like talking to people. . . . There is nothing to
disturb you. . . . etc.

Think also about why you should be good to people and how much you
will like it, when people are nice to you. . . . Go into a deeper. . . . etc.

If you feel sad or angry, think of something nice that you can remember
that happened to you. If you cannot remember anything nice, then think of
something nice or good that you wish would happen to you. While you are
thinking about these nice things, the sadness or anger is leaving you and you
will feel nice, calm and good. . . . Go into a deeper. . . . etc.

---

*From *Clinical Hypnosis: Principles and Applications* by H. B. Crasilneck and J. A.
Hall, New York: Grune & Stratton, 1975. With permission.

I want you to listen to me some more. From today, you are going to think and dream about why you should learn in school and at home. You feel also that you want to learn and this will make you feel good. You feel that you are as good and smart as the other children and you can learn and read just as they can learn and read. When you are reading, you will feel nice, good and calm inside. Go into a deeper and deeper. . . . etc.

As soon as you start to learn anything, you will feel good and like reading and learning more and more. Remember, as soon as you start to learn, you will only think about the words and letters in front of you. Go into a deeper and deeper. . . . etc. [p. 90]*

At each session, the teacher rated every child for the presence or absence of "relaxation," manifested by eye closure and motionless behavior, with the appearance of sleep. There was no measure of hypnotic responsiveness, and the authors themselves questioned whether relaxation and hypnosis should be equated.

Teacher ratings of improved self-confidence correlated positively with the number of sessions attended by each pupil but correlated negatively with the percent of sessions in which each pupil was judged to be relaxed. Ratings of relaxation were positively correlated with improved attention in class but were not related to five other academic and behavioral variables. The authors urged caution in interpreting the data because of teacher bias, lack of a control group, and lack of any real indication of hypnotic responsiveness.

Noting the emphasis on eye closure in the induction, the young age of the children, and the fact that the sessions were supervised by teachers with whom the children may have had a relationship marked by failure and negative attitudes, we too doubt the validity of equating relaxation with hypnosis, and are really not surprised at the paucity of positive results. In the last analysis, this study really tells us very little about the value of hypnotherapy for learning-disabled children with behavior problems in school.

Reading Disability

Illovsky (1963) studied the effect of group hypnotherapy with five nonpsychotic adolescent boys confined to a state hospital because of delinquency and severe behavior disorders. Five similar adolescent patients served as no-treatment controls. All subjects were nonreaders, with reading skills at or below first-grade level at the beginning of the study. Every day, before class began, the experimental group listened

---

*Reprinted from the April 1976 *International Journal of Clinical and Experimental Hypnosis*. Copyrighted by the Society for Clinical and Experimental Hypnosis, April, 1976.

to a hypnotic induction followed by several suggestions for increased motivation, concentration, and performance in reading. While no standardized hypnotizability scale was administered, these boys all responded to several informal measures similar to items from the Stanford Scales. One boy in this group cooperated minimally and was not included in the data analysis. After 6 months, the four remaining boys in the hypnotherapy group had gained an average of 2 years and 3 months in reading skills; the no-treatment controls had gained an average of 9 months. The author concluded that "hypnosis through its well-known hypermnesia can maintain and even enhance the reading ability of the hypnotized subjects" (Illovsky, 1963, p. 65). Such a conclusion seems unwarranted, in view of uncontrolled factors such as attention. At follow-up 2 months later, two boys in the experimental group showed no further improvement.

Jampolsky (1975) reported his hypnotherapeutic work with a small group of third- and fourth-grade children who were having difficulty learning to read. In a unique effort to overcome the negative reinforcement to which such children are repeatedly subjected, Jampolsky also used imagery techniques with the teachers and parents, encouraging them to visualize the children as successful readers. The research included a control group of poor readers who apparently received no treatment but were tested at the beginning and end of the study.

The experimental group participated in an eight-step program over a period of three 45-minute sessions: (1) since the children had already demonstrated problems with traditional visual learning, the group hypnotic induction minimized suggestions for visualization and focused instead on kinesthetic techniques such as feeling a weight pull their arm down or feeling fur on their face; (2) the children then imagined being in a pleasant place of their own choosing and concentrated on rhythmic breathing; (3) they were encouraged to get rid of painful associations to learning by mentally washing such bad feelings, dirt, and grime out of their brains; (4) they imagined themselves writing a small book about their favorite subject; (5) they used suggested tactile, auditory, and visual imagery to picture themselves on a motion picture screen reading their books with fluency, success, confidence, and joy, thus creating an ego ideal; (6) they climbed into their images on the screen, merging with the ideal self; (7) they imagined the new self permeating all body tissues; and (8) they were asked to repeat this process daily for 5 to 10 minutes before going to school and before going to sleep. Jampolsky emphasized that this is a holistic approach to learning rather than the bit-by-bit process usually employed.

Over a 1 month period, the experimental group averaged an increase in reading skill of 1½ years, while the control group gained only 1 month. Self-esteem was markedly increased in the experimental group, and the parents and teachers reported decreased tension and increased energy. When the experimental group was retested 1 year later their progress continued to be excellent, as compared to that of the control group. Jampolsky's results are encouraging, although the study contains methodological problems similar to those of the Illovsky study. Jampolsky presented no evidence that the subjects were really in hypnosis and, if so, that hypnosis and not some other variable accounted for the results.

Krippner (1966) studied 49 children, age 8 to 17 years and generally of average intelligence, enrolled in a 5-week remedial reading program. Hypnotherapy was utilized adjunctively with nine children whose parents specifically requested it. The median amount of reading improvement for the entire group was 5 months, as measured by a standardized reading test. In the hypnosis group, eight children scored above the median and one at or below the median; in the control group, 16 children scored above the median and 24 at or below. The difference between the two groups was statistically significant, although the difference in actual amount of improvement (6 months versus 5 months) was too small to be of much practical value.

For the hypnosis group, Krippner tailored the induction to the expectations and needs of each child. The suggestions pertaining to reading focused on three areas: reducing tension and anxiety, enhancing motivation to read, and increasing concentration and attention span.

Tension: As you relax, you begin to stop worrying. You stop worrying about reading. You begin to think how much you would like to read better. You begin to think how much you would like to improve your reading ability. You know that you can read better if all the muscles of your body are relaxed. If all of your muscles are relaxed, you will be able to pay closer attention to what you read. You want very much to relax your muscles while you read and to be completely at ease. You want very much to relax all the little muscles in your eyes while you read. This will help you to read with your eyes wide open so that you will not miss any of the letters. If your eyes are wide open, you will not miss any of the words. If your eyes are wide open, you will read much, much better.

Motivation: Every time you read a word or a sentence correctly, you will feel very good inside. You will feel proud of yourself because you read so well. You will enjoy the feeling that reading well gives you. You will want to read some more words and sentences. You will become interested in reading books and magazines and newspapers. Every time that you read something correctly, and understand what you read, your interest will increase. You will want to read another book, or another magazine, or another newspaper.

Sometimes you will make mistakes while reading. These mistakes will not bother you because we all make mistakes. None of us is perfect. However, when you read a word or a sentence very well, you will be pleased and happy. You will want to read more and more.

Concentration: When you open your eyes, you and your clinician will select a story in a book that interests you. After looking it over for a few minutes to make certain that it is really interesting, you will start to read the story. You will find that you are able to pay very close attention to the story. You will pay close attention for many, many minutes. It will be just as if your eyes are glued to the page. In fact, you will not want to take your eyes away from the story until you have read several pages. Perhaps you will even finish the whole story. When you have trouble with a word, your clinician will help you out. But this will not affect your attention which will be very, very strong. At the same time, your concentration will be better than it has been for a long, long time. You will think about nothing but the characters in the story and what is happening to them. You will understand what you are reading. You might even see the characters in your mind's eye. You will enjoy what you are reading. Your concentration and attention will be so good today that you will find it even easier to concentrate and to pay attention tomorrow. [pp. 263–264]*

In discussing his results, Krippner noted the need for cautious interpretation. It is possible that parents in the hypnosis group were especially cooperative and optimistic about the entire remedial program, with unknown effects on their children's progress. The effect of special attention from the hypnotherapist in the experimental group is also unknown. Finally, it is possible that the suggestions might have been equally effective in the absence of any hypnotic induction.

Although Crasilneck and Hall (1975) have not attempted a research study, their clinical results are optimistic, yielding moderate to marked improvement in approximately three-fourths of their child patients presenting with dyslexia. They do not mention the length of required treatment, although they mention one adolescent with very severe dyslexia, previously diagnosed as retarded, who appeared to them to have normal intelligence and no severe emotional problems. "After extensive hypnotherapy lasting a few years, she graduated from high school, passed both the written and practical part of her driver's license test, and has become more functional" (Crasilneck & Hall, 1975, p. 190). Presumably most of their dyslexic patients were not this severely affected. In their hypnotherapeutic work with dyslexia patients, suggestions include the following:

---

*From "The Use of Hypnosis with Elementary and Secondary School Children in a Summer Reading Clinic" by S. Krippner, *The American Journal of Clinical Hypnosis*, 1966, 8, 261–266. With permission.

Your vision is simply going to improve. . . . You can recognize words with much more ease. . . . Once you have learned the word, it will make an impression upon your unconscious brain and mind, and recall of this word in the future will be much easier. . . . Your memory for words that you learn will become implanted in your mental processes and will be recalled in a smooth, coordinated fashion. There will be an excellent coordination between your eyes, your brain, and your memory . . . and your reading capabilities will continuously improve until they return to normal. . . . You will be much less anxious and much less afraid in your reading and learning habits. . . . Your reading is going to improve consistently. [p. 190]*

We have heard some therapists say the material "will burn itself into your brain." Because of the hypnotized patient's tendency to take words literally, we prefer the more neutral phrase "make an impression" as used by Crasilneck and Hall.

Number Reversals

Jampolsky (1970) studied 10 children in grades one to three, age 6 to 9 years, who manifested number reversals. All the children had abnormal EEGs and various signs of minimal brain dysfunction. The five children in the experimental group had a single hypnotic induction focusing on kinesthetic and tactile imagery and including suggestions that they would learn to write numbers properly. There was no determination of whether these children were actually in hypnosis. The single hypnotic session was followed by 2 weeks of remedial training in writing numbers, using a variety of special techniques for learning-disabled children. The five control children received no hypnotic induction and no remedial training. After 2 weeks, number reversals were entirely eliminated in the experimental group; the control group showed a slight increase in reversals. The design of the study makes it impossible to determine whether the difference was due to hypnotherapy, to remedial training, or to other factors.

Test Anxiety

We sometimes see children whose IQs are at least average, whose study skills are adequate, and whose teachers insist that they have mastered classroom material as evidenced by workbook assignments, learning games, and other classroom activities. Yet, when these children are confronted with a formal test of their knowledge, they be-

---

*From *Clinical Hypnosis: Principles and Applications* by H. B. Crasilneck and J. A. Hall, New York: Grune & Stratton, 1975. With permission.

come markedly anxious and perform at a level much lower than would be expected.

When children with test anxiety come to our office, they usually are quite aware that their anxiety is unwarranted, and they are highly motivated for help. Sometimes the test anxiety is a clue to a more pervasive problem requiring intensive psychotherapy; careful diagnostic assessment is essential. Often, however, the problem can be treated quite directly, usually with gains then spreading to other areas of the children's lives. Our approach includes the following steps:

Step 1. Having established the children's understanding of the irrationality of their anxiety and their motivation for help, we teach them to go into hypnosis by whatever method seems most appropriate.

Step 2. In hypnosis they visualize themselves in some activity, unrelated to school, in which they know they are competent and perform with minimal anxiety.

Step 3. Having achieved a feeling of competence, they then let go of the specific content of the imagery, retain the feeling, and visualize an ideal self with the same good feelings in a classroom.

Step 4. They then experience a series of images, in a manner similar to systematic desensitization beginning with a very brief and simple performance task such as distributing homework sheets. They move through images of more difficult tasks, culminating in an image of taking a major test or final examination, always retaining the feeling of confidence and competence, and merging with each positive image as it becomes clear. If at any point anxiety develops, they drop back to an easier image before progressing.

Step 5. They are informed that this kind of rehearsal in fantasy often carries over into the actual situation.

Step 6. They are given a posthypnotic suggestion that, when actually required to perform, they can recall and reexperience the same good feelings as in the therapeutic session; they can do the same when preparing for the examination.

Step 7. They are taught self-hypnosis, with the suggestion to review the positive images at an appropriate time and place, preferably twice daily for 5 to 10 minutes.

Step 8. Finally, they are reminded that no one performs perfectly all the time, and they are encouraged to set realistic expectations and to perceive failures as opportunities for new learning.

We find that two to five sessions are usually sufficient to master the problem, provided there is no significant psychopathology in the patients, their families, or the school situation itself.

CONCLUSIONS

Clearly, research and clinical reports are rife with methodological problems that prevent us from concluding anything about the value of hypnotherapy for enhancing learning and performance. Some of the more detailed approaches contain therapeutic suggestions that are interesting and might indeed prove valuable, but both clinicians and researchers must distinguish between "interesting" and "valuable." It is unfortunate to find this distinction lacking in some of the research reports. For example, Woody and Billy (1970) begin their paper with a brief literature review, including the statement that "Krippner (1966) successfully used clinical suggestion and/or hypnosis to decrease tension and increase motivation with children enrolled in a reading clinic" (p. 268). Our own evaluation of Krippner's (1966) research found no basis for such a conclusion.

At the same time, it has not been shown that hypnotherapy is not helpful in learning and performance problems in children. We, therefore, suggest that clinicians continue to treat such problems with hypnotherapy, with proper modesty in the claims they make to prospective patients. In the future, we hope that both clinicians and researchers will consider methodological issues more carefully; otherwise, we will continue the present state of working in a context of ignorance and sometimes making "much ado about nothing" in published reports.

REFERENCES

Crasilneck, H. B., & Hall, J. A. *Clinical hypnosis: Principles and applications.* New York: Grune & Stratton, 1975.

Gardner, G. G. Use of hypnosis for psychogenic epilepsy in a child. *The American Journal of Clinical Hypnosis,* 1973, *15,* 166–169.

Illovsky, J. An experience with group hypnosis in reading disability in primary behavior disorders. *The Journal of Genetic Psychology,* 1963, *102,* 61–67.

Illovsky, J., & Fredman, N. Group suggestion in learning disabilities of primary grade children: A feasibility study. *The International Journal of Clinical and Experimental Hypnosis,* 1976, *24,* 87–97.

Jacobs, L. & Jacobs, J. Hypnotizability of children as related to hemispheric reference and neurological organization. *The American Journal of Clinical Hypnosis,* 1966, *8,* 269–274.

Jampolsky, G. G. Use of hypnosis and sensory motor stimulation to aid children with learning problems. *Journal of Learning Disabilities,* 1970, *3,* 570–575.

Jampolsky, G. G. Hypnosis in the treatment of learning problems. Paper presented at the 27th annual scientific meeting of the Society for Clinical and Experimental Hypnosis, Chicago, 1975.

Krippner, S. The use of hypnosis with elementary and secondary school children in a summer reading clinic. *The American Journal of Clinical Hypnosis*, 1966, *8*, 261–266.

Lazar, B. S. Hypnotic imagery as a tool in working with a cerebral palsied child. *The International Journal of Clinical and Experimental Hypnosis*, 1977, *25*, 78–87.

London, P. *Children's Hypnotic Susceptibility Scale*. Palo Alto, Calif.: Consulting Psychologists Press, 1963.

Sternlicht, M., & Wanderer, Z. W. Hypnotic susceptibility and mental deficiency. *The International Journal of Clinical and Experimental Hypnosis*, 1963, *11*, 104–111.

Watkins, J. G. Hypnotherapy. American Psychological Association Post-Doctoral Institute course, Brooklyn, New York, August, 1962.

Woody, R. H., & Billy, H. T. Influencing the intelligence scores of retarded and nonretarded boys with clinical suggestion. *The American Journal of Clinical Hypnosis*, 1970, *12*, 268–271.

Woody, R. H., & Herr, E. L. Mental retardation and clinical hypnosis. *Mental Retardation*, 1967, *5*, 27–28.

10

Hypnotherapy for Pain Control

Historical accounts of hypnotherapy include many reports of its use for pain control. Given that children generally have more hypnotic talent than adults and that ability to control pain with hypnotic suggestion is positively correlated with hypnotizability (Hilgard & Hilgard, 1975), it should come as no surprise that children have been found to be more adept than adults in using hypnotherapy for control of pain (Wakeman & Kaplan, 1978).

While these findings are true in terms of group comparisons, of course there are individual differences. It would be more accurate to say that some children in some circumstances benefit from some hypnotherapeutic approaches to control some kinds of pain. The following case report illustrates these complexities; it also illustrates the power of the spoken word in a hypnotherapeutic context.

Frank L., age 13, suffered electrical burns over much of his body after trying to retrieve a kite that had landed on a high voltage wire. In the course of his hospitalization, he was taken to the department of physical medicine for a special test to determine the extent of nerve damage to his hand. During the test, he reported to the hypnotherapist a pain level of 8, on a 0 to 10 scale, in his right arm and back. He responded very well to suggestions for reduction of the pain in his arm, lowering it to a 0 level in a minute or so. He could not, however, do anything about the pain in his back. When questioned about this, he said that he did not want to relax and lie down on his back because his back would then stick to the sheet and he would have to go through the severe pain of getting unstuck in order to get back to his own room and back to his bed. This pain was so severe that Frank could not use hypnosis at all to modify it. The therapist agreed with his logic and casually remarked, "That's okay. I'll go back upstairs with you and you can get rid of the back pain after you are in your room and back in your own bed."

Since the therapist knew that Frank had had little success using self-hypnosis for severe pain, of course she intended to communicate that she would help him. She accompanied Frank back to his room. A few minutes after he was in bed, she told him that he could now begin work to get rid of the pain in his back. He smiled and said that, as soon as he got into bed, the back pain disappeared. He had indeed taken the therapist's casual remark as a posthypnotic suggestion. Interestingly, he then reported return of pain in his arm, which disappeared after a brief session of about 5 minutes. He was possibly responding to the demand characteristics of the therapist's seeming expectation that he would still have pain when he got into bed.

Hypnotherapists sometimes approach the problem of pain in children in a trial-and-error fashion, randomly trying hypnoanalgesic techniques with which they are most familiar, with little thought as to why one method might be preferable to another in a particular instance. Although we know of no research which specifically addresses this issue, we think that some techniques might be preferable to others when one considers the biological, psychological, and social contexts in which pain occurs. The following material deals with aspects of a child's experience of pain that might influence choice of technique.

VARIATIONS IN THE EXPERIENCE OF PAIN

Age

The neonate cannot distinguish pain from other unpleasant experiences such as hunger or cold. Moreover, because of incomplete cortical development, there is probably no memory of painful experiences in the neonatal period. By the end of the first year of life, the child can identify and localize pain, and by the end of the second year there is clear evidence of memory. Small children quickly learn to avoid painful stimuli such as a hot bulb on a lamp or Christmas tree, and they may begin to cry at the mere sight of a doctor who has previously given some painful treatment. Since most children as young as 2 have developed skills in imagery and in receptive language and can perceive adults as sources of help, these factors together with motivation to avoid pain should make young children receptive to hypnotherapeutic techniques for pain control. The main problems involve a poorly developed sense of time and of cause and effect. Thus a 2-year-old probably could not benefit from a statement such as, "If you will do this or think about that, then the pain might go away." However, more naturalistic techniques, such as story telling, which capture the child's attention and therefore focus attention away from pain will often be successful. Generally, a child of 4 or 5 should be able to utilize hypnotic suggestions for pain control unless past or present experience has taught a contrary expectation.

Individual Differences in Tolerance

Children vary greatly in terms of ability to tolerate pain. Given three children who have apparently equal amounts of pain, the first will continue playing, the second will ask someone to "kiss it and make it all better" and will then continue playing, and the third will experience complete disruption of play and behave as if a catastrophe had occurred. In Petrie's (1967) terms, these children represent reducers, moderates, and augmentors, and they tend to distort perceptions in other areas (e.g., size) in the same way that they distort perceptions of pain. In a study of adolescents and adults, Petrie (1967) found that juvenile delinquents and youngsters involved in contact sports tended to be reducers. Alcohol and aspirin, both of which are associated with increased tolerance of pain, significantly lessened pain for augmentors but had little or no effect with reducers. Likewise, we would speculate that hypnotherapy for pain control might be more effective for augmentors than for reducers. However, the moderates might prove to be the most responsive to hypnotherapy, especially if the augmentors have some emotional investment in experiencing or expressing the experience of pain. It is not clear whether the differences among Petrie's groups reflect biological or psychological differences or both.

Emotional Significance

For some children, pain has little emotional significance and is perceived mainly as a nuisance or a bad experience to be terminated as soon as possible. For other children, pain may have a variety of meanings and may serve a variety of psychological functions: (1) punishment for real or imagined sins; (2) getting attention and love, especially for children who tend to be ignored when "everything is okay"; (3) identification or merging with a loved one who has had similar pain, especially if there has been real or threatened abandonment by that person; (4) avoiding feared or unwanted situations that would be inevitable if the child were not in pain; (5) remaining close to a loved one whom the child feels a need to protect or in whose absence the child does not feel secure (most school-phobic pains fall into this category); (6) gaining status in certain families or cultural contexts where expressions of pain are socially acceptable and highly valued; (7) unconscious expression of hostility toward parents or siblings ("I'll make you feel bad to see me in pain"); (8) controlling others, especially for children with passive–aggressive tendencies ("I'll make you stay home with me. I'll ruin your day, and you can't get mad at me because you have to feel sorry for me because I'm in pain"); (9) assuring continuation of life, especially in sick children who have been taught that God uses death to take away pain; and/or (10) fulfilling the will of God, especially in children who have been taught that people must suffer for their sins and that continued suffering makes one somehow special in the eyes of God.

These are only a few of the ways in which pain can have emotional meaning; one must always be on the alert for other idiosyncratic kinds of significance. Hypnoanalgesic suggestions are likely to have no effect if the therapist has not dealt with the emotional significance of pain, either directly or indirectly.

Context of the Pain

Many aspects of the child's reality affect the extent to which pain will be tolerated. Previous painful experiences may have shaped the child's expectations that the present experience will be dreadful. Certain coexisting bodily states such as fatigue or physical discomfort will probably reduce pain tolerance. Coexisting psychological states are also important. Anxiety and depression usually reduce pain tolerance. Excitement and anticipatory joy, such as at the time of a birthday, will often enhance pain tolerance.

A child's response to pain may depend partly on understanding of its purpose: (1) no understanding in a very small child; (2) no purpose, e.g., an accident; (3) an unjust purpose, e.g., a wound resulting from a fight; (4) a logical purpose, e.g., a dressing change for burns. When a child understands the purpose or source of pain, reaction may also be influenced by the response of others. A parent who responds with anxiety and confusion will elicit a more negative reaction in a child than will a parent who responds with acceptance and with clarity about what needs to be done.

Children's reactions to pain are often influenced by the context of their expectations concerning adult response as much as by the response itself. Helen H., age 9, sustained a small laceration of her hand after a mischievous fight on the school playground. Frequently ridiculed and punished by her parents, the child was terrified that she would be punished for her misbehavior. She made no effort to report the accident and hoped to conceal it entirely by wiping the blood on her red dress. Although blood loss was minimal, she fainted a few minutes later. The fainting probably was an unconscious expression of her need to avoid "facing the consequences." The child was frankly disappointed when the pediatrician, after some deliberation, decided that sutures (painful punishment) would not be necessary. We would expect that this child would not have responded to hypnoanalgesic suggestions, had they been offered, despite her good imaginative skills.

In general, we would expect children to benefit less from hypnotherapy for pain which occurs in a negative context as compared with pain which occurs in a more neutral context. Therefore, we recommend that pediatricians and other child health specialists counsel parents regarding optimal ways of responding to pain in their children. Of course, doctors and other medical staff also play an important role in creating or modifying the reality context of pain in children. The doctor who communicates that pain is inevitable and may become even more severe will tend to have patients who experience a great deal of pain. On the other hand, if all members of the medical team approach the child with a calm and positive manner, then the child may well be able to fulfill the expectation that the situation is manageable and may even be enjoyable. Because children lack the preconceptions of adults, because they may be influenced positively or negatively, and because their future perceptions concerning pain may be permanently affected, it is incumbent on all adults to choose words related to pain very carefully when speaking to children.

TOWARD UNDERSTANDING HYPNOANALGESIA

Most researchers and virtually all clinicians in the field of hypnosis agree that the phenomenon of hypnoanalgesia is real, that patients and subjects are not faking in order to please the experimenter or for some other reason. While it is possible to deny the limited pain involved in a laboratory experiment, the idea of faking becomes far-fetched in severe clinical pain such as one sees in surgical procedures or in advanced cancer. Some skeptical researchers have deemphasized the role of hypnotic suggestion in favor of such constructs as role playing or expectation (e.g., Barber & Hahn, 1962; Stam & Spanos, 1980). We agree that role playing and expectation can enhance one's ability to modify pain, but we also believe that these factors are neither necessary nor sufficient for hypnoanalgesia. For example, Crasilneck and Hall (1973) demonstrated hypnotic pain reduction with naive children and with culturally unsophisticated subjects not acquainted with the expectations of the hypnotherapist. We have had similar clinical experiences.

It is one thing to accept the phenomenon of hypnoanalgesia as real; it is another thing to explain the mechanism by which it occurs. Two lines of research, one psychological and the other physiological, offer promising leads.

A Psychological Lead: Alternative Cognitive Controls

It is often the case in science that new ideas occur almost by chance, beginning in unrelated areas and finding new direction by virtue of the creative ability of the scientist. Thus the contribution of Hilgard and Hilgard toward explaining hypnoanalgesia began with a demonstration of hypnotic deafness that had nothing at all to do with pain. In a classroom demonstration, a subject who had been given suggestions for hypnotic deafness failed to respond to loud noises or to questions from classmates. Another student, noting that nothing was wrong with the subject's ears, asked if there might be some part of him that actually did hear. When the subject was asked to lift one finger, if some part of him other than the hypnotized part knew what was going on, he lifted one finger and then asked the instructor to explain this involuntary movement. The "hypnotized part" continued in ignorance, while the "other part" was able to give a full account when it was in ascendance following a signal (touching the arm). In the waking state, the subject was given a cue for release of hypnotic amnesia, at which point he remembered everything (Hilgard & Hilgard, 1975).

It occurred to the Hilgards that a similar mechanism might be operating in the case of hypnotic pain control, and a series of subsequent experiments demonstrated this to be true. Subjects who were capable of hypnotic pain control were asked if some "other part" of them knew more of what was going on than the hypnotized part. In about half the cases, while the hypnotized part reported low levels of pain, the "other part" reported pain at higher levels. The Hilgards described the "other part" as a "hidden observer," emphasizing that it is "a metaphor for something occurring at an intellectual level but not available to the consciousness of the hypnotized person. It does not mean that there is some sort of secondary personality with a life of its own— a kind of homunculus lurking in the shadows of the conscious person" (Hilgard & Hilgard, 1975, pp. 168–169).

In attempting to explain their findings, the Hilgards postulated alternative cognitive controls, which may or may not be in ascendance at any given time. These ideas also offer an explanation for the fact that subjects who are hypnotically analgesic demonstrate physiological signs of pain (e.g., increased heart rate) while reporting no felt pain. The theory of alternative cognitive controls, also called neodissociation theory, is further explicated in a more recent book by E. R. Hilgard (1977) that we recommend to those interested in broader theoretical developments related to hypnosis and to human consciousness.

A Physiological Lead: Endorphins

In recent years, the discovery of endorphins—endogenous morphinelike peptides—has produced a large number of new studies relating to pain control. When these substances are released from various body sites into the blood, there is an analgesic effect sometimes lasting 2 or 3 hours. Researchers are now trying to identify particular circumstances (e.g., stress) and/or special populations (e.g., schizophrenics) in which endorphins are most likely to be released. Owing to problems of measurement and other methodological pitfalls, reported findings are tentative and sometimes contradictory. The question, for our purposes, is whether endorphins are somehow related to hypnotic analgesia.

Olness, Wain, and Ng (1980) reported a pilot study of blood endorphin levels in four chronically ill children trained to use self-hypnosis for control of pain in a clinical setting. At initial training, the age range was 6 to 8 years. At the time of the research study 2 to 7 years had elapsed, during which all children practiced their pain control skills in regular group review sessions. Each child underwent venipuncture, first in the waking state, then following induction of self-hypnosis with suggestions for arm analgesia and subjective reports from each child that analgesia had been achieved. Results of radioimmunoassay revealed no detectable blood endorphin levels in any of the children either in the waking state or in hypnosis. Explanations relate to (1) difficulties in measuring endorphins, (2) the possibility that these well-trained children were actually in hypnosis during both blood drawings, (3) the possibility that hypnotic analgesia is not mediated through opiate receptor sites, and (4) the possibility that the relaxation associated with hypnosis actually diminishes endorphin levels rather than increasing them.

Goldstein and Hilgard (1978) approached the problem somewhat differently, using naloxone, a drug known to reverse the analgesic effect of morphine and of endorphins. They reasoned that if hypnotic analgesia were mediated by endorphins, then naloxone should negate the analgesic effect. They found, however, that naloxone did not interfere with hypnotically achieved analgesia in their adult subjects.

In spite of the negative results of these two studies, we do not think this area of inquiry should be abandoned, at least not until there are advances both in the measurement of hypnotic responsiveness and in the measurement of endorphins.

GENERAL PRINCIPLES FOR TEACHING HYPNOANALGESIA

In working with several hundred children who have learned hypnotic pain control for various conditions, we have found the following principles to be useful.

• Children may not always want to use their pain control skills. Some children sail through a bone marrow aspirate with no chemical anesthesia 1 month and refuse to do so the next month. Likewise, some children make frequent requests for chemical analgesics, say the first and third postoperative day, but none on the second day. The variation may reflect some physiological factor, perhaps related to endorphins. It may simply mean that the child prefers to lean on someone else on some days and not on other days. Depending on the secondary gain available, a child may prefer to have some complaints on any given day. As hypnotherapists, we encourage our patients to use their hypnotic talent, but we also recognize that sometimes to do so might interfere with other more pressing needs. We let the children be their own guides, occasionally to the consternation of parents or other staff who wish we would be more forceful.

• When children ask to learn hypnoanalgesia, we focus on mastery, expressing confidence in their abilities, giving them choices regarding when and how much they wish to practice, letting them decide what imagery they wish to use. In order to accomplish these goals, it is necessary to spend time with child patients, becoming familiar with likes, dislikes, and interests.

• The therapist needs to analyze his or her own attitude toward discomfort. Most of us, by the time we reach adulthood, because of our childhood experiences and our training, have certain negative notions about pain which we may project onto our patients. A therapist who lacks faith in a child patient's ability to overcome pain is unlikely to succeed in helping the child.

• Expectations of parents regarding discomfort are important variables, and parents may also benefit from self-hypnosis exercises. In fact, in certain situations it may be preferable for the parent to learn concurrently with the child. Children are less conditioned to the necessity for pain, suffering, and mental anguish if not overwhelmed by the negative expectations of their parents concerning pain.

• Expectations of other members of the treatment team must be considered. How does the oncologist, the neurologist, the dentist, feel about the necessity for routine anesthetics? What are their expectations about the inevitability of pain in various circumstances? A wise hypnotherapist can often do much to avoid inadvertent sabotage from colleagues.

• The initial discussion of hypnotic pain control should be tailored to the child's interests and developmental level, the parents' wishes, and the therapist's strengths. For some adolescents, explanations may be lengthy and involve descriptions of the nervous system and pain pathways. For most younger children, briefer explanations are preferable. Some preschoolers benefit from watching a videotape of children of similar ages who are demonstrating hypnotic pain control. Children of grade school age understand the concept of similar sound signals being interpreted differently by the brain. For example, the sound "b" may be interpreted by the brain as "bee," "be," "b," or the sound "c" may be interpreted as "see," "c," "sea." Similarly, the signal from the entrance of a needle into the skin may be interpreted in multiple ways and the child is capable of learning such control.

• It is helpful to have the child describe the pain, recognizing that descriptive words used by adults may not be meaningful. If the child cannot be more specific than to say "it hurts," the therapist might offer several alternatives such as a pecking bird, a whirling tornado, a scratch from a rose bush, a raging fire. The child's description may then be incorporated into a therapeutic suggestion, for example, "If you like, you can let that pecking bird fly away." Concrete images are preferable to abstract terms. Sometimes it is useful to ask a child to give current pain a numerical rating, where 0 indicates no pain at all and 10 is very severe or the worst ever for this kind of problem. Like adults, children are quite good at comparing pain from one time to another, and they often enjoy the concrete numerical evidence of change.

• When possible, it is important to go beyond suggestions for hypnotic relaxation and to include specific suggestions for hypnoanalgesia. Research has shown that relaxation alone may produce some reduction in felt pain, especially if anxiety is a significant component, but that greater pain reduction is associated with suggested hypnoanalgesia (Hilgard & Hilgard, 1975). Some children are so frightened or upset that they cannot cooperate with analgesic suggestions. In these cases a simple hypnotic induction may have a distracting effect and be better than nothing at all.

• Hypnotherapy for pain control may have a variety of side benefits, especially in the case of children with chronic or life-threatening illness. These include reduction of anxiety, enhancement of mastery and hope, increased cooperation, and increased comfort among family members and among other members of the health care team.

• Some children have difficulty believing that hypnotic pain control is possible. In these cases, it may be helpful first to demonstrate some other form of altered body sensation. Techniques such as hand catalepsy or arm levitation usually impress the child and arouse sufficient curiosity to proceed to explore pain control.

• The therapist should avoid being too specific about when and how the pain will go away. One can rapidly back oneself into a corner by such statements as, "The pain will be gone in 10 minutes" or "The hurting will go away when I count to five." If the prophecy is not fulfilled, the therapist loses credibility, and then even appropriate suggestions may have no effect.

• It is important to avoid a situation in which the therapist or patient must either demonstrate successful hypnotic pain reduction or run the risk of disappointing or losing respect from others such as colleagues or family. This attitude of challenge or "I'll show you" creates anxiety in both therapist and patient and runs counter to the relaxed and confident attitude that is fundamental to acceptance of hypnotic suggestions. We think it is important to defer demonstrations until it is clear that the child can succeed. If parents or colleagues are present during the initial hypnotherapy session, the therapist should clarify that the purpose of the session is to see which hypnotic methods will be most helpful.

TECHNIQUES OF HYPNOANALGESIA

The following techniques represent methods we have used with our patients. We often use several in combination. Every technique involves suggested dissociation, either directly or indirectly. For instance, notice how the phrase "that arm" rather than "your arm" facilitates dissociation. As with induction techniques, our list is by no means complete. Other hypnotherapists will prefer variations of our methods or will develop other methods.

Direct Suggestions for Hypnoanesthesia

Request for numbness. "You know what a numb feeling is. How does numbness feel to you? [Child responds.] Good, just let that part of your body get numb now. Numb like a block of ice [or whatever image the child has used]."

Topical anesthesia. "Just imagine painting numbing medicine onto that part of your body. Tell me when you're finished doing that."

Local anesthesia. "Imagine injecting an anesthetic into that part of your body. Feel it flow into your body and notice the change in feeling as the area becomes numb."

Glove anesthesia. "First, pay attention to your hand. Notice how you can feel tingling feelings in that hand. Then let it become numb. When it is very numb, touch that hand to your jaw [or other body part] and let the numb feeling transfer from the hand to the jaw."

Switchbox. The therapist explains the idea that pain is transmitted by nerves from various parts of the body to the brain, which then sends a "pain message" back to the body. The therapist can describe nerves and their pathways or can ask the child to provide a color for nerves. The importance of accuracy varies with the age and needs of the child. Then the child is asked to choose some sort of switch that can turn off incoming nerve signals. The therapist can describe various kinds of switches, such as flip, dimmer, pull, or even a television computer push-button panel or control panel of lights. Having chosen a switch, the child is asked to begin practicing turning off the switches or the lights that connect the brain and certain areas of the body. It is useful to ask the child to turn off the incoming nerve signals for defined periods of time (e.g., 10 minutes, 15 minutes, or 90 minutes). The success of the exercise is judged by touching the child with a small gauge needle or some other sharp object and asking for a comparison with feelings on the other side where the nerve signals are unchanged.

Distancing Suggestions

Moving pain away from the self. "Imagine for a while that that arm [or other body part] doesn't belong to you, isn't part of you. Think of it as part of a sculpture or a toy or picture it just floating out there by itself." Some patients comfortably imagine having only one arm; others imagine three arms, one of which is dissociated.

Transferring pain to another body part. "Imagine putting all the discomfort of the spinal tap into the little finger of your right hand. Tell me how much discomfort is in that little finger. Give it a numerical rating and let me know if it changes. Good. Now let it float away."

Moving self away from the pain. "You said you like to go to the mountains. Imagine yourself there now. Let yourself really be there. Just leave all the discomfort and be in the mountains. See the trees and flowers. Watch the chipmunks playing. You can give them some of your food if you like. Smell the fresh air and the pine trees. Listen to the gentle wind. Listen to the running stream." In one study of adults (Greene & Reyher, 1972), it was suggested that body-oriented imagery (e.g., feeling the warmth of the sun) was less effective for hypnotic pain control than imagery that was not body oriented (e.g., looking at scenery or skiing). We do not know if these results are applicable to children.

Suggestions for Feelings Antithetical to Pain

Comfort. "Recall a time when you felt very comfortable, very good. Then bring those good comfortable feelings into the present. Let your body feel comfortable here and now. You can let comfortable feelings fill your whole body and mind completely, until there is just no room for discomfort. You can be completely comfortable, and you can keep these good feelings for as long as you like."

Laughter. "Laughing helps pain go away. Think of the funniest movie you ever saw or the funniest thing you ever did or your friend did. Each time you imagine laughing, your pain becomes less and less. You may find yourself really laughing and feeling very good."

Relaxation. "Concentrate on breathing out, for that is a relaxing motion. If you relax completely when you breathe out, you can reduce the pain. Follow your breathing rhythm. Relax more each time you breathe out. You may find that you can cut the pain in half. And then in half again. Use your energy where it will help you feel better and get better."

Distraction Techniques

Focus on unrelated material.   Young children often obtain some pain relief if the therapist tells a story, either in its original form or with ridiculous variations such as changing the characters ("Once upon a time there were three little wolves and a big bad pig") or their roles ("Once there was a wolf who cried 'Boy, boy' "). Older children may be distracted by discussion of areas of interest such as sports or music.

Focus on procedure or injury.   This method is especially useful for children for whom cognitive mastery is a major coping mechanism. The therapist asks the child to describe the injury in detail, how it occurred, how others reacted, and so on. In the case of a painful procedure, the therapist describes various instruments and asks the child to assist by holding instruments or bandages, counting sutures, or checking the time at various points.

Focus on lesser of two evils.   If a child feels both pain and cold, the therapist can focus on the cold. If a child is having a spinal tap and also has an IV running, the therapist can focus on the IV.

Directing Attention to Pain Itself

For various reasons, some children refuse or are unable to focus attention on anything but the experience of pain. The therapist can utilize this behavior to the child's own advantage. By joining with the child and asking for a detailed description of the pain, the therapist can offer subtle suggestions for change and relief. Confusion techniques also help.

Lighted globe.   "Imagine you are inside a lighted globe and you can see yourself walking around on the inside of a map of your discomfort. Notice that discomfort very carefully. See it right now in a color you don't like. I'll ask you to check it again later. Notice what size it is. It might be the size of a grapefruit or a grape or a lemon. Even a pinhead has a size. We'll check the size again later. And notice the shape. What shape is it right now? And what is it saying to you now? How loud is it right now? Later we'll see if you can still hear it. Look again. What color is it now? That's interesting. It seems to be changing. I wonder how you did that. How small is it now? Can you change the size too? Yes. You are really in charge there in that lighted globe. You are a good mapmaker. You can go wherever you want. Feel whatever you want. What shape is the discomfort now? Can you still hear it?"

Reinforcement

We encourage—but not demand—our patients to practice their skills in hypnotic pain control, using variations or new methods as they see fit. The more confident children are of their ability to use these skills, the more likely it is that they will use them whenever it is appropriate to do so. Other methods of reinforcement include selected use of audiotapes, videotapes, parents acting as therapeutic allies, group meetings, and communication with other patients who have successfully used hypnotherapy for pain control.

CONCLUSIONS

Although pain control is one of the oldest uses of hypnotherapy, understanding of the process remains in its infancy. The next several years can be expected to produce exciting research findings that will clarify many difficult issues and allow therapists greater precision in selecting hypnoanalgesic techniques for individual patients.

REFERENCES

Barber, T. X., & Hahn, K. W., Jr. Physiological and subjective responses to pain producing stimulation under hypnotically-suggested and waking-imagined "analgesia." *Journal of Abnormal and Social Psychology*, 1962, *65*, 411–418.

Crasilneck, H. B., & Hall, J. A. Clinical hypnosis in problems of pain. *The American Journal of Clinical Hypnosis*, 1973, *15*, 153–161.

Goldstein, A., & Hilgard, E. R. Lack of influence of the morphine antagonist naloxone on hypnotic analgesia. *Proceedings of the National Academy of Sciences*, 1975, *72*, 2041–2043.

Greene, R. J., & Reyher, J. Pain tolerance in hypnotic analgesic and imagination states. *Journal of Abnormal Psychology*, 1972, *79*, 29–38.

Hilgard, E. R. *Divided consciousness: Multiple controls in human thought and action.* New York: John Wiley & Sons, 1977.

Hilgard, E. R., & Hilgard, J. R. *Hypnosis in the relief of pain.* Los Altos, Calif.: William Kaufman, Inc., 1975.

Olness, K., Wain, H. J., & Ng, L. A pilot study of blood endorphin levels in children using self-hypnosis to control pain. *Developmental and Behavioral Pediatrics,* 1980, *1,* 187–188.

Petrie, A. *Individuality in pain and suffering.* Chicago: University of Chicago Publishing Co., 1967.

Stam, H. J., & Spanos, N. P. Experimental designs, expectancy effects, and hypnotic analgesia. *Journal of Abnormal Psychology,* 1980, *89,* 751–762.

Wakeman, R. J., & Kaplan, J. Z. An experimental study of hypnosis in painful burns. *The American Journal of Clinical Hypnosis,* 1978, *21,* 3–12.

11

Hypnotherapy for Pediatric Medical Problems

A growing body of clinical and research data attest to the effectiveness of hypnotherapy in pediatric medicine. In many instances, children can utilize their hypnotic talent adjunctively to reduce or eliminate disease symptoms. Hypnotherapy is sometimes a primary therapeutic modality, apparently capable of altering the disease process itself. In some conditions, such as migraine, it is difficult to be precise in determining if hypnotherapy is an adjunct or a principal therapeutic tool.

When many children with medical problems successfully use hypnotherapy, their expressions of victory are obvious and justified. They have less need for medications that, at best, are a nuisance and, at worst, have harmful side effects such as stunting growth, damaging other body organs, and clouding consciousness. They spend less time in hospital wards and emergency rooms, and suffer fewer unpleasant medical procedures. They enjoy the physical and psychological benefits of normal activity. They move beyond the constricting role of "the sick one" in their families, developing a fuller sense of self based on more balanced expression of needs and abilities. In every way, they are healthier.

For some children with chronic or life-threatening disease, hypnotherapeutic accomplishments may be limited. These children often develop behavior disorders or experience severe anxiety and depression, usually associated with helplessness, hopelessness, and low self-esteem. Such difficulties may limit capacity for constructive fantasy and preclude the positive aspects of a doctor–patient relationship which seem to underlie successful use of hypnotherapeutic skills. For example, Donald R., an adolescent boy with sickle cell anemia, initially seemed enthusiastic that hypnotherapy might allow better pain control and possibly reduce the length of hospitalizations. He had good imagery skills and enjoyed hypnotic tennis games during which his pain and depression vanished. However, he could not overcome 16 years of being infantalized by his parents and living with the assumptions that the safest place was a hospital and that comfort came from narcotic drugs. In spite of obvious relief from hypnotherapy, he refused to use his skill in the absence of the therapist. As soon as she left his hospital room, he called the nurse to request more narcotics. Repeated efforts to help him met with continued resistance, and the therapist eventually terminated visits.

For some children, recent advances in medical management have extended life spans or achieved cures. But new problems arise that challenge us to develop new hypnotherapeutic approaches. Children who would have died a decade ago now live only to have to cope with permanent disfigurement or with guilt because others did not survive or with continuing pressure to feel deserving of having received an organ transplant at the risk of harming another person. We know relatively little about these problems of survival except that we can expect them to occur with increasing frequency unless therapeutic approaches that focus on prevention are developed. The possible role of hypnotherapy as a preventive tool needs exploration.

Therapeutic methods that enhance a sense of mastery and competency are most likely to help children cope with medical problems and with the complications of being cured. Children who successfully develop mastery skills may carry these skills into adulthood, becoming more able to prevent certain diseases and to reduce morbidity when illnesses occur. Hypnotherapeutic interventions seem ideally suited to these ends.

We will now discuss the uses of hypnotherapy in a wide variety of medical problems, based on the existing literature and on our own experiences. There are many other medical problems in which hypnotherapy might be useful, and we urge the reader to extrapolate accordingly.

ALLERGIES

Asthma

Asthma is a condition in which airways of the lower respiratory tract are obstructed either by bronchospasm, excessive sputum production, or mucosal edema. Such obstruction is manifested clinically by wheezing. It is helpful to distinguish *extrinsic asthma*, that triggered by external stimuli such as allergy, from *intrinsic asthma*, that not provoked by external stimuli. Extrinsic asthma is believed to occur as a result of inhalation, or occasionally ingestion, of an antigen that reacts with an antibody in the gamma globulin fraction of plasma (an IgE antibody). Intrinsic asthma, which is more common, may also reflect immunological mechanisms, but presently its pathogenesis is unclear (Snider, 1978). Hormonal, autonomic nervous system, and neurotransmitter imbalances have been postulated as involved. For example, Henderson, et al. (1979) reported experiments in which asthmatic patients were compared with normal controls and with patients who had allergic rhinitis. The pupils of the asthmatic patients required significantly less phenylephrine to dilate than did the pupils of the other two groups. This difference suggests greater autonomic sensitivity and/or responsiveness in the asthmatic patients.

Psychological factors have long been known to play a role in asthma, especially of the intrinsic type. Patients are often described as anxious, shy, dependent; they often see themselves as passive victims of their disease. They are convinced that they must rely on medications for control of wheezing, and some patients conclude that a hospital is the only safe environment. These children will enter the emergency room dramatically and do not respond to drugs or psychological intervention until they are safely admitted and assured of remaining in the hospital.

The symptoms of asthma are powerful weapons, and children can use them consciously or unconsciously to control their families or to satisfy a variety of emotional needs. Many clinicians have seen children stop wheezing within hours after being hospitalized, thus escaping from pressures and pathological interactions at home. Such observations often lead to recommendations for residential treatment, sometimes at a great distance from home. The problem with this approach is that, while patients may improve as a result of the separation, they eventually go back to the same environment; then the vicious cycle begins anew. It seems more effective in some cases to work with the child in the context of family treatment, perhaps including hypnotherapy for the entire family (Kohen, 1980a; Moore, 1980). At times, we encourage children to lead relaxation sessions with their parents, thus giving them the opportunity to control parents in a more positive way.

Other psychological factors in asthma are expectation and suggestibility. Clinical observations of child and adult asthmatics have demonstrated both increased and decreased wheezing in response to placebos coupled with appropriate suggestions. Laboratory studies have further documented this finding. Luparello et al. (1970) found that adult asthmatics not only demonstrated increased airway resistance when given a placebo antigen but also reversed their bronchospasm when given a saline solution placebo. Thorne and Fisher (1978) found that adult asthmatics experienced changes in physiological measures of respiratory efficiency following hypnotically suggested asthma, provided they were responsive to hypnotic induction. The same phenomena have been reported in children, both on the basis of clinical observations (Reaney, Chang, & Olness, 1978) and on the basis of laboratory research including pulmonary function studies (Khan, Staerk, & Bonk, 1974). The latter study included 20 asthmatic children, age 8 to 13 years. Positive response to hypnotically suggested asthma occurred in four children, all of whom scored high on the Barber Suggestibility Scale. Seven other high scorers, however, showed no change in pulmonary functions following the hypnotic suggestions. Moreover, some children reacted positively to sham allergens but not to hypnotic suggestion of bronchospasm, and vice versa. These data indicate that psychological aspects of asthma are complex and that simplistic treatment approaches are likely to have a limited effect.

Hypnotherapeutic Approaches to Childhood Asthma

Although there are several reports of hypnotherapy with asthmatic children, most with positive results, the actual methods used vary greatly from one study to another, making comparisons difficult. Treatment techniques have included hypnoanalytic and other insight-oriented methods, general ego-strengthening suggestions, relaxation training, teaching patients to increase and decrease wheezing, other suggestions aimed at enhancing the child's sense of control, training in self-hypnosis, and direct suggestions for symptom relief. Before reviewing this literature, we present two case reports representative of our current approaches to the problem. Generally we emphasize increased mastery and control, and we urge patients to extend hypnotic skills by training in self-hypnosis. While we attempt to understand underlying dynamics, insight-oriented techniques often play a relatively minor role. Sometimes, however, intensive psychotherapy is necessary before change occurs.

Sam M. was hospitalized at age 6 for treatment of status asthmaticus. He had experienced multiple hospitalizations in another state for asthma, which had begun at age 4. He was hospitalized four times in rapid succession before being referred for hypnotherapy. It was noted on the fourth admission that the patient "enjoys the hospital environment." There were significant family stresses: the parents had been divorced approximately 1 year previously, the mother had a new baby by her second husband, and the parents were fighting over custody of Sam.

Sam was seen as an outpatient six times in a period of 6 weeks for hypnotherapy. First, he and his family were given information about the disease, aided by drawings of the airway as "an upside down tree" with comparison of relaxed (dilated) and tight (constricted) branches. He was asked to prepare his own drawings of the asthmatic and nonasthmatic bronchial trees, again to reinforce his knowledge and mastery of the situation. In hypnosis, he enjoyed visualizing himself on a flying blanket, going where he chose, in control, and loosening up his airways. He also visualized himself in the future, free of his asthma and enjoying an active game of football, his favorite sport. In between sessions, he was encouraged to practice self-hypnosis at home. It was noted during the third visit that the patient came in with active wheezing and a respiratory rate of 36 over a 4-minute period. While in hypnosis, his respiratory rate reduced to 16 and wheezes were no longer heard on auscultation. A few minutes later, in the waiting room, he was heard to ask his mother if he could go home to play. She said that he would have to clean his room. Within 5 minutes, severe wheezing occurred that was again relieved by hypnosis exercises. Shortly after treatment began, Sam's father noted that, while at home, he was able to "stop a bad attack in 20 minutes" using his self-hypnosis. Subsequently he was seen approximately once a month for 6 months during which time, in spite of frequent attacks at home, he had no emergency room visits and no hospitalizations. Thirteen months after beginning hypnotherapy, he was hospitalized and during his hospitalization refused hypnosis. At this time, he seemed very upset over the conflict between his parents regarding his custody. His admission seemed to have been triggered by being grounded at home by his mother. He did not want to go home and repeatedly refused to practice hypnosis. Subsequently, he was followed by phone only. His father stated that the patient clearly could use his self-hypnosis and did so frequently. However, the family conflict remained unresolved.

The parents refused a recommendation for psychotherapy.

Hugh N. was first seen for hypnotherapy at age 7. His asthma had progressed to the point that he frequently had to stay home from school, and his pediatrician was about to begin steroid therapy. A cute redhead, Hugh's eyes sparkled at the idea of learning hypnotic skills. When he described his problem as not being able to get enough air into his lungs, the therapist explained that the problem in asthma is really not being able to get trapped air out of the lungs. Following good response to hypnotic induction involving progressive relaxation and hand levitation, the therapist asked, "What color are your lungs today?" When Hugh said he didn't know what color his lungs were, the therapist—with a twinkle—told him to stop talking like a grown-up and to answer the question. Grinning, Hugh said his lungs were green. Then the therapist said, "Good. Now what color is the air for you today?" Still grinning, Hugh said the air was orange. The therapist then said, "Fine. Now take a nice deep breath. Watch that orange air go all the way down to the very bottom of your lungs until all you see is orange. Then breathe out and watch all the orange air come up so that your lungs are all green again, from top to bottom." After Hugh successfully used this imagery, the therapist remarked that she hadn't ever heard him wheeze and asked him to imagine a beginning asthma attack. He produced a barely audible wheeze. The therapist said, "That's not much of a wheeze—can't you do better than that?" When Hugh wheezed more clearly, the therapist said, "Good. Now you have shown us that you really can control your wheezing. You can make it worse. Now control it the other way and make it go away." He did. This conversation led to further discussion of mastery, following which Hugh was taught self-hypnosis. The therapist suggested that he practice the color exercises daily and that he also use his hypnotic talent at the first sign of any wheezing. In the office, Hugh demonstrated his skills to his mother, and they agreed that he would be responsible for practice. One week later, Hugh's mother reported marked improvement, and treatment was terminated after three more sessions. About 1 year later, Hugh requested another appointment, stating that he had forgotten his skills and that his asthma was getting worse again. One hypnotherapeutic review session was sufficient to put him back in control, and follow-up some months later revealed continuing gains. Steroids were never begun. In the initial sessions, Hugh's mother admitted that she feared he might die or get into serious trouble and that she knew she was overprotective toward him. However, she refused the therapist's suggestion that she obtain psychotherapy for herself. The family eventually moved to another state.

Results of Hypnotherapy with Asthmatic Children

Review of research literature reveals that widely disparate hypnotherapeutic techniques result in similar dramatic improvement both in extrinsic and intrinsic asthma, though the emphasis is more on the latter. Clearly, we don't yet understand the mechanisms of change. Possibilities include enhancement of mastery, reduction of anxiety that may have some physiological effect, direct effects in relaxing bronchial smooth muscle, changes in parental attitudes and behavior, and resolution of unconscious conflicts. In any study, it is important to realize that the postulated mechanisms of change, derived from theoretical positions and related technical approaches, may or may not actually be responsible for an improved medical condition.

Diamond (1959) used hypnoanalytic techniques with 55 asthmatic children who had no positive findings on skin testing or had not responded to vaccine therapy. Five children did not respond at all to hypnotic induction, and another 10 achieved only a modest response. Of the remaining 40 patients, all achieved complete remission of symptoms and remained symptom-free during a 2- to 4-year follow-up period. These children experienced hypnotic age regression to the time of the first asthmatic attack, associated with emotional trauma such as severe guilt or fear of loss of parental love. They then responded to insight-oriented approaches in which they no longer needed to use their asthma as a way of getting positive parental attention and developing feelings of emotional security.

Smith and Burns (1960) used direct hypnotic suggestions for immediate and progressive symptom relief with 25 asthmatic children, age 8 to 15 years. All responded satisfactorily to hypnotic induction and some claimed subjective improvement over the 4-week treatment period. However, repeated pulmonary function tests revealed no significant change in any of the children. The authors concluded that they had failed to demonstrate any value of hypnotic suggestion for asthmatics. It surprises us that not a single child responded with improved pulmonary functions. We wonder whether the experimenters expected negative results and communicated a subtle bias. We also wonder whether the "strongly suggested" relief was expressed in a very authoritarian way in this clinic, perhaps circumventing the children's egos and unwittingly supporting passivity.

Diego (1961) taught five asthmatic boys, age 11 to 13, to precipitate and stop asthmatic attacks in hypnosis. He then gave them posthypnotic suggestions that they would be able to stop future attacks by hypnotic relaxation. All five patients reported rapid subjective improvement, and four continued improved for several months' follow-up. One boy relapsed after a month but improved again following a year of insight-oriented psychotherapy.

Aronoff, Aronoff, and Peck (1975) studied the efficacy of hypnotherapy in aborting acute asthmatic attacks in 17 children, age 6 to 17 years. Subjects were given direct hypnotic suggestions for chest relaxation, easy breathing, and reduction of wheezing. In most cases, they experienced immediate improvement, as measured both by pulmonary function tests and subjective reports. The authors noted that anxiety may aggravate asthma by stimulating the autonomic nervous system, and they speculated that "hypnosis, by promoting general relaxation, diminishes vagal stimulation and consequently diminishes release of mediators felt to be responsible for the bronchospasm" (Aronoff, Aronoff, & Peck, 1975, p. 361). Though the method in this study is similar to that of Smith and Burns (1960), we suspect that the general approach may have been more permissive and ego supportive.

Collison (1975) reported a retrospective analysis of 121 asthmatic patients treated with hypnotherapy. This report included six patients under age 10 years and 39 under age 20 years. Collison developed four categories of response: "excellent" when there was complete freedom from asthmatic attacks without medication in the follow-up period; "good" when there was a reduction of attacks with continuation of medications; "poor" when there was less than 50 percent improvement in frequency of attacks or need for medication; and "nil" when there was no change from the pretreatment assessment. Of the six youngest patients, four had excellent or good responses. Of 39 patients in the 11- to 20-year category, there were 32 excellent or good responses. In the older age groups, there were significantly fewer satisfactory responses. Since the youngest groups also were most responsive to hypnotic induction, there was some question as to whether age or depth of trance would be a better predictor of success in a prospective study. Severity of disease was also an important variable. Patients whose asthma was not so severe as to require steroids generally responded best to hypnotherapy. Collison's techniques included suggestions for ego strengthening and for general relaxation, together with exploration of psychological factors related to the disease. He deliberately avoided direct suggestions for symptom removal, fearing that such suggestions might serve only to mask medical problems and ultimately have a harmful effect. He noted the inherent difficulties in retrospective analysis and the need for prospective studies that control the multiple variables involved.

Barbour (1980) reported preliminary results of the use of self-hypnosis in adolescent asthmatics. A study of six patients, over a 5-month period, indicated that the use of self-hypnosis was associated with a reduction in the severity and frequency of asthma attacks. Before self-hypnosis training, skin tests with local inhalant antigens were done in four patients and demonstrated positive reactions to 14 antigens; skin tests were positive for only 7 antigens after 5 months of self-hypnosis. The same four patients also had skin testing done in a hypnotic state, and no reactivity to antigens occurred in any of the patients. This finding encourages the possibility that immune responses may be modified via appropriate uses of hypnotherapy and that hypnotherapy may not only reduce morbidity from asthma but, in fact, be curative in certain patients.

While we do not recommend the use of hypnotherapy in childhood asthma as a substitute for usual medications, we do believe that it can reduce the need for visits to emergency rooms and hospitalizations, and, in some children, the requirement for certain medications.

Although we are not attempting a complete review of psychological approaches to childhood asthma, we want to mention that several studies involving biofeedback training have reported positive results (Feldman, 1976; Kahn, 1977; Scherr & Crawford, 1978). Spevack and associates (1978) have reported that asthmatic children responded well to training in "passive relaxation." We wonder about the extent to which these children may have been responding to unintended hypnotic suggestion, especially since some of the studies included training in progressive relaxation. As we have said before, hypnosis can occur without hypnotic induction. At the same time, when studies purport to relate hypnotherapy to relief from asthma but fail to measure trance responsiveness, it is not clear that children who improve were actually in hypnosis. We have already seen (Kahn, Staerk, & Bonk, 1974) that some children with documented hypnotic talent do not respond to suggestions related to their disease. We need much more research before we can untangle the possibilities in this complex area.

Recurrent Hives

We have noted clinically that children suffering from recurrent generalized hives or massive reactions to bee stings have had fewer difficulties and more rapid recoveries when using adjunct hypnotherapy. Suggestions given have included those for general relaxation, mastery, and imagery of the patient without the swellings. It is possible that the state induced by hypnosis does reduce the allergic response. It may be directly through effects on a mediator of immune reactions, such as the mast cell (cell which stores granules containing potent inflammatory and repair materials released upon injury to the organism) or indirectly through reduction of heart rate, blood pressure, and/or respiratory rates. Preliminary studies of the effects of suggestions given under hypnosis on immune processes were conducted by Good (1979) in the late 1950s. Because of the important implications for patients with specific allergies and immunodeficiencies, these studies need expansion.

Specific Allergies

Perloff and Spiegelman (1973) reported the use of hypnotherapy in treating a 10-year-old girl's allergy to dogs. The child, acutely sensitive to dog dander, but wishing to have a dog, was taught a visual desensitization while in hypnosis. Thereafter, her sensitivity to dog dander disappeared. Barbour's (1980) study with adolescents lends credibility to this clinical report.

DERMATOLOGICAL PROBLEMS

Itching, Scratching, and Picking

Hypnotherapy provides a useful adjunct in management of many skin conditions including atopic eczema, psoriasis, and acne. In these conditions hypnotherapy may serve to reduce scratching or picking and therefore interrupt the vicious cycle of scratching-picking, discomfort, scratching-picking, exacerbation, and more discomfort. Suggestions that encourage general relaxation, a sense of mastery in controlling the disease progress, and images of coolness and wetness seem most helpful in these situations.

Mirvish (1978) reported a case history in which hypnotherapy led to relief of symptoms and improved behavior in a 10-year-old boy with chronic eczema.

Olness (1977) reported a case of intractable itching in a 9-year-old boy hospitalized for evaluation of possible rheumatoid arthritis. The pediatric resident caring for the boy considered teaching the boy hypnosis but had not yet begun when a social worker came to request urgent help. The boy was, at that moment, clawing at himself frantically. Olness established that the social worker had good rapport with the boy and asked her to sit down with him and talk about something cool like a swimming pool or a lake. The social worker said, "He's afraid of water. In fact he won't get in the bathtub here." Olness then suggested the concept of snow and ice and winter sports. An hour later, the social worker returned, elated. She had discovered that snow sliding was a great joy for this boy. They sat together, imagining a particular hill, its particular bumps, and they felt the snow spray as they slid down the hill. The incessant scratching stopped. Two days later, when a resident asked the patient's private physician about starting steroids, the physician, watching the boy racing down the hall, said, "He doesn't need them now. Since he started that hypnosis, he's doing fine." One might question whether or not formal hypnotherapy was used. Certainly rapport with an interested caring therapist, imagery, and suggestion of a feeling to counter pruritis were parts of the successful outcome for this patient.

As is true in conditions associated with uncomfortable symptoms, it is often helpful to teach self-hypnosis to children who itch and to recommend that they practice when they are comfortable in order to have more facility in self-control when symptoms recur.

Hyperhidrosis

Ambrose (1952) reported a case of a 13-year-old boy with excessive sweating that responded to hypnotherapy. The condition had begun at age 8, when the boy was evacuated during the second World War. While hypnotically regressed to age 8, he remembered being beaten up by a gang of boys while on his way to his new school. The boy became quite tense while describing these events, which he also recalled out of trance. Following six visits, he had no further problems in control of sweating. Ambrose postulated that hypnotherapy cut off the increased release of acetylcholine at the postganglionic nerves that had previously caused excessive sweating. At this time, this hypothesis has been neither confirmed nor denied, but studies of chemical mediations coincidental with hypnotherapy are essential for comprehension of mechanisms involved in such dramatic resolution of autonomic response problems.

Warts

Warts are reported to respond to many interventions. Left to its own devices, the half-life of a wart is about 1 year.

Surman, Gottlieb, and Hackett (1972) reported the successful hypnotic treatment of a 9-year-old girl who had 31 warts on her hands and face that had failed to respond to four attempts at conventional treatment. She was told that first one side would be treated for five sessions and, if the warts went away, the other side would be treated. She chose her left hand and left side of her face for initial wart removal. Hypnotic induction included eye closure, simulated stair descent, and hand levitation. The patient was then told she would feel a tingling sensation in all the warts on the left side. The left-sided warts began to disappear after the first session. By the fifth visit, she had lost 26 warts. After 3 months of follow-up, only two small warts remained.

Tasini and Hackett (1977) reported the use of hypnotherapy in three immunosuppressed children all of whom had developed numerous warts. Each of the patients had been repeatedly treated with standard wart regimens for several years prior to the successful use of hypnotherapy. Hand levitation was used for induction. The patients were asked to think of doing something they enjoyed and to relax more each time they breathed out. While in trance, the patients were told that the warts would feel dry, then turn brown and fall off. Patients were seen for three to five sessions. Dramatic regression of warts began within a few weeks in each child, eventuating in complete disappearance. There was no evidence of recurrence in follow-ups that ranged from 4 to 8 months.

Following an appropriate induction, one can ask children to give themselves the message that they are cutting off the food supply to the wart or warts. This suggestion may be included in the course of a routine physical examination, and the child is asked to reinforce the suggestion twice daily at home. We recall cases in which warts were treated topically in routine office practice only to have patients return with wart recurrences. Since adopting hypnotherapy as the primary mode of wart therapy, our patients have not required further topical chemicals.

In commenting on studies reporting disappearance of warts following hypnotherapy, Thomas (1979) emphasized the potential value of understanding what goes on when a wart disappears in association with hypnosis. He recommended further investigation in this area. Clawson and Swade (1975) speculated that the mechanism involved in wart removal via hypnotherapy is the constriction of capillary sites to the warts. Whether the mechanism is vascular or immunological, it would seem that its understanding might relate eventually to treatment of other tumors and skin diseases.

DIABETES

The psychological components of diabetes are well known (Ehrlich, 1974). Parents feel guilt about genetics and resent their lack of control. Family members are anxious about possible insulin reactions or episodes of ketoacidosis. Patients resent the intrusion of urine tests, diets, and drugs. Some children develop fears over injections. The daily injection of insulin may become a cause célèbre in the family unit. Hypnotherapy, presented in the context of patient mastery, can provide a solution for some of the difficulties. We have taught self-hypnosis to many diabetic children in individual and group sessions.

Paul B. was referred for hypnotherapy to overcome his fear of needles when he was 6 years old. A year earlier, he had been diagnosed as having diabetes. Insulin injections were given for a few weeks and stopped as he entered the honeymoon phase of the disease. When insulin was required again nearly 1 year later, this naturally aggressive, active, and rather dominating child was crushed. He struggled to avoid injections, screamed throughout them, and was generally depressed. His mother, father, and younger brothers were upset, torn by their sympathy for Paul's predicament and their need to cooperate with the treatment regimen. When Paul was seen initially in the office, he sat sullenly next to his young, intelligent, and obviously concerned mother. He responded with interest when handed a 50-cent piece to hold but made no comment as his mother briefly described the onset of diabetes and his fear of needles. The therapist said, "I once knew a 5-year-old boy who had diabetes and was so mad that he had to have those shots every day. He was mad at his doctor and at his parents and at his brother, who didn't need to get the shot. But then he learned something that they didn't know about how to handle needles himself. He knew, but his brother didn't." Paul asked, "What was it?" The therapist answered, "It was a way to turn off switches between his skin and where the needle went in and his brain — except in the beginning I couldn't tell him that because he was too young to know what a brain was." "I know what a brain is," said Paul. "Do you know what a nerve is too?" "Yep" he said proudly. "Well, you're already way ahead of this younger kid." Paul then learned the coin technique of induction, followed by favorite place imagery, suggestions about his switch system, and how he could use it. Throughout, the therapist stressed his ability, his control, his choice to use his skill when he wished, and to share with his family as he wished. At the conclusion of the first session, Paul was comfortable when touched with an insulin needle. He agreed to practice at home daily and to return in 1 week. His mother reported that injections no longer posed problems. He turned off his switch before each one, and the rest of the family didn't know how he did it. Subsequently, Paul attended group sessions where he was a good teaching assistant and very helpful to children with similar problems.

It is possible that the use of hypnotherapy to enhance mastery in diabetics, particularly as they approach adolescence, will indirectly affect morbidity from the disease. Children who are actively participating in their therapy may also be more likely to follow recommendations regarding urine testing, eating, and insulin with fewer complications and hospitalizations.

EPISTAXIS

Edel (1959) reported the case of a 10-year-old boy who had been referred for reading difficulties. After eight sessions using hypnotherapy, his reading problem disappeared and he no longer required tutoring. Two months later, he was brought into the physician's office because of a severe nosebleed. The use of bilateral anterior nasal packs with vasoconstrictors was to no avail. The physician gave instructions for posterior nasal packing and decided to add hypnotherapy as an adjunct. He told the patient that he could stop the bleeding himself, that he should hold his head way back and relax. Within minutes, the bleeding stopped and the boy breathed easily. When his head was placed forward, no blood spilled out. The next morning the parents reported there had been no further bleeding.

Although this was a patient previously familiar with hypnosis, it would be reasonable to give similar suggestions to any child with life-threatening bleeding from any source.

HEMOPHILIA

The monk Rasputin used hypnosis to aid the hemophiliac czarevitch in the control of bleeding. In the 1950s, hypnosis was reported to be effective in control of bleeding and pain during dental surgery in hemophiliacs. In 1975, LaBaw taught a group of hemophiliacs self-hypnosis and encouraged them to use this technique when faced with anxiety-provoking situations, particularly bleeding episodes. His 4-year study documented a significant reduction in the number of units of blood products required by 10 adult and child patients who practiced self-hypnosis on a regular basis.

Gustke's pilot work (1973) suggested that some hemophiliac patients were able to raise Factor VIII levels in association with hypnosis. However, there are no controlled studies to support the idea that hypnotherapy consistently reduces bleeding in hemophiliacs. As routine adjunct therapy, hypnotherapy may be as valuable for its enhancement of mastery as for what it can do to reduce pain, relieve anxiety, or reduce the frequency of bleeding episodes.

Olness & Agle (in press) have reported group practice sessions for hemophiliac patients and their families for 6 years. Although individual practice sessions are available to the hemophiliac patients, most become comfortable and prefer the group format. Sessions last 1 hour. During the initial 10 minutes, patients share experiences, ask questions, and explain to newcomers. Thirty minutes of hypnosis exercises include suggestions for general relaxation, pain control, and reduction of bleeding. Following this, adults are invited to participate in self-hypnosis exercises. Children join parents if they wish or go to another room for play or movement exercises with another therapist. In recent years, children have been offered the option of practice in thermal biofeedback. Graphic evidence of control of skin temperature seems to have encouraged many children to pursue their self-hypnosis exercises more regularly. A typical account of such a group session is as follows:

J. K. had taught his family to do relaxation exercises during the summer. His mother was, for the first time with his help, able to have major dental work done without general anesthesia. T. is doing very well with his intravenous injections. One morning, while he was at the Art Institute, he experienced pain associated with the eruption of a molar. His mother was concerned that they would have to leave because T. was so miserable. She asked him to sit down and turn off his switches, which he did promptly. He and his family were happy and comfortable during the rest of their visit. D. D., age 4, has been doing well in turning off his switches for IVs and has amazed the nursing staff.

When we asked the children about the sort of imagery they were using, J. K. reported that he imagined antique cars running about his bloodstream to stop bleeds especially in his ankle. He said this was effective. K. K. imagines planes full of bombs of Factor VIII that he dispatches to parts of his body that need them as well as a special glue named Super-Clot that he squeezes out in bleeding areas. The group went through a review of the switch-off technique, a coin induction also using favorite place imagery, and an exercise in which each child visualized a package containing a special gift for that child. Dr. D. guided the parents through a general relaxation using the image of a walk along a beach. The children also participated with their parents and expressed pleasure in the experience.

It is our perception that younger children learn best from older children in the group setting. If not threatened by much individualized cajoling and attention, they seem to learn by osmosis. Some younger children (age 2 to 3) merely sit quietly observing for one or two sessions without giving overt evidence of participation. Parents often report evidence of their learning at home before they show co-operation in the group sessions.

The children have provided many subjective reports of decreased bleeding. For example, Lanny L. said he awakened at midnight with a stiff arm, turned off the bleeding, and that his arm was fine by morning. His parents confirmed the report. Tom H., age 3, said he had a stiff arm (confirmed by his parents) but "I unstiffed my arm today."

Parents involved in the hemophiliac group have reported perceived benefits associated with the relaxation exercises for themselves. Not only have they learned specific pain control techniques, which they have invoked during dental procedures or surgical experiences, but they also state they have found themselves calmer in stress situations related to the hemophilia. One father attributes reduction of blood pressure (20 millimeters diastolic) over a period of several months to his regular practice of self-hypnosis.

Over this 6-year period, the hemophiliac boys have decreased their average use of Factor VIII replacement therapy. They have also become more mobile with less use of splints, crutches, and fewer days lost from school because of bleeding episodes. However, they have also become older and perhaps more careful about activities that might result in bleeding. Several have moved from hospital to home administration of replacement therapy, and two had major surgery which required large amounts of replacement therapy over a short period.

GASTROINTESTINAL DISORDERS

Recurrent abdominal pain is a common symptom among pediatric patients and one for which organic causes are often not found (Apley, 1977; Berger et al., 1977; Dodge, 1976). As a last resort, these patients are sometimes referred for hypnotherapy to relieve symptoms. While hypnotherapy may be helpful in these situations, its use simply to relieve pain is less likely to be successful than in children with known organic reasons for pain. A typical case history follows:

Linda, age 15, was referred by a pediatrician for symptomatic relief from abdominal pain that had been present for 6 months. The pain was recurrent, intermittent, and not associated with any specific time of day or situation. The parents had divorced 2 years earlier, and both had remarried. The patient's mother had custody, and the patient visited her father and his new family on weekends. Evaluation had included numerous laboratory and radiological studies, the results of which were normal. The patient was losing weight, which increased uneasiness in the referring pediatrician who was concerned about an undetected malignancy. At the time of the first visit for hypnotherapy, the patient and her mother were uneasy. They spoke very little to one another and demonstrated little affect. The patient was told that she would learn a self-hypnosis exercise that she could review at home, that she would be in control, and that she could practice pain control if she wished. The patient indicated her wish to learn hypnosis but responded mechanically to the initial induction. When she returned, she claimed to have practiced but said there was no improvement. During this session, she used hypnotic age regression to recall an event that she had enjoyed and in which she had felt in control; she enhanced the feeling of joy and mastery by squeezing her right fist. She was then asked to become aware of things that were irritating her or worrying her and to decide if she could let go of any of them. Following this session, she spontaneously said that she felt better but did not reveal any of her possible concerns. She then refused a recommendation for psychotherapy. She said she would practice self-hypnosis at home and that she was feeling better. A week later, she left her mother's home and moved into her father's home. All symptoms abated, she gained weight, and continued to come for follow-up appointments for review of hypnotherapy during the next 2 years. While she continued to refuse psychotherapy, she had no recurrence of abdominal pain and no indication of substitute symptoms.

Williams and Singh (1976) reported the case of an 11-year-old boy hospitalized for the third time in 16 months because of recurrent abdominal pain. The results of laboratory and x-ray studies were normal. Eighteen months earlier, he had undergone surgery to correct a right hydronephrosis. Subsequent recurrences of pain triggered gastrointestinal, neurological, and metabolic evaluations with normal results. There was a strong family history of abdominal disorders. After psychiatric evaluation, hypnotherapy was recommended. The boy was an excellent subject and, while in trance, repeated the following statements after the therapist: (1) "Cooped-up feelings can cause tension," (2) "Tension can cause physical pain," and (3) "By relaxing, I can reduce tension and eliminate the pain." The patient reported disappearance of pain during the exercise and was taught self-hypnosis to maintain his clinical improvement. In 20 months of follow-up, he had only one transient recurrence of abdominal pain, which was possibly due to gastroenteritis. The authors noted that this child, as is true of most with abdominal pain, no longer had any need to continue self-hypnosis exercises once the presenting symptom had resolved. We have also found this to be the case.

We have used hypnotherapy as an adjunct in management of children with ulcers, chronic hepatitis and varices, regional enteritis, and ulcerative colitis. Controlled studies are needed to assess effects of hypnotherapy on morbidity and mortality in these diseases. It is our impression that the enhancement of mastery and reduction of pain contribute to more rapid improvement in these patients.

JUVENILE RHEUMATOID ARTHRITIS

Juvenile rheumatoid arthritis (JRA) is well known as a disease of exacerbations and remissions. Conventional treatment deprives the patient of many controls and may in itself trigger emotional problems. The loss of free movement associated with the disease process invariably leads to some degree of depression in both children and families.

We often recommend hypnotherapy as an adjunct with these patients not only for relief of symptoms but to enhance self-mastery and enable the patient to control a portion of therapy. The complexities of psychogenic components of this disease are demonstrated in the following case history.

Mary F., a 10-year-old girl, came with her 12-year-old sister and mother to "learn hypnosis for pain control." Both girls had been diagnosed as having rheumatoid arthritis and eczema and were under the care of rheumatologists. They suffered intermittent pain, particularly in the knee and ankle joints, and they often missed school. In addition to the problems of arthritis and eczema, the 10-year-old girl was obese. She had attended one session of a group meeting for weight control but had refused to return.

Mary said she had been taught some hypnosis by a 14-year-old friend. Her sister and mother also said they had used self-hypnosis exercises for general relaxation. When asked about her interests, the patient said she liked singing, painting, and handicrafts. Her favorite colors were blue and red. Her mother described her as very creative and added that she often wrote stories and poems for fun.

Following progressive relaxation exercises, Mary rapidly appeared comfortable. When she confirmed via ideomotor signals that she was ready to go on, she imagined herself in a favorite place, doing what she liked, enjoying the feeling of being comfortable. After 2 minutes she appeared to be asleep. Then she became upset and began crying. The therapist told her she was safe, that she need not continue to feel upset, that she could leave her favorite place if she found it upsetting and come out of trance when she was ready. Almost immediately she stopped crying, opened her eyes and said that her favorite place was in bed, that she had fallen asleep, and that she had what she had once or twice a week while sleeping—a night terror. Her mother confirmed that she frequently had night terrors. The patient was asked to think about a scene in which she could be very comfortable without falling asleep and then to describe what it was when she returned for her next visit. Her 12-year-old sister went through the identical progressive relaxation and imagery exercise with no evidence of discomfort and subsequently demonstrated good evidence of pain control.

A follow-up appointment was made but not kept because of a death in the family. The sister required hospitalization and she was able to use self-hypnosis and pain control suggestions very well. When Mary returned 1 month later, she explained that she wished to use imagining herself floating in water for an induction, to focus on pain control and weight reduction. She seemed enthusiastic, did well in the hypnotherapy session, and agreed to practice twice daily. Subsequently she lost weight, demonstrated pain control, and returned for monthly group practice sessions for children with chronic pain problems.

This patient demonstrates some of the problems that can develop in hypnotherapy. Although it is often appropriate to allow a child his or her "own favorite place" without the necessity to reveal its whereabouts, it clearly would have been better to have known in this instance. Mary's choice of her bed as a favorite place suggests depression, which would also be consistent with her obesity and other chronic problems. An additional problem was the previous uncontrolled practice of self-hypnosis at home. This practice, while possibly leading to rapid trance induction, may also have made her less responsive to heterohypnosis. She did, however, seem to be highly motivated to have some personal part in her treatment and was very pleased with her subsequent excellent response.

Whether psychogenic components of JRA are causal or reflect the disease process and its treatment is not clearly understood at this time. Although much is known about immune factors and chemistries that reflect changes in those factors, the trigger for those changes remains elusive.

Cioppa and Thal (1975) reported a fascinating account of a 10-year-old girl in whom JRA had been diagnosed by a rheumatologist. She responded minimally to large doses of salicylates and physical therapy. Prior to a trial of steroids, hypnotherapy was recommended. At the time of the first hypnotherapy session, the patient was confined to a wheelchair and appeared severely depressed. The hypnotherapist taught her ideomotor responses and asked, "Does some part of your mind know why you have arthritis?" The ideomotor response was in the affirmative and the patient appeared visibly upset. The hypnotherapist then gave her a general suggestion that her legs would feel better. The patient and her mother were upset by this approach and disconcerted that the session was held in the department of psychiatry, since they did not believe that the arthritis had a psychological component. They did not want to return. That evening the girl spontaneously remarked that her legs felt different. One month later, the patient could walk with difficulty but deep depression persisted and the pediatrician asked that the child undergo a second hypnotherapy session. The patient was told that she did not have to tell the therapist the problem as long as she knew what it was and as long as she was certain that it would quickly resolve itself if she really wanted it to resolve. She was given hypnotic suggestions that her joints would feel much better, that she would feel happier, and that she would be able to play with her friends soon. Four hours later, the patient rode her bicycle for the first time in 3 months. Ankle swelling and pain subsided rapidly over the next few days, and, for the first time in several months, the patient could wear shoes. At that point, her depression began to lift. She was seen for three additional sessions. Improvements in her condition included being able to jump up and down with no pain, return of her sense of humor, and loss of fear of both injections and the hospital. Four months later, aspirin was stopped, and a 31-month follow-up revealed no recurrence of symptoms. It was of interest that the hospital staff, at a follow-up conference, implied that she had not had JRA in the first place but merely a conversion reaction with concomitant laboratory findings suggestive of JRA. Prior to her remission, a conversion reaction had not been mentioned in the differential diagnosis. We have seen this phenomenon repeatedly among medical personnel who feel uncomfortable about "coincidental" cures that occur in conjunction with hypnotherapy in "organic" diseases.

Cioppa and Thal noted that a number of diseases could be considered to represent the conversion of a chronic tension state into an organically manifest disease state. Factors of spontaneous remission are poorly understood although the writings of Norman Cousins (1976) have triggered much interest in the effects of attitude changes on remissions. Cioppa and Thal noted that, to be therapeutically effective, a reversal of attitude apparently must occur at a subconscious level. This may be brought about through hypnotherapy.

MALIGNANCIES

Since cancer remains one of the leading causes of death in children, we have deferred discussion of studies of hypnotherapy with cancer patients to a separate chapter (Chapter 13) on terminal illness. We want to emphasize here that since 1960 there has been a dramatic increase in survivors. While these children become free of disease, they often pay dearly in terms of psychological trauma resulting from diagnostic and treatment procedures and from the expectation of death. Hypnotherapists must begin to attend more to the problems of survival.

It is also important that hypnotherapists consider themselves, their feelings, responses, and perspectives from time to time. Transference and countertransference problems can be particularly intense in a therapeutic relationship with a child with a life-threatening illness. Moreover, it is possible that therapists' attitudes may affect morbidity and eventual therapeutic outcome. Although this area is fraught with problems for the researcher, we hope to see answers take shape. Specifically, we wonder whether or not patients can use specific hypnotherapeutic techniques to facilitate biochemical, immunological, nutritional, and/or psychological interactions that lead to cure.

NEUROLOGICAL PROBLEMS

Hypnotherapy has been associated with disappearance of migraine headaches, postencephalitic headaches, tics, hiccoughs, cyclic vomiting, and urine retention. It has also been used as adjunct therapy to help children with seizures, chronic muscle disorders, cerebral palsy, and to facilitate rehabilitation after severe neurological injuries. Its use in children with so-called MBD (minimal brain dysfunction) was discussed in Chapter 9.

Headaches

Recurrent headaches, like recurrent abdominal pain, are often of psychogenic origin. However, they may also have well-known organic origins such as encephalitis, ingestion of monosodium glutamate, carbon monoxide poisoning, or malignancies. A careful and reasonable evaluation to rule out some of these causes is essential before embarking on a course of hypnotherapy. If an organic cause of the headache is clear, it is reasonable to begin hypnotherapy for pain control fairly rapidly. Children usually respond quickly (Kohen et al., 1980). If the headache is likely to reflect psychogenic antecedents, successful hypnotherapy usually includes helping the patient relax and become aware of unconscious irritants. It is not always essential that the therapist know what those are, but it is critical that the patient is given the opportunity, in hypnosis, to consider worries or conflicts, to consider whether these really belong to the present or are habitual reactions carried over from the past and can now safely be jettisoned. In the latter case, it may be useful for the patient to imagine holding the problems in one hand and then releasing the grip and letting them float away. However, if the problems still have dynamic significance, more extensive psychotherapy—with or without hypnosis—is indicated.

In the case of recurrent headaches with a known cause, such as migraines, it is useful to teach self-hypnosis and to encourage the patient to practice on a daily basis at home for 4 to 6 weeks with calendar recording of practice. Most children are unlikely to practice regularly much longer, but they do cultivate a conditioned response during the practice period that they can invoke at the beginning of a subsequent headache. An example of such a patient is Nancy, age 10.

Nancy K. was referred by a pediatric neurologist for hypnotherapy in the management of intractable migraines that were handicapping her life in many areas. Excessive drug therapy was required and results were not ideal. Nancy and her family were depressed over her chronic illness and its interference with family activities as well as school. At the first visit, Nancy was told that she could learn a method of headache control that she could use later to treat herself. The therapist explained that it would be important for her to practice regularly for at least 6 weeks so that she would be sure of her skills. Then the therapist drew diagrams of the nervous system, explained the theory of vascular changes which trigger migraines, and explained the concept of using imaginary switches to control pain. Nancy was delighted at the idea of having her own method, and she learned rapidly. On the third visit, she was taught the jettison technique for letting go of worries. Within 1 month, she was off all medications and in complete control of her headaches. When she sensed an aura of a migraine, she was able to stop its progression.

Seizures

Hypnotherapy has been reported to be successful not only for psychogenic seizures (see Chapter 7) but also for seizures whose etiology is primarily organic. Crasilneck and Hall (1975) reviewed the literature concerning adults and concluded that "although the mechanism for such effect is not always clear, it may often be usefully conceptualized as a change in the balance of facilitating or inhibiting neural impulses" (pp. 205–206). They noted further that reported improvement of epilepsy after hypnotherapy "may involve some change in the excitability of the cortex around the epileptogenic focus, although experimental validation of this hypothesis is lacking" (p. 206).

Williams, Spiegel, and Mostofsky (1978) reported five case histories in which children and adolescents with chronic seizure disorders responded well to a combination of psychotherapy and hypnotherapy. They emphasized that uncontrolled seizures produce psychological trauma for any patient and that treatment that enables the patient and family to deal with this trauma more effectively might contribute to the breaking of a cycle of seizure-inducing psychophysiological activation.

We employed hypnotherapy with a patient who had nocturnal epilepsy that was unresponsive to conventional anticonvulsants. Although the patient had significant psychological problems and was being seen concurrently for psychotherapy, the fact that seizures occurred primarily during sleep suggests an organic basis for her epilepsy. We present the case in some detail in order to underscore the difficulty of understanding both etiology and treatment mechanisms.

Katie Q. was first referred for hypnotherapy as adjunct management of nocturnal seizures at age 15½ years. The patient had first developed seizurelike activity at age 12. She was hospitalized and found to have EEGs with abnormal foci in left anterior and frontal regions of the brain. She was placed on phenobarbital and Dilantin. During a subsequent hospitalization for seizure control, her EEG was found to be normal (a finding that does not rule out organic etiology) and medications were discontinued. Her "spells" continued, usually at night and rarely during the day. She would awaken with severe muscle spasms, lasting about 2 minutes, followed by the feeling of paralysis of all of her body except her left arm and head. She frequently urinated, and felt a loss of control. After many months' trial of anticonvulsants and psychiatric treatment, with little change in seizure control, the patient was referred for hypnotherapy.

Katie was seen six times for hypnotherapy. During the first session, efforts were initially made to determine her hobbies, interests, dislikes. She indicated a preference for rock and jazz music and enthusiasm about horseback riding, bicycle riding, and walks. The therapist went on to discuss sleep stages and how they are reflected in EEG patterns. Rapid eye movement and nonrapid eye movement sleep were discussed. Katie was told that it would be useful if her subconscious mind could give information to her about the stage during which the seizures were triggered (i.e., from medium to deep sleep or from light to medium sleep).

Hypnosis was achieved via eye fixation on one of many rings she had on her fingers. She then focused on breathing out and coordinating that with progressive relaxation. She was given the option of closing her eyes and visualizing numbers in sequence until she found a favorite place in her mind. She used a lifted finger to signal when she felt as though she were actually in a favorite place. She rapidly indicated she was there and was given the option of relaxing even more deeply by horseback or bicycle riding in an area of her choosing. She chose horseback riding. She was asked to ride until she was so relaxed that her body recognized she could identify the sleep phase in which her seizures occurred. Although she appeared very relaxed, she did not, over a 10-minute period, give any further finger signals. Recognizing possible resistance, it was suggested that she perhaps would need more practice before she was ready to obtain this information and that she should, nonetheless, program herself to turn off the trigger to the seizure as she was passing from one stage of sleep to another. She accepted this and, when out of trance, agreed that she would practice the exercise twice a day.

Two weeks later, Katie seemed eager to go into hypnosis. Induction was similar and once again she was asked to continue relaxing until she was ready to identify the sleep phase in which her seizures occurred. Repeatedly, her right and left thumbs raised slightly, and after 12 minutes the right pointer finger lifted. When asked if that was her "yes" finger, she again raised the right finger and signaled that the left pointer finger was "no." Further inquiry about sleep stages revealed no new information. The therapist reinforced the suggestion that, at an unconscious level, she had all the information she needed to control the seizures and that she could turn off the trigger as she passed from one sleep stage to another.

On the third visit, Katie seemed more relaxed than in any previous session and went through the initial induction without verbal cues. After 5 minutes, she raised her right index finger signaling that she was relaxed enough to program her autonomic nervous system to control body functions in a way that was good for her. The therapist said, "It's all right. If you wish to have pleasant dreams instead of seizures,—to enjoy those dreams, let those dreams be satisfying and pleasant. When you control the seizures, you will be a stronger and happier person. Sunshine always follows rain." Following this session, Katie was relaxed, good humored and said she thought the time was 5 minutes instead of the actual 25 minutes.

During the month before beginning hypnotherapy, Katie had 15 seizures. During the next month, there were only four seizures. Between the third and fourth sessions, Katie had two nocturnal seizures, possibly associated with anxiety concerning a planned 20-mile charity walk. At the fourth visit, the therapist added positive future imagery, asking Katie to imagine feelings of physical and emotional well-being at a future time when she was seizure-free. She was then asked if she would be willing to determine her seizure aura. She agreed and went rapidly into a trance with very few verbal cues. She indicated with an ideomotor signal when she was prepared to determine the aura. After 5 minutes she opened her eyes, said it was weird and she didn't enjoy the part when she was getting information about her aura. She said she felt as though both legs were moving rapidly up and down. She said in the fifth session that she did not want to pursue the aura. She was taught a jettison technique after focusing on a happy memory amplified with a clenched fist. On coming out of trance, she said she enjoyed this. Ability to jettison problems was reinforced in the sixth session. Subsequently she improved remarkably in school and home relationships. There were no further seizures over a 2-year follow-up.

Urine Retention

Williams and Singh (1976) reported positive response after a single session of hypnotherapy in the case of a 10½-year-old girl with psychogenic urinary retention. This followed a herpes zoster infection in her inguinal area and placement of a suprapubic cystostomy. Urinary infections followed, and life-threatening sepsis was a possibility in this patient with compromised immunological defenses. The psychiatrist noted that this patient had been traumatized and terrified by numerous bodily invasions that deprived her of autonomous control of body functions. While in a trance state he had her repeat the following statements out loud: (1) "When people are very scared and upset they stop making pee-pee," (2) "By relaxing, I can overcome my scared and upset feelings," and (3) "The sooner I can make pee-pee, the sooner they will take the tube out." The three points were written down on a card for the patient to review during self hypnosis. Within a few hours, after this single session, she began voiding.

Olness has often written reminder affirmation statements for children to use during self-hypnosis. This may be important especially in children who have stronger visual than auditory images. The following case history concerns an adolescent patient with acute neurological handicaps, including urinary retention, who developed his own creative imagery to overcome the problems.

Neal C., age 17, was admitted to the hospital for the sixth time in relapse with Hodgkin's disease, stage IV-B. He was referred for hypnotherapy to control severe back pain, headaches, and nausea. At the time of the initial hypnotherapy session, he was pleasant, interested but frequentlyly complaining of pain and anorexia. After some discussion about his interests, likes, dislikes, and habits, the therapist chose an induction method related to his interest in electronic circuitry. He imagined himself constructing a radio until he was ready to accept suggestions for relief of symptoms. At the first visit, he was given suggestions to recall a happy meal time and enjoy feelings of pleasant hunger. At the conclusion of the first hypnotherapy session, he volunteered that his headache was "almost gone," and he added, "strange, now I feel hungry." Chemotherapy was begun on the following day. Although the patient had expressed prior fears about vomiting, no nausea or vomiting occurred. When seen 2 weeks later in outpatient follow-up, he reported having had no nausea or vomiting throughout the recent course of treatment. He also volunteered that he used self-hypnosis to enable him to sleep easily each night. At that visit, hypnotherapeutic techniques reviewed included progressive relaxation, and imagery of computer construction. It was recommended that the patient read Norman Cousin's article in *The New England Journal of Medicine* (1976) concerning personal mastery in the face of chronic illness.

Neal did well for 9 months until he was admitted to the hospital with severe neurological symptoms including diplopia, loss of balance, absent gag reflex, and urinary retention. Consultants in neurology and oncology were unable to explain the symptoms. Results of EEG studies, computerized tomography (CT) scans, analysis of spinal fluid, and other laboratory studies were normal. Because of the patient's inability to care for himself after a week of hospitalization, plans were under way for nursing home placement. Happily, the patient dramatically improved. His dictated account, requested from him on the day following his recovery follows:

Early afternoon the doctors came into my room and said that unless I improved in the next 48 hours they would begin an experimental drug called ARA-C in order to remove or help restore my double vision, dizziness, bladder control, balance, and gag reflexes. ARA-C was an experimental drug and both of them agreed that it didn't provide much hope so that night I was going to try to program my own and restore all or release some of these reflexes.

The reflex that I missed most was stereo vision and if I was going to have one eye covered in order that I would not get these headaches and nausea and see double. That was the first one I concentrated on. At 7 P.M. that night, I virtually closed off my room to the public, had a dose of Tylenol and laid back, uncovered my left eye, and looked at the ceiling at a cat poster, which had been put there a day earlier. This cat was going to be my object and the focus for the next 12 hours while I concentrated on obtaining my vision without the headaches, nausea, and dizziness and try to regain control of my bladder.

The way I went about relaxing or restoring these functions was very simple. I simply lowered the head on the bed back to a comfortable position, opened both eyes and immediately I would see two cats spread apart approximately two feet and they were throbbing and coming in and out at me. This was confusing but with the Tylenol the headache was tolerable. I continued staring at the cat for a period of 10 to 15 minutes when I would have to shut both eyes in order to relax for awhile because I could feel the headache coming on and felt that if I pushed it too far to begin with the headache might become unbearable and I would give up. After resting my eyes for a period of 3 to 5 minutes, I would begin opening my eyes and again concentrate on the cat, trying to maintain a single image in my mind where there was two. I would think of a single cat, and sometimes the cats would be closer together and sometimes a little farther apart. To this method, I would go through over and over and whenever I needed a rest I'd shut both eyes in order that they both would get the same effect.

After 3 or 4 hours I began to notice that the cat was a bit closer and maybe not throbbing as much, which was encouraging, and I would rest and I would get my Tylenol in order to help relax and relieve the headaches. After about 6 to 8 hours, at about 3:30 in the morning, I could maintain a single cat without really trying very hard but the pulsating was still there and I fell asleep for about 2 hours. At 6:30 that morning, I again was staring at the cat; this time it was much easier to maintain a single image and the throbbing had virtually disappeared. The pain had subsided enough that the next day I did not take Tylenol at all and the doctors, because of this, postponed the ARA-C another 24 hours.

Also during the night that I was concentrating on my cat, I was concentrating on bladder control. I had not been able to control my bladder for about 7 days. I thought that was another function that I would be able to return to myself. The way I went about doing that was, as I concentrated on the cat, I concentrated on having my bladder turned off, as an on-and-off faucet, and the faucet was turned all the way off. I felt that if I could keep the faucet off for 12 hours and then turn it on and concentrate just on going on after 12 hours, the bladder would have to be full of enough liquids that no matter what, it would go. This method proved effective except that when I turned the on back it took about 10 minutes for the first stream to flow. Once again, the doctors thought this was encouraging, therefore, they would let the drug slip by for 1 more day.

I myself felt much happier and was in brighter spirits that day because I feel like I accomplished much more than I could have with the drug. All Saturday, with my stereo vision restored and not having to wear a patch and my partial bladder control restored, the main worry was having headaches and there was still the reflex or the gag reflex and more control of the bladder. I turned the bladder off in my mind and just concentrated that it was in the off position for a full 12 hours before I'd even try to go. This proved to be effective, as this time when I let my mind turn the bladder on, I went to the bathroom almost immediately. The gag reflex I had no idea about how to go about getting this small reflex back. I had something I would try and that was just to imagine that everytime I swallowed that swallowing is like a wave coming on an ocean, and this would go down my throat and when the wave would break it would hit my stomach. This I repeated over and over and over, and it seemed that that night that I was even able to swallow water. I just imagined a wave and that it would break on my stomach.

Sunday morning, I continued to show improvement in all areas, and I believe the doctors were much happier. One doctor was finally smiling and the other didn't come in. I had gotten control of most of my functions, more control, felt weak, unbalanced, unsteady with standing up, but this may be due to being in bed for a week straight. I was in much greater spirits and I feel that I can have a quicker recovery rate, and Sunday afternoon my NG tube was removed and I was able to swallow clear liquids on my own.

Unfortunately, I will begin chemotherapy in another hour. I am very nervous. I will try to use relaxation. I feel that I can give better answers if I were posed questions as I am a terrible dictator. I've been very brief and I have been unable to put into words exactly how, what, when, why, whatever happened.

Subsequently the patient underwent 5 days of chemotherapy without difficulty, and was discharged. Discharge diagnosis was (1) Hodgkin's disease, stage IV-B, in partial remission, and (2) acute brain syndrome, cause unknown. The patient remained in good health for 4 months. He then developed influenza complicated by pneumonia and died after 48 hours.

Cyclic Vomiting

We are unable to find any reports in the literature of hypnotherapy for cyclic vomiting. We have worked with two of these patients, both of whom achieved some degree of symptom relief through hypnotherapy. In each case, however, we referred the patient to medical subspecialists for further evaluation, and eventually organic explanations for the vomiting were found. This is a reminder, especially in difficult and uncertain areas, that one should be wary of the grab-bag diagnosis of "psychogenic."

Karen I., age 10, was referred for hypnotherapy after 60 hospitalizations for rehydration necessitated by cyclic vomiting. She had previously undergone extensive evaluations and 1 year of psychotherapy. Shortly before the onset of the vomiting, 3 years earlier, she had been frightened by a description of the movie, *The Exorcist*. Karen had been informed by one group of consultants that the symptom would resolve at the time of puberty and that there was no cure. In the initial hypnotherapy session, Karen was taught progressive relaxation and given general ego-strengthening suggestions. In subsequent sessions, she was given suggestions to counter nausea. Although she managed to abort her attacks when the therapist was present, she could not use self-hypnosis for this purpose, and the frequency of hospitalizations did not decrease. The therapist asked that she be evaluated by a pediatric neurologist and endocrinologist who, after 1 year of intricate testing, defined a urea cycle abnormality and found that the patient could eliminate the attacks by controlling her intake of protein. They later tested the hypnothesis by giving her a protein load and following the rise in her blood ammonia levels. Subsequently, she did well. Although self-hypnosis helped her symptomatically, while the cause was being elucidated, it did not substitute for a thorough evaluation.

Neurologically Mediated Intractable Reflexes

Both intractable hiccoughs and sneezing may be treated successfully with hypnotherapy. Patients may be taught progressive relaxation and given diagrams of the involved reflex with suggestions to control the switch between the brain and the reflex. Daily reinforcement through self-hypnosis is recommended.

Cerebral Palsy

Lazar (1977) described her treatment of a 12-year-old boy with athetoid cerebral palsy and mild mental retardation. After induction using imaginary television, treatment included observation of the self with relaxed and controlled hands, recall of previous relaxing experiences, suggestions designed to increase hand function, and focus on feelings about independence and anger. Sessions were reinforced with cassette tapes. While the boy reached only a light hypnotic state, he nonetheless achieved good results. His teachers noted improvement in his handwriting and in his ability to work in shop class. Lazar postulated that teaching such a patient self-hypnosis encourages independence and a sense of accomplishment, so important in handicapped patients. She suggested that hypnotherapy might be most effective with these children if begun at an early age when there is the best chance of minimizing secondary emotional problems and maximizing motivation for optimal motor functioning.

Secter and Gelberd (1964) also advocated hypnosis as a relaxant for patients with cerebral palsy. In a brief study of 12 cerebral-palsied children, they found that 8 responded to hypnotic induction; intelligence levels ranged from "subnormal" to normal.

The successful use of hypnotherapy in maximizing performance of athletes encourages its trial in any problem involving muscle function. Rehearsal of correct movements mentally is associated with measurable changes in catecholamine responses (Landsberg & Young, 1978). The adjunct use of hypnosis would seem reasonable in rehabilitation following injuries and muscle disuse.

Reflex Sympathetic Dystrophy

One of our colleagues (Lewenstein, 1981) shared with us the following case history; so far as we know, it is the first report of successful hypnotherapy with reflex sympathetic dystrophy.

A 15-year-old girl "felt something snap" in her right knee while standing still on a basketball court. Subsequently, she developed pain in her right lower leg distal to the knee and involving the entire lower leg. The pain was described as maximal behind her leg and on the right sole. The entire lower leg distal to the midthigh turned purple.

She obtained several medical consultations. Torn ligaments and/or thrombophlebitis were diagnosed. She was hospitalized and given anticoagulants. When x-rays and a venogram were normal, and she did not improve, she was transferred to another hospital for further evaluation and treatment.

On admission she was found to have a mottled, cool right leg from the midthigh down and was unable or unwilling to bear weight on the right leg because of intense pain. There was circumferential hyperesthesia with pain on light touch in the lower leg and an area of numbness over the right thigh. In spite of aggressive physical therapy with hydrotherapy, the patient did not improve. She was referred for hypnotherapy 2 weeks after admission.

During the first hypnotherapy session, she was asked to imagine a tree, with multiple branches, growing and blossoming in the spring sunlight. She was told that she could imagine the blood vessels in her legs as similar to the branches of the tree.

She was told that the nerves and blood vessels to her legs had been confused at the time she injured her knee and that she could correct this problem by focusing on the imagery of the healthy tree in her self-hypnosis practice. Since she recognized that she had injured her right arm a number of years ago and it had healed completely, it was likely that her right leg would also heal completely.

The patient noted subjective improvement by the following day and walked without crutches 2 days later. The patient was seen every 2 to 3 days for an additional 10 days and was encouraged to continue self-hypnosis practice. She was discharged to home and was doing well 5 months later.

Rehabilitation Following Central Nervous System Injury

Crasilneck and Hall (1970) reported the successful use of adjunctive hypnotherapy in the treatment of a 10-year-old boy who suffered cerebral contusion, concussion, and edema following a 15-foot fall. Three and one-half months after the fall, he was discharged to home in a fetal position, with a fixed stare, no evidence of recognition, and no speech. He was also incontinent. The mother then requested a trial of hypnotherapy. In the first session, the therapist told the patient that he could be helped if he could cooperate and then asked him to close his eyes. When the boy did not respond, the therapist gently closed his lids manually and gave him repeated suggestions that he could achieve deep hypnosis. When he was thought to be in trance, he was told that he could get well and that he could communicate by blinking his eyes, once for no and twice for yes. He immediately responded to questions with appropriate eye blinks. He was seen for hypnotherapy once weekly for 1 year. Each time, suggestions were made for return of essential functions. Gradually the patient improved, eventually developing normal speech, ability to walk assisted, and ability to read normally. The authors postulated that the therapist's attitude and persistence, combined with the structured hypnotherapy situation, led to a changed expectation for recovery by the family and facilitated positive motivation and behavior change in the boy. This case also points out the importance of speaking to noncommunicating patients as if they are hearing and as if response is expected.

PELVIC EXAMINATIONS IN ADOLESCENT FEMALES

Kohen (1980b) reported the successful use of hypnotherapy to aid adolescent girls through their first pelvic examinations. The anxiety of this event can be reduced by gentle, sensitive physicians. The use of hypnotherapy can foster a sense of competency and control in the teenager undergoing her first pelvic examination as well as reduction of anxiety prior to future similar examinations.

Prior to the pelvic examination, the physician should allow the patient time to acknowledge her concerns and express his or her willingness to help her be comfortable through the examination. It is explained to the patient that she can use her imagination to facilitate comfort. If she has previously stated that she enjoys skiing, for example, the physician suggests, "Go ahead and let yourself imagine that you're skiing" and continues to give suggestions for progressive relaxation. The physician must explain each part of the procedure as he or she also reinforces the suggestions of relaxation and comfort. A posthypnotic suggestion is given to relax even more easily and quickly during future pelvic examinations.

If patients have negative expectations based on uncomfortable previous examinations, the physician may ask, "Would it be okay if it doesn't bother you this time?" This question may represent the beginning of an indirect hypnotic induction, causing the patient to pause and reflect on the idea that there is a choice in this matter. It is important that the therapist understand how the patient believes things will be different or better because of hypnotherapy. The teenager must be reminded of her own skills and responsibility for success in achieving comfort and control. Time spent in adding hypnotherapy as an adjunct to pelvic examinations makes it possible to do better examinations more quickly, thus saving time in the long run.

SPORTS MEDICINE

Morgan (1980) reviewed potential applications of hypnosis in sports medicine research and practice. Appropriate uses of hypnosis in this area include management of excessive precompetition anxiety and analysis of factors involved in "slumps," long periods when athletes inexplicably perform well below previous levels. Athletes may become aware of errors in body movement that they do not recognize in their usual cognitive state. In some cases, hypnosis may properly be used to help an injured athlete perform, but the therapist must be keenly aware of the signal value of pain and must not put the athlete in a situation where he or she is likely to become further disabled. Facilitation of performance by hypnosis should be attempted only when such an approach is not contraindicated at a medical, physiological, or psychological level.

Morgan (1980) concluded that evidence for positive effects of hypnosis on muscle strength and endurance is equivocal, although negative hypnotic suggestions often result in performance decrement. These findings lead us to question the validity of the many popular books which state that imagery and relaxation exercises—possibly involving hypnosis—can enhance performance in individual sports such as tennis and skiing (e.g., Gallwey, 1974; Gallwey & Kriegel, 1977). Certainly, attempts to "psych up" an athlete to perform at record-breaking levels are not likely to be helpful and may be dangerous.

Morgan further reported that hypnotically suggested exercise alters cardiac rate, respiration rate, total ventilation, oxygen consumption, and cardiac output in the nonexercise state. Observed metabolic changes often approximate responses reported for actual exercise. The application of this finding to actual performance, however, is unclear.

Our clinical experience in using hypnotherapy for sports problems has been limited to its use for preperformance anxiety.

Jane P., age 11, was referred because she had severe anxiety for several days prior to solo ice-skating competition, and this was adversely affecting her performances. She had been skating since age 4 and had been in competition many times with no difficulty until 6 months prior to referral. After discussion of her interests, likes, and dislikes, she entered a hypnotic state easily by imagining herself reading a favorite story. She was taught ideomotor signals and asked if she would be willing to review past skating competitions. When she readily agreed, the therapist asked her to regress to a competition at age 8, age 9, and age 10. She had positive recollections of the earlier competitions but recalled an unpleasant comment from a peer at the competition after which her excessive anxiety began. While still in hypnosis, she was asked if she would be willing to get rid of this comment, which was still bothering her. When she agreed, she was given the option of sending the comment off in the distance via pony express, airplane, or train. She chose the pony express and let the horse gallop into the distance until she could no longer see it. Following this, she was asked to focus on the image of herself successfully completing the next competition, doing well, and feeling pleased with her performance and her control. She then practiced self-hypnosis once daily until the next competition. She was calm and happy thereafter, did well in her next public performance, and called the therapist to express her pleasure.

GENERAL RECOMMENDATIONS

In a paper on hypnotherapy with pediatric cancer patients, Olness (1981) made several recommendations to therapists who work in this area. Since these recommendations are applicable to many pediatric medical problems, we have adapted them here.

- Child health care professionals should be encouraged to learn and use self-hypnosis for themselves. Proper use of this modality can lead to reduction of personal stress, which is an inevitable factor in working with children who have medical problems. The heightened ego receptivity of the hypnotic state (Fromm, 1977) may also facilitate creativity in considering diagnostic issues and developing treatment plans. In some cases, health care professionals can participate in group sessions with patients and their families (e.g., groups for children with cancer or hemophilia). The shared experiences may be of benefit to all.

- Hypnotherapists must be willing to spend time with child patients, getting to know them as individuals and planning treatment accordingly. Standardized or "canned" approaches are likely to fail, given the fact that there is no such thing as a standardized or "canned" patient.

- When hypnotherapy may be appropriate for a medical problem, children should be exposed to this possibility soon after diagnosis. Progress is slower among children who have developed secondary emotional problems or who have well-established negative conditioned reflexes from months or years of accumulated fears of procedures and drugs.

- Hypnotherapy sessions should occur frequently during the first weeks of diagnosis, and children should be encouraged to practice on their own. Children with chronic illnesses should be invited to attend group practice sessions on a monthly or twice-monthly basis in order to avoid loss of hypnotic skills during long symptom-free or medication-free periods.

- Every hypnotherapy session should enhance the child's sense of mastery and should be conducted at the child's speed. Practice efforts of children should be facilitated, not forced.

- The effects of parental attitudes and mental health status on the evolution of childhood diseases must be considered carefully, and techniques must be developed to meet parental mental health needs. Parents and siblings can be encouraged to learn self-hypnosis and to participate in group sessions.

- For children who are discouraged or uncertain of their hypnotic skills, the use of thermal biofeedback—with its visual proof of control over physiological processes—should be considered as an adjunct.

CONCLUSIONS

Hypnotherapy is useful as a primary or adjunct tool in the management of a wide range of childhood medical problems. It is of particular value in the enhancement of mastery in children who have chronic diseases, especially if the focus is on early intervention and prevention.

For many medical problems, several different hypnotherapeutic approaches have been reported to be successful. Prospective studies are needed to determine which approaches are most successful and to assess the particular value of hypnotherapy in relation to other kinds of treatment. Long-term follow-up studies of children with hypnotic skills will allow us to note enhancement or waning of those skills as well as possible relationships to ability to cope with medical problems in adulthood.

REFERENCES

Abboud, F. M. Relaxation, autonomic control, and hypertension. *The New England Journal of Medicine*, 1976, *294*, 107–109.

Agle, D. Psychological factors in hemophilia: The concept of self care. *Annals of The New York Academy of Sciences*, 1975, *240*, 221–225.

Ambrose, G. Nervous control of sweating. *Lancet*, 1952, *1*, 926.

Apley, J. Psychosomatic aspects of gastrointestinal problems in children. *Clinics in Gastroenterology*, 1977, *6*, 311–320.

Aronoff, G. M., Aronoff, S., & Peck, L. W. Hypnotherapy in the treatment of bronchial asthma. *Annals of Allergy*, 1975, *34*, 356–362.

Barbour, J. Medigrams: Self hypnosis and asthma. *American Family Physician*, 1980, *21*, 173.

Benson, H. *The relaxation response*. New York: William Morrow, 1975.

Berger, H. G., Honig, P. J., & Liebman, R. Recurrent abdominal pain: Gaining control of the symptom. *American Journal of Diseases of Children*, 1977, *131*, 1340–1344.

Clawson, T. A., Jr., & Swade, R. H. The hypnotic control of blood flow and pain: The cure of warts and the potential for the use of hypnosis in the treatment of cancer. *The American Journal of Clinical Hypnosis*, 1975, *17*, 160–169.

Cioppa, F. J., & Thal, A. D. Hypnotherapy in a case of juvenile rheumatoid arthritis. *The American Journal of Clinical Hypnosis*, 1975, *18*, 105–110.

Collison, D. R. Which asthmatic patients should be treated by hypnotherapy? *Medical Journal of Australia*, 1975, *1*, 776–781.

Conners, C. K. Application of biofeedback to treatment of children. *Journal of the American Academy of Child Psychiatry*, 1979, *18*, 143–153.

Cousins, N. Anatomy of an illness (as perceived by the patient). *The New England Journal of Medicine*, 1976, *295*, 1458–1463.

Crasilneck, H. B., & Hall, J. A. The use of hypnosis in the rehabilitation of complicated vascular and post-traumatic neurological patients. *The International Journal of Clinical and Experimental Hypnosis*, 1970, *28*, 145–159.

Crasilneck, H. B., & Hall, J. A. *Clinical hypnosis: Principles and applications*. New York: Grune & Stratton, 1975.

Diamond, H. H. Hypnosis in children: The complete cure of forty cases of asthma. *The American Journal of Clinical Hypnosis*, 1959, *1*, 124–129.

Diego, R. V. Hypnosis in the treatment of the asthmatic child. *Bulletin of the Tulane Medical Society*, 1961, *20*, 307–313.

Dodge, J. A. Recurrent abdominal pain in children. *British Medical Journal*, 1976, *1*, 385–387.

Edel, J. W. Nosebleed controlled by hypnosis. *The American Journal of Clinicial Hypnosis*, 1959, *2*, 89–90.

Ehrlich, R. M. Diabetes mellitus in childhood. *The Pediatric Clinics of North America*, 1974, *21*, 871–884.

Feldman, G. M. The effect of biofeedback training on respiratory resistance of asthmatic children. *Psychosomatic Medicine*, 1976, *38*, 27–34.

Fromm, E. An ego-psychological theory of altered states of consciousness. *The International Journal of Clinical and Experimental Hypnosis*, 1977, *25*, 372–387.

Gallwey, W. T. *The inner game of tennis*. New York: Random House, 1974.

Gallwey, T., & Kriegel, B. *Inner skiing*. New York: Random House, 1977.

Good, R. A. Hypnosis and delayed hypersensitivity reactions. Personal communication, 1979.

Gustke, S. S. Alterations in *in vitro* coagulation during hypnosis in hemophiliacs. Paper presented at the annual meeting of the American Society of Clinical Hypnosis, Toronto, October, 1973.

Heimel, A. Use of hypnosis in pediatric clinical practice: A report of 68 patients. *Proceedings of the Northwestern Pediatric Society*, September 28, 1978. (Abstract)

Henderson, W. R., Shelhamer, J. H., Reingold, D. B., Smith, L. J., Evans, R., III, & Kaliner, M. Alpha-adrenergic hyper-responsiveness in asthma. *The New England Journal of Medicine*, 1979, *300*, 642–647.

Khan, A. U. Effectiveness of biofeedback and counter-conditioning in the treatment of bronchial asthma. *Journal of Psychosomatic Research*, 1977, *21*, 97–104.

Khan, A. U., Staerk, M., & Bonk, C. Hypnotic suggestibility compared with other methods of isolating emotionally-prone asthmatic children. *The American Journal of Clinical Hypnosis*, 1974, *17*, 50–53.

Kohen, D. P. Hypnotherapy in a child with asthma. Videotape presented at the annual meeting of the Ambulatory Pediatric Association, 1980.(a)

Kohen, D. P. Relaxation-mental imagery (hypnosis) and pelvic examinations in adolescents. *Journal of Behavioral and Developmental Pediatrics*, 1980, *1*, 180–186.(b)

Kohen, D. P., Olness, K., Colwell, S., & Heimel, A. Evaluation of hypnotherapy in 500 child behavior problems. Paper presented at the annual meeting of the American Society of Clinical Hypnosis, Minneapolis, November, 1980.

LaBaw, W. L. Autohypnosis in hemophilia. *Haematologia*, 1975, *9*, 103–110.

Landsberg, L., & Young, J. B. Fasting, feeding, and regulation of the sympathetic nervous system. *The New England Journal of Medicine*, 1978, *298*, 1295–1301.

Lazar, B. S. Hypnotic imagery as a tool in working with a cerebral palsied child. *The International Journal of Clinical and Experimental Hypnosis*, 1977, *25*, 78–87.

Lewenstein, L. N. Personal communication, January, 1981.

Luparello, T., Leist, N., Lourie, C. H., & Sweet, P. Interaction of psychologic stimuli and pharmacologic agents on airway reactivity in asthmatic subjects. *Psychosomatic Medicine*, 1970, *32*, 509–513.

Mirvish, I. Hypnotherapy for the child with chronic eczema: A case report. *South African Medical Journal*, 1978, *54*, 410–412.

Moore, C. Hypnotherapy with parents of asthmatic children. Paper presented at the annual meeting of the American Society of Clinical Hypnosis, Minneapolis, November, 1980.

Morgan, W. P. Hypnosis and sports medicine. In G. D. Burrows and L. Dennerstein (Eds.), *Handbook of hypnosis and psychosomatic medicine*. New York: Elsevier/North Holland Biomedical Press, 1980.

Olness, K. In-service hypnosis education in a children's hospital. *American Journal of Clinical Hypnosis*, 1977, *20*, 80–83.

Olness, K. Imagery (self-hypnosis) as adjunct therapy in childhood cancer: Clinical experience with 25 patients. *American Journal of Pediatric Hematology/Oncology*, 1981, *3*, 313–321.

Olness, K., & Agle, D. The enhancement of mastery in the person with hemophilia via relaxation-imagery exercises (self hypnosis) or biofeedback techniques. *The National Hemophilia Foundation*, in press.

Perloff, M. M., & Spiegelman, J. Hypnosis in the treatment of a child's allergy to dogs. *The American Journal of Clinical Hypnosis*, 1973, *15*, 269–272.

Reaney, J., Chang, P., & Olness, K. The use of relaxation and visual imagery in children with asthma. *Proceedings of the Ambulatory Pediatric Association*, 1978.

Scherr, M. S., & Crawford, P. L. Three-year evaluation of biofeedback techniques in the treatment of children with chronic asthma in a summer camp environment. *Annals of Allergy*, 1978, *41*, 288–292.

Secter, I. I., & Gelberd, M. B. Hypnosis as a relaxant for the cerebral palsied patient. *The American Journal of Clinical Hypnosis*, 1964, *6*, 364–365.

Smith, J. M., & Burns, C. L. C. The treatment of asthmatic children by hypnotic suggestion. *British Journal of Diseases of the Chest*, 1960, *54*, 78-81.

Snider, G. L. The treatment of asthma. *The New England Journal of Medicine*, 1978, *298*, 397–399.

Spevack, M., Vost, M., Maheux, V., & Bestercezy, A. Group passive relaxation exercises in asthma. *Pediatric News*, 1978, *12*, 14.

Surman, O. S., Gottlieb, S. K., & Hackett, T. P . Hypnotic treatment of a child with warts. *The American Journal of Clinical Hypnosis*, 1972, *15*, 12–14.

Tasini, M. F., & Hackett, T. P. Hypnosis in the treatment of warts in immunodeficient children. *The American Journal of Clinical Hypnosis*, 1977, *19*, 152–154.

Thomas, L. *The medusa and the snail*. New York: Viking Press, 1979.

Thorne, D. E., & Fisher, A. G. Hypnotically suggested asthma. *The International Journal of Clinical and Experimental Hypnosis*, 1978, *26*, 92–103.

Williams, D. T., & Singh, M. Hypnosis as a facilitating therapeutic adjunct in child psychiatry. *Journal of the American Academy of Child Psychiatry*, 1976, *15*, 326–342.

Williams, D. T., Spiegel, H., & Mostofsky, D. I. Neurogenic and hysterical seizures in children and adolescents. *American Journal of Psychiatry*, 1978, *135*, 82–86.

12

Hypnotherapy in Pediatric
Surgery

The use of hypnosis as the sole anesthetic in major surgery is quite rare, probably because of the relative safety and convenience of chemical anesthetics. Hypnosis has been used infrequently for this purpose with adults (Kroger & DeLee, 1957; Wangensteen, 1962; Winkelstein, 1959). We know of no similar published accounts with children.

Hypnotherapy is useful in pediatric surgery to facilitate emergency room procedures, preoperative comfort, induction of anesthesia, and postoperative comfort and cooperation. It is also used for a variety of minor surgical procedures in such areas as burn therapy and dentistry.

We know of no instances in which pediatric surgical patients have used hypnosis inappropriately to mask symptoms, such as pain, when awareness is necessary for prompt diagnosis and treatment, although we have heard fears to the contrary. We remind our patients to give themselves suggestions that are in the best interests of their body and good health in order to offset the possibility that the signal value of symptoms will be ignored. The following case history is an example of a child's ability to use judgment in applying hypnotic skills.

Joe T, age 10, came into the emergency room with severe periumbilical pain and a history of preceding nausea and vomiting. He also had a history of migraine headaches for which he had successfully learned to use self-hypnosis. While in the emergency room, awaiting

222

the surgery consultant, he was clearly uncomfortable. Nursing staff reassured him, saying he could probably have a medication for pain following the surgeon's visit. The surgeon made the diagnosis of appendicitis and scheduled the patient for surgery within the hour. When offered preoperative analgesics, the patient refused, saying, "It's going to be fixed, now I can turn off my switch." He visibly relaxed and was comfortable until induction of general anesthesia. Following surgery, the patient used self-hypnosis to counteract pain and nausea and to facilitate healing.

EMERGENCY SITUATIONS

Modifying Attitudes

If hypnotherapy is going to be successful during pediatric emergency room procedures, one must realize that children bring more to the situation than a laceration or fracture. They bring their own feelings, mixed in unknown ways with attitudes of parents, teachers, and others who have witnessed the current crisis or discussed previous crises with them. Kelly (1976) has pointed out that fear, pain, and guilt are characteristic of virtually every emergency situation. There is the fear of the process of the accident or problem and its outcome, fear of the unknown, and fear of losing control. Pain may include recall of past pain coupled with whatever the present sensation is and anticipation of future pain. Guilt may be real or conditioned by family or friends. In a study of children's emergency room visits, Alpert (1977) concluded that the majority had psychogenic antecedents, for example, a death in the family, a family quarrel, a move, or a serious illness in a parent. Emergency room staff should consider such possibilities, even though the reason for admission is, on the surface, an accident.

Successful hypnotherapy is also dependent on the attitudes of the emergency room staff. That is, if the staff expects a negative experience for all concerned, then negative suggestions will almost guarantee fulfillment of those expectations. For example, the use of a mummy or papoose board or other restraints conveys an expectation that the child is going to resist. Likewise, requiring parents to leave the scene of repair conveys an expectation that they cannot be of help to the child. When properly prepared, many parents can reinforce suggestions not only in the emergency room but later at home. Allowing them to observe the induction of hypnosis and the procedure may be relaxing, desensitizing, and a good learning experience for them.

There are exceptions, but most parents can be helpful in emergencies that involve children. Therapists gain more by expecting parents to be helpful and supportive than by expecting them to hamper procedures.

Modifying the Child's Experience

A hypnotherapist usually does not have much time to get to know a child who comes to the emergency room. The situation often precludes opportunities to explain hypnosis and to determine the value of several different induction techniques. However, these circumstances do not rule out the use of hypnosis or of hypnotic techniques without any formal induction. Precisely because of the emergency, children may be highly motivated to respond to positive suggestions.

Occasionally, direct or indirect hypnotic suggestions can be given before a child even reaches the emergency room. If a parent makes a preliminary telephone call, the doctor can suggest specific phrases that might be helpful. One of us (author Olness) found such techniques helpful when her daughter cut her forehead while being chased through the house by her sister. When the child felt the blood on her face, she started screaming. Her mother's first comment was "What beautiful, healthy red blood you have. Let's go into the bathroom to get a better look at it." The child immediately stopped screaming. As she left for the emergency room, she leaned out the car window and yelled at her sister, "And I have strong, healthy blood. Mama said so."

When the physician first greets the child in the emergency room, it is important to convey understanding of the situation and its attendant feelings. One might say, "It's scary to be in a new place like this and to have that cut. It's bleeding a lot and it might bleed some more." When the doctor acknowledges the child's reality, the child is more ready to believe other statements and follow other suggestions.

Erickson (1958) has pointed out the value of commenting on certain aspects of the child's reality in order to turn apparently negative behavior to advantage. For example, one can comment that a child's tears are beautiful or that loud yelling reveals very healthy lungs.

The child needs reassurance, but vague statements that everything is going to be all right are usually of little value. A clearer, more specific comment may allow the child to be more hopeful that the present situation will change. The doctor who says, "I wonder if it will stop bleeding in 1 minute or 2 or 4" not only suggests hope but also arouses curiosity that modifies anxiety and enhances cooperation.

Compare this approach with the negative implications of "I've got to try to stop this bleeding. Now you just have to be still."

After gaining rapport, the physician needs to explain what will happen to the child. Here again, current approaches are often at variance with successful use of hypnotic techniques. It is very common to hear people tell a child, "It is going to hurt." For two reasons, we believe that physicians may have become dishonest in their efforts to be honest with children. First, it is difficult to predict the extent to which a child will experience the sensory and suffering components of pain. Second, children—as much or more so than adults—can use various techniques to reduce pain, and so-called honest statements about feeling pain may limit the child's creativity by imposing negative expectations. At the same time, one should not tell a child, "It won't hurt," for such a remark can undermine credibility and trust, both now and in the future. Erickson (1958) found the middle ground with comments such as "Now this could hurt a lot, but I think maybe you can stop a lot of the hurt or maybe all of it." Or, one might say, "This might hurt some, but it just may not bother you very much. Some people say this feels like pressure, some like a kitty scratching, some like a baby chick pecking, some like buzzing. I wonder what it will feel like for you." Here the child's curiosity is again aroused, and willingness to cooperate is enhanced.

Some children benefit from distraction. Others, for whom cognitive mastery is a major coping mechanism, prefer to watch every detail of a procedure. The physician can ask whether the child wants to learn about how doctors treat injuries or prefers to engage in some other enjoyable activity. Either way, the child achieves dissociation from pain. For example, Gardner (1978) reported a case in which a 4-year-old chose to play with his cat and cheerfully described his play while the pediatrician placed four sutures in a thigh laceration without any anesthetic. In such cases, the physician might say, "Thank you for telling me what you would like to be doing. Go ahead and imagine you're doing it. I'll fix this while you're doing your favorite thing. You can help me by telling me what you're doing now." Many children readily accept these indirect suggestions for control and cooperation.

For the child who wants careful descriptions of the treatment, one can use relatively soothing words. Injection of local anesthetic is "a squeezing feeling." Antiseptic solution is "cool or cold." A fractured arm or leg is "like a block of wood." Burns can feel "more and more cool and comfortable." Children can be asked to time the procedure, to count stitches, to estimate blood loss, to hold bandages or instruments—generally to provide assistance in such a way as to enhance mastery, minimize anxiety, and indirectly reduce pain.

Distraction may be used in the context of cognitive mastery by asking the child to observe body parts that are not involved in the injury. For example, if the injury involves the left knee, the physician might also check the right knee carefully and say, "How does your right knee feel? Is it warm? Is there pressure here? Keep feeling that. I need to know if the feeling changes." Direct techniques for pain control, as described in Chapter 10, may also be used. It may also be helpful to include suggestions to stop bleeding (e.g., "It's bled enough. It would be okay to stop bleeding now"), to send "fighter cells" to take away germs, and to start healing immediately. Postprocedure suggestions should focus on ego strengthening, comfort, easy cooperation with future procedures (e.g., bandage changes, suture removal), and rapid healing.

Andolsek and Novik (1980) reported successful use of hypnotherapy for emergency treatment of two 3-year-old and two 4-year-old children. Procedures included suturing lacerations, treatment of a hematoma underneath a fingernail, and incision and drainage of a thumb abscess. Trance states were induced by encouraging the child to pick a topic of conversation and to focus on the most vivid sensory details of the chosen topic. Goals were to direct attention away from fear and to give the children a feeling of control over a potentially traumatic situation. Parents were encouraged to reinforce the positive suggestions. Following the procedures, the children and parents were encouraged to express their feelings about the experience.

PREOPERATIVE VISITS

When a child is admitted to the hospital for surgery, a hypnotherapist usually has time to get to know the patient and, it is hoped, to help coordinate attitudes and approaches of the family and the various hospital staff involved in the case. It is indeed unfortunate when a hypnotherapist helps a child develop positive attitudes toward surgery only to be sabotaged by the negative suggestions of someone else who may have had a previous unpleasant surgical experience. It is sometimes helpful to warn children of this possibility and to suggest that they can remember positive images even if someone else suggests something to the contrary. If possible, all members of the treatment team should focus on mastery, reinforcing the concept that the child can be an active participant in the treatment process.

In many hospitals, children are encouraged to see short movies or engage in puppet plays describing events that will occur before, during, and after surgery. A hypnotherapist may use imagery techniques to facilitate good adaptation through rehearsal in fantasy. Since hypnotherapy does not involve any standardized equipment, it may be especially useful in dealing with individual surgical problems and psychological needs. For example, amputation of a limb is one kind of experience following an accident and another kind of experience following discovery of a malignant tumor.

In general, hypnotherapeutic suggestions may focus on comfort and calm, easy return of normal body functions, and rapid healing. Since many children fear death as a result either of anesthesia or of surgery, imagery concerning the immediate and long-term future is important. A sample set of hypnotherapeutic suggestions follows:

You know the nurses who get food for you and fix your bed. You know the doctor who will do the operation. He is helping too. I'd like to teach you a way of helping us and helping you. You can help yourself get better faster and no one else can do that as well as you. You can learn how to help yourself faster than grownups can. . . . You have learned many ways to control your body. You know how to use your muscles to walk, to write, to eat, to ride a bicycle. Now you can ride a bicycle without thinking about how you do it. You taught yourself, so it became automatic. You keep many parts of your body running automatically. Your food enters blood and goes to all parts of your body. Your heart beats strongly to push that food around. You breathe in good pure oxygen which your body needs. You're doing it right now. You just keep all those automatic systems moving smoothly and easily, the same way you ride your bicycle or the same way you write your name. . . . You can do the same things after your operation. Your body can automatically remember nice hungry feelings and you can enjoy your favorite foods. What is the first thing you will want to eat? And your body can remember how to feel comfortable . . . how to move and walk . . . how to relax your bowel and bladder when you need to go to the bathroom . . . how to enjoy playing with toys and games. The doctors and nurses can help you as much as you need, and you can help yourself. Soon you will be well enough to go home. What is the first thing you want to do when you get home? Good. Think about that now.

Although the focus is on positive suggestions, we are careful not to suggest that the child must deny appropriate feelings of anxiety, depression, or anger. In the course of therapeutic interviews, we listen carefully for evidence of these feelings in conversation, play, hypnotic fantasy, and reports of dreams. Then we help the child recognize and integrate the feelings.

ANESTHESIA

It is well known that patients who approach surgery with a high degree of fear and agitation require larger amounts of chemical anesthesia, thus increasing the risks of complications. The postoperative course is also likely to be more difficult from both a surgical and a psychological standpoint.

As anesthesiologists have appreciated the significance of the preoperative psychological state in pediatric surgical patients, they have made efforts to allay fears of general anesthesia by use of such techniques as stroking, story telling, or rubbing a pleasant scent of strawberries, perfume, or bubble gum inside the inhalation mask. Although many anesthesiologists have had no formal training in hypnosis, they may use the analogy of a space trip, talking to the child about a space mask and about breathing special air like astronauts.

Since the 1950s, there have been several reports of use of hypnosis with children as an adjunct to chemical anesthesia (Antitch, 1967; Betcher, 1960; Cullen, 1958; Daniels, 1962; Marmer, 1959; Scott, 1969). These reports describe several advantages of hypnotherapy and of the resulting alliance between the child and the anesthesiologist. By becoming more active participants, children cope better with the psychological trauma of surgery. They adjust more easily to the hospital environment and formulate more positive attitudes about the hospital experience. Preoperative sedation can be reduced or omitted altogether; this is particularly valuable for children who respond to partial clouding of consciousness by becoming more agitated rather than less so. With the child in hypnosis, it is easier to induce general anesthesia, and it is often possible to reduce the amount given. Many anesthesiologists note a smoother course both during surgery and in the postoperative phase.

The techniques of hypnotic induction used by anesthesiologists vary with the age of the child. With infants and very young children, a soothing voice is sufficient even if the child does not understand the words (Cullen, 1958). Techniques reported for older children include story telling, television games, suggestions for eye heaviness and sleep, eye fixation, and progessive relaxation.

Some anesthesiologists give suggestions for postoperative comfort and return of normal body functions during the operative procedure. Simple suggestions may encourage the child to shift from negative to positive attitudes about the healing process. For example, one might say, "The sensations you have in the area of the incision are reminders that healing is taking place in that area." These suggestions may be aided if the child has, preoperatively, seen a drawing or diagram that explains the procedure. Some authors (e.g., Cheek, 1959) believe that anesthetized patients may hear comments in the operating room and respond accordingly to intended or unintended suggestions. Others (e.g., Trustman, Dubovsky & Titley, 1977) have found methodological flaws in studies on this topic and have questioned the validity of the conclusions. In any case, it seems reasonable to be guided by the dictum that operating room staff members should not say anything they don't want the patient to hear.

Bensen (1971) reported the use of postanesthetic hypnosis in surgical patients in the recovery room. This report included 30 children and adolescents posttonsillectomy and 1 11-year-old boy postcircumcision. Among 16 children, age 5 to 12, only 1 child needed pain medication during the first day posttonsillectomy. Of 14 older patients, age 12 to 18 years, 3 required one dose of analgesic prescription a few hours postoperatively. The author pointed out the need for a reliable and accurate laboratory method to assess and measure the effectiveness of posthypnotic suggestion.

It is unfortunate that anesthesiologists often do not continue their postoperative visits beyond the recovery room. A child can benefit from frequent reinforcement of positive suggestions following surgery. A cassette tape can be helpful in this regard as can reinforcement by well-trained nurses or parents (Olness, 1977).

Gaal, Goldsmith, and Needs (1980) reported a controlled pilot study of the effect of hypnotic suggestion on expressions of anxiety and pain in a group of 10 children, age 5 to 10, undergoing tonsillectomy. No child had previous experience with either hospitalization or surgery. Each child met with the experimenter before surgery, at which time the experimenter answered questions truthfully and engaged in pleasant conversation designed to put the child at ease. In the 10 minutes immediately prior to surgery, the experimenter continued in the same way with the control group, asking about interests, hobbies, favorite TV programs, and so on. For the experimental group, this 10-minute period was devoted to a hypnotic induction using television game/visual-imagery technique with suggestions for strenuous activity followed by fatigue, relaxation, and desire to sleep. After induction of anesthesia, the experimental group received tape-recorded suggestions for postoperative feelings of calm, comfort, ease of swallowing, and trust; the control group heard a tape-recorded nonsense story.

Assessment of anxiety and pain was made by independent observers who did not know to which group each child belonged. Anxiety was rated by behavioral indicators such as level of motor activity, tearfulness, verbalization of fear, and physical resistance. There were no differences between experimentals and controls prior to the preinduction conversation; both groups were relatively calm and cooperative. After surgery was completed, the control group was significantly more anxious ($p = .05$). The experimental group was as calm as at the first measure of anxiety. Postsurgical intergroup comparisons showed the controls to be significantly more anxious and uncooperative than the experimentals ($p = .01$).

Assessment of postoperative pain was based on the children's own reports and on their needs for chemical analgesics. Both measures showed significant differences between the two groups. That is, children in the experimental group complained less frequently and of less severe pain, and they required only one-fifth as much analgesic medication as the controls. The authors planned to extend the study to include 60 children.

As we review these reports, we are not certain whether it is best to utilize hypnotic suggestions with pediatric surgical patients before, during, or after surgery or at all these times. Further, one cannot be certain if the patient responds to deliberate positive suggestions or to the absence of negative suggestions such as "I'll bet this kid is going to vomit a lot." Controlled studies could clarify these issues.

BURNS

Children who are severely burned face multiple problems: pain, anxiety, depression, anorexia, insomnia, physical disability, itching, and cold. They also have to deal with significant changes in body image and with reactions from other people in the hospital and at home. These problems can interact in a vicious cycle of pain-anxiety-depression-anorexia-poor healing secondary to inadequate nutrition-more grafting-more pain.

Bernstein (1963, 1965) and LaBaw (1973) have published anecdotal reports describing successful use of hypnotherapy for several of these problems, especially pain, anxiety, and anorexia.

Wakeman and Kaplan (1978) reported a controlled prospective study in which patients, age 7 to 70, who learned hypnosis, as compared to controls who received supportive psychotherapy, used significantly lower percentages of maximum allowable analgesics. Among the patients who used hypnosis, the youngest group, age 7 to 18, used significantly less analgesics than did two adult groups, age 19 to 30 and 31 to 70. In addition to suggestions for pain control, these patients were also given suggestions for general ego strengthening, improved body image, and ability to cope effectively after discharge from the hospital.

In our work with burned patients, we prefer to begin hypnotherapy on the first day of admission, before the patient has been negatively sensitized to whirlpool therapy or debridements or is lethargic from narcotics. It is expecially true with burned patients that suggestions must be individualized and revised from day to day in order to keep pace with the child's changing condition. We explain our approach to other members of the burn team and encourage them to reinforce specific hypnotic suggestions. In addition to suggestions for symptom relief, we sometimes give suggestions that the child can use hypnotherapy to facilitate healing directly. As yet, there are no data to support this hypothesis, but we think it a reasonable one in light of other indications that children can successfully use hypnotherapy for treatment of dermatological problems (Mirvish, 1978; Tasini & Hackett, 1977) and that they can control their peripheral temperatures and, presumably, blood flow to extremities (Dikel & Olness, 1980).

The following case report is an example of our approach with burned patients. In this case, the problem was relatively circumscribed, namely pain and poor cooperation during whirlpool therapy.

Tammy S., age 4, was hospitalized with second-degree burns on her chest, sustained when a pot of coffee overturned on her at home. One week later, she was referred for hypnotherapy to control her discomfort during whirlpool therapy. She was a bright, active child who related well to hospital staff except at the moment of whirlpool baths.

Initially the hypnotherapist sat by Tammy's bed and looked at drawings she had made that morning. She explained the figures in the drawings, including a girl with a bandaged chest. That provided the entry for discussion of her burns. She seemed relieved when the therapist said her burns were getting better every day and wondered if she had decided what she would do first when she got home. Then the therapist said she knew Tammy didn't like whirlpool baths and she could teach her what to do so they wouldn't bother her. She added that she knew Tammy could learn easily and that she would need to practice her skills regularly. Leaving the decision to the child, the therapist played a game with her and then left with the comment that she would return when Tammy asked to learn these new skills. As she walked down the hospital corridor, Tammy came running after. "When will you teach me?" "Whenever you're ready." "Now."

In the office visit that immediately followed, trance was induced using eye fixation on a coin. Then the therapist explained about nerves, how they carry feelings of cold, wet, warm, burning, sticky, soft, and many other feelings to her head. She was then taught the switch off technique for pain control. She seemed very pleased at the conclusion of the session. When the therapist asked if she could go with Tammy for her whirlpool therapy the next day, the child agreed. She reviewed the hypnotic procedures and turned off the switch for her chest until the whirlpool therapy was over. In complete contrast to the previous day, she did not struggle, kick, scream, and cry. The nurse's notes said, "She tolerated the whirlpool therapy well." On the following day, Tammy said she didn't need the therapist to show her how to turn off her switches, and she did well. On the third day, she was discharged.

It is often inappropriate to use tape-recorded hypnotic suggestions for burned children in the early phases of treatment when problems are changing from day to day and even from hour to hour. However, a tape may be useful in the later stages of treatment when the child's condition is stable and problems are more predictable, at least for a few days at a time. The following material is a typescript of a tape recording made for one of our 11-year-old burned patients several years ago, when the therapist was going to be out of town for 4 days. Suggestions covered a variety of problems on which the child was then working. Wording was quite flexible since the child might use the tape at any time of day or night, with or without other patients present. We have made no changes from the original except to alter the child's name. If we were to make such a tape today, we would omit the word "try" in the suggestions, since this suggests the possibility of failure. The patient, however, reported no problems, saying she listened to the tape nine times during the therapist's absence and found it helpful in a variety of ways.

Hi Sherry. This is the tape recording that I told you I would make, and while you're getting ready to listen to it, try to get yourself in as comfortable a position as you can. Just fix your bed or wherever you are so that you are as comfortable as you can be. And then just as we have done before, think about the ways and the many many times we have helped you get more and more relaxed. That's what we are going to do on this tape. We are going to think about helping you relax more and more. And we are going to think about the many positive things, the many things you can do now that you couldn't do before. How much better you are now, than you were before, knowing that you are getting better and better. You are getting well.

So try to make yourself just as comfortable as you possibly can and just listen to my voice on this tape. You can put the earphone, the ear plugs in your ears if you like, or you can just listen without them, whichever feels more comfortable. And just try to imagine me there with you, imagine me sitting close to you. If you close your eyes and think very hard you can almost see a picture of me in your mind. You can hear my voice more and more clear, almost as if I were really there. And it will be almost as if I am there. Even though I am away for a little while, you know I am thinking of you. You know I still want you to get well. You know how very much I like you. You and I are pretty good friends. Sometimes we can get mad at each other, but we both know that's okay, and we can still be very good friends.

And now as you have this picture of me in your mind, more and more clear, just let your whole body begin to relax, listening to everything I say. First, think about your head relaxing and your face, beginning at the very top of your head, and your forehead relaxing, and your eyes feeling very relaxed and maybe a little heavy, and if you feel like closing your eyes, you can do that. And your whole face feeling very relaxed and very comfortable. And think of your neck feeling relaxed and comfortable; your neck is going to get well. You have had grafting on your neck and it is going to get better and better. So any worries you have about it, you can just let them go, knowing it's going to get better. And your shoulders can become more and more relaxed, and your arms and hands. Put your hands in a nice comfortable position. Your right hand and left hand. And think a minute about your hands, how much better they are, how much more you can do with your hands. Opening your mail, feeding yourself, making pizza in OT. So very many things—writing; and each day there will be more and more things you can do. More and more, so that your hands can feel very comfortable now and very relaxed, and you can feel more and more good. And let those very nice feelings go down and down deeper and deeper through your whole body. And down and down through your legs, and all the way down through your feet, knowing that your legs and your feet are getting better too.

All of you is getting well little by little. And I want you to think of that thought that you are getting better. And every time that thought begins to slip away from you, you can catch it with your mind and bring it back, bring it back. Just like we focus a camera, you can focus your mind on that idea. Focus that thought. You are getting better, more and more safe, more and more deeply relaxed, through your whole body now.

And we know that there are times when you have some pain or some itching somewhere. And we don't like that, but we know that it is going to happen from time to time. But we also know that more and more you can control the pain and the itching, because you can let the pain or itching, whenever it begins, be like a signal for you to relax deeper and deeper down and down until comfortable feelings fill you up more and more. And there is no room left for bad feelings or scary feelings, or painful feelings. Whenever there is any pain or itching it will be like a signal for you to focus and bring into your mind those nice relaxed feelings, immediately and completely until you are deeper and deeper relaxed, and comfortable feelings fill your whole body and your whole mind. And you know that more and more you can control any kind of feeling. Letting the scary feelings and the pain and the itching drift away, and letting the comfortable feelings fill you more and more. Fill you more and more with comfortable feelings, until there is no room left for any other kind of feelings.

And you know that this is getting to be more and more automatic; it happens without your even thinking about it. So that more and more you are able to sleep, you are able to sleep as much as you need to. And you may find that when it's time to go to sleep at night, you just let those relaxed and comfortable feelings, just come to you closer and closer. Filling you more and more, because you know you are getting better. So you will have a good night's sleep, when it's time to go to sleep. And just as you will be able to sleep as much as you need to, you will also have nice hungry feelings and enjoy the things you eat. And you will find that more and more you're interested in getting up and doing things. All the activities on the ward, you will like those activities more and more. Because you will be able to do them more and more. So you can sleep, you can eat, you can do all the activities, but most important, you can let yourself know you are getting better, because you deserve to get better. You're a good person, Sherry. You have worked very hard to get well.

And we will continue to work. When I see you, we will work more, as much as you need. And you will listen to this tape, Sherry, as much as you need to, as much as you want to. It will be just up to you how much you listen to it. But when you do, you may find more and more each time, that you can let yourself become very relaxed. Just as if I'm there talking to you. Feeling very safe, and very good. Knowing that if you need any medication for pain or itching, you can ask the nurses for it. But knowing that more and more you are getting to be able to control these problems yourself. And each time you listen to this tape, just as we practiced together, you will be more and more able to relax deeper and deeper. So that the pain and the itching and all the scary feelings will drift away and you will have comfortable feelings, more and more.

Now I am going to count up to five, and as I count, you can get just as awake as you would like to. If you want to, you can get very wide awake, and then you can do whatever would be good to do. Whether it's getting up, or eating or doing some activity, or just drifting off to sleep. Whatever would be good for you to do now, you can do. You can wake up as much as you like, as much as you need to as I count to five. So that if there are activities you want to do, or things like eating, or getting up, you'll be very wide awake. But if you want to go to sleep, you can be nice and relaxed, and drift off to sleep. Even if you wake up you can stay nice and relaxed but you'll be wide awake. I'm going to count now, and when I get up to five, you can turn off the tape recorder, by pushing where the little square is, and that will turn off the tape recorder. Now I am going to count, one . . . two . . . three . . . four . . . five . . . feeling very good, feeling very good, and I'll see you soon. Turn off the tape now.

Because burned patients have extensive practice in using hypnotherapeutic techniques, they often develop considerable confidence in their abilities. Betcher (1960) capitalized on this confidence in his work with a 10-year-old girl who had suffered third-degree burns and had used hypnosis successfully for dressing changes. Six months later, the child was readmitted for surgery in order to release severe flexion contractures of her neck which had forced the chin onto the sternum with complete inability to extend the head. Initially it was planned to do the operation under general anesthesia. However, the position of the child's head combined with the depressive effect of the chemical agent to compromise her respiration to such an extent that she rapidly became cyanotic. The surgery was cancelled and it was decided to reschedule it later using hypnosis as the major anesthetic agent until the contractures were released. Betcher (1960) gave the following account of the second surgical attempt:

Two weeks later the child was readmitted a few days before surgery. The patient and her parents were given an explanation of the method of anesthesia and since they were familiar with its use for the changing of the painful dressings during her first admission, they agreed readily. Two rehearsal sessions were performed on the days prior to surgery. Suggestions were given that her left arm was becoming numb. When the numbness was complete she was to place it across her neck for transference of the numbness. Complete analgesia to pinprick was achieved at each session. The operation was rehearsed step by step using a blunt instrument and demonstrating how the surgeon would do the procedure. No pre-medication was given to the patient. On the operative day, the patient was again hypnotized in her room and taken to the operating room. Afer the patient was placed on the operating table, the hypnosis was deepened. Numbness was achieved in her left hand and was transferred to her neck.

During the preparation by the surgeon, constant reassurances were given to reinforce the numbness in the region of the neck. Although analgesia to pinprick was complete, the patient began to whimper softly at the incision of the scalpel. The face had been covered by the sterile drapes since the operative area was from the mandible to the sternum. This draping was utilized to fashion a tent over the face and an anesthetic tube was placed in this area to allow the gases to flow over her face. The analgesia proved sufficient to allow the surgeon to proceed without any objection from the child. As soon as the neck was opened wide, the anesthetic mask was attached to the tubing and was applied to the face. Total chemical anesthesia was then produced. It was simple to introduce an endotracheal tube with the head now fully extended. The surgeon then completed the necessary surgery including skin grafting in two and a half hours. Only small increments of cyclopropane anesthesia were necessary for the smooth conduct of the anesthesia. Since posthypnotic suggestions had been given, the postoperative period was completely without discomfort even though the child was placed in a plaster of Paris shell from the head to the waist. [pp. 818–819]*

DENTISTRY

Bernick (1972) reported a variety of applications of hypnotherapy in children's dentistry including (1) raising the pain threshold, (2) reducing the resistance to local anesthesia, (3) assisting in the adaptation to orthodontic appliances, (4) reduction of the gag impulse during the taking of impressions or x-rays and during general operative dentistry, (5) relieving general apprehension, (6) breaking habit patterns for thumb sucking and myofunctional problems, (7) motivating the child and parents to accept treatment and to improve oral hygiene, (8)

---

*From "Hypnosis as an Adjunct in Anesthesiology" by A. M. Betcher, *New York State Journal of Medicine*, 1960, 60, 816–822. With permission.

relaxation of facial muscles, (9) control of saliva and capillary hemor-rhage, (10) maintenance of patient comfort in long procedures, and (11) as a premedication for general anesthesia.

Both Bernick (1972) and Shaw (1959) emphasized the importance of using nonhypnotic suggestion to help the child perceive the dental experience in a positive way. They suggest positive and pleasant communications from parents and dental office staff, getting to know the child's interests, allowing the child to experiment with various in-struments, modeling behavior, behavior shaping, and giving careful explanations at a level the child can understand.

Pediatric dental patients respond to a variety of hypnotic tech-niques to achieve pain control. Bernick (1972) used glove anesthesia with a 13-year-old boy who had developed a morbid fear of injections. This child used hypnosis as the sole anesthetic agent for several dental visits. In later visits, he used hypnosis to facilitate acceptance of injec-tions of local anesthetic for more extensive work. Shaw (1959) reported his use of the "switch technique" in which the child is asked in hyp-nosis to turn off pain switches to various parts of the mouth. He also described other methods, including glove anesthesia and direct sug-gestions for numbness. All these methods may be used with or with-out additional local anesthesia, depending on the child's needs.

Neiburger (1976, 1978) reviewed patient reactions to dental pro-phylaxis for 150 children, age 3 to 12, with and without waking sug-gestions that they would experience a tickling feeling and would want to laugh during the procedure. He found that the children were more cooperative when these "sensory confusion" suggestions were used than when no suggestions were given.

Hypnotherapy has been particularly helpful to control bleeding in hemophiliac patients who require dental work (Lucas, 1965). The mechanism by which bleeding is controlled is not yet understood, al-though Lucas emphasized the factor of emotional stress.

Crasilneck and Hall (1975) used hypnotherapy to help a 10-year-old boy overcome extreme apprehension about dentistry. Therapeutic procedures included abreaction of past dental trauma and posthyp-notic suggestions for feelings of relaxation and well-being during fu-ture dental work. The boy subsequently remained calm and coopera-tive during several visits for extensive dental work.

Thompson (1963) reported use of hypnotherapy with a 12-year-old girl who had an hysterical fear of dentistry. Suggestions focused on this child's ability to let go of fears that belonged to earlier experi-ences. Thompson heightened motivation for treatment with the "three crystal balls technique" in which the child was asked to imagine her teeth (1) in their present state, (2) in the future without dental correction, and (3) in the future with dental correction. She then focused on the third image. Although the child achieved only a light hypnotic state, she did become sufficiently cooperative for dental work to be accomplished.

OPHTHALMOLOGY

Browning et al. (1958) compared 9 children treated with hypnotherapy for suppression amblyopia with 10 who did not receive hypnotherapy. In hypnosis, the nine children were told that they would be able to see clearly with the amblyopic eye. Immediately following the hypnotherapy sessions, eight of the nine experimental subjects improved in near vision compared with only one of the control group who received "nonhypnotic persuasion techniques." Distance vision was unchanged in both groups. A few days following hypnotherapy, some of the experimental subjects regressed in near vision. This led the authors to question whether emotional factors might play a role in suppression amblyopia. At a 3-year follow-up (Smith et al., 1961), eight of the nine experimental subjects showed regression, although not always to the original prehypnotic level. A second hypnotherapy session produced improvement in near vision in six of these subjects, again suggesting a functional component in suppression amblyopia.

Look et al. (1965) published a case report of a girl who had undergone unsuccessful surgery for strabismus at age 22 months. In spite of orthoptic training for several years, at age 12 the patient had no binocular fusion. Hypnotherapy was then begun. Over the next 5 months her visual acuity without glasses became normal, and binocular fusion was developed. Orthoptic training and hypnotherapy continued regularly, and her gains were maintained over 3 years. This success suggests that long-term hypnotherapy is necessary to maintain gains as is generally true of all methods used to treat suppression amblyopia.

Williams and Singh (1976) reported used of hypnotherapy in an 8-year-old girl with hysterical amblyopia. Two hypnotherapy sessions over a 3-day period resulted in full visual restoration with no recurrence of symptoms in 14 months of follow-up.

Olness and Gardner (1978) reported the successful use of hypnotherapy to facilitate comfortable insertion of contact lenses in a 2-year-old boy. When this patient developed bilateral cataracts, he and his mother were faced with two surgical procedures, followed by having to adjust to contact lenses in addition to glasses. The patient's mother sought anticipatory hypnotherapy for herself and her son to allow them to cooperate with each other when she inserted the contact lenses. In two sessions of hypnotherapy, the mother and child learned imagery techniques in which they associated the contact lenses with feelings of quietness, gentleness, and mastery. The boy participated in the imagery exercise and, although he sometimes engaged in anticipatory fretting, he never had to be held down. His participation in this experience allowed him the opportunity to make a positive growth experience out of a potentially traumatic situation.

Lewenstein (1978) used hypnotherapy as the sole anesthetic with two children, age 6 and 11, for postoperative evaluation and adjustment of sutures placed in the extraocular muscles during strabismus operations. Accurate adjustment is possible only when the patient is fully alert and cooperative. In one child, measurement of ocular alignment in hypnosis revealed that no further adjustments were necessary after initial surgery. In the other child, examination aided by hypnosis revealed that the initial correction was inadequate; adjustment was made while the child remained in hypnosis, thus obviating the need for reoperation under general anesthesia.

NEUROSURGERY

In some neurosurgical procedures it is important to have the patient conscious and cooperative so that the surgeon can make decisions concerning ablative procedures. Crasilneck, McCranie, and Jenkins (1956) reported the use of hypnotherapy, combined only with local anesthesia in a 14-year-old girl who was having an epileptogenic focus removed from her cortex. The patient had two or three seizures daily, in spite of anticonvulsant medications, since a head injury which had occurred 4½ years earlier. She underwent four hypnotherapy sessions prior to surgery before undergoing a 9-hour neurosurgical procedure. She remained cooperative and was comfortable throughout except for mild pain while the dura was separated from bone. Of special interest is the fact that she awakened from trance twice when the hippocampal region was stimulated.

ORTHOPEDICS

Jones (1977) reported the use of hypnosis as an adjunct to the anesthetic protocol in 23 children, age 11 to 16, having the Harrington procedure for idiopathic scoliosis. This procedure necessitates the operative placement of one or two metal rods for correction of the spinal curve. A risk of paraplegia exists. If the patient can be awakened during the surgery to demonstrate voluntary motor ability, the surgical team can check for the complication of paralysis and achieve immediate decompression if necessary. Patients in this study were seen by the anesthesiologist on a daily basis for 1 week prior to surgery. Hypnosis was explained and induced several times. The sequence of events in the operating room was rehearsed in hypnosis, and the patients were also taught self-hypnosis for relief of postoperative symptoms, especially secondary muscle spasm. About 4 hours after the beginning of surgery, the anesthetic depth of chemical anesthesia was lightened to the point where the patients could blink their eyes on command. The patients were then asked to bend their toes and ankles. If they did so easily, they were reassured and reanesthetized. Postoperatively, the prearranged signals for relaxation were begun as soon as the patients began to awaken. A general decrease in the need for postoperative analgesics, increased cast tolerance, and decreased nausea were observed postoperatively.

Hypnotherapy can be useful both before application of splints and casts and during the recovery period for relief of muscle spasm and for preparation for cast removal and reestablishment of normal movement. It can also be useful in the postoperative period following amputation. Two representative case histories follow.

Mark C., an obese 8-year-old boy, suffered a fractured femur while playing football in a neighborhood lot. Following operative reduction, he was placed on oral codeine for treatment of the pain associated with quadriceps spasm. Three days later, he had developed nausea as a side effect from codeine, and his frequent vomiting episodes necessitated complicated bed changes (he was in traction) and more discomfort. He had also developed constipation as a side effect of the codeine, and defecation in his bed-ridden position became exceedingly difficult. At this point, he was referred for hypnotherapy.

We asked him if he would be willing to make himself feel better without the medicine and he agreed immediately. When asked what he would like to be doing rather than being in the hospital bed, he said he would like to be riding a bicycle down a hill. We asked him to imagine himself doing that, and he quickly entered a trance. We taught him the concept of nerves and central switches and encouraged him to find his own switches and turn them off for the area of the femur. We also gave suggestions for rapid healing and restoration of normal body functions. These suggestions were reinforced daily for 1 week. He had no further complaints, no further requirement for codeine, and was very pleased with his personal success. Following discharge, we asked him to practice visualizing normal leg motion in walking and running in preparation for removal of his cast. Rehabilitation was accomplished rapidly and the patient again was pleased with his participation in therapy.

Nancy S., age 11, developed pain in her right leg. Bone biopsy revealed a Ewing's sarcoma and amputation above the knee was performed. She was first seen by the hypnotherapist in the recovery room where suggestions were given for comfort and normal sensations of hunger. Following return to her room, she experienced no vomiting and requested only oral medication for pain. On the first postoperative day, she was somewhat depressed. She asked to be hypnotized before attempting to move from her bed to a chair. She said she wanted to imagine taking a nap at home. After the therapist assisted her with this imagery, she moved to the chair and then back to bed with only minimal discomfort. The next morning, she was markedly depressed and expressed fear of pain during a physical therapy session scheduled later in the day. She consented to using hypnotic imagery to facilitate ambulation, but involved herself only half-heartedly. In physical therapy, she was markedly anxious and cooperated poorly. However, the therapist continued to give informal suggestions for easy return of ambulation. The third day she was in better spirits and stood up with the aid of parallel bars. The staff gave much praise for each bit of improvement. By the fifth postoperative day, she was walking easily with crutches, clearly proud of her independence. The surgery and physical therapy staffs were very impressed with her progress. She was discharged 2 days later. This patient demonstrates the fact that significant depression and anxiety may interfere with optimal response to hypnotherapy but that, nonetheless, hypnotic suggestions may have a positive delayed effect, especially if other staff members approach the patient positively.

OTOLARYNGOLOGY

There are few reports of specific applications of hypnotherapy to otolaryngological problems in children. Edel (1959) reported the case of a severe nosebleed controlled by hypnosis (see Chapter 11), and Bensen (1971) has noted the successful use of hypnotherapy in children and adolescents following tonsillectomy. The following reports describe successful hypnotherapy to overcome otolaryngological problems.

Susan, age 10, had been unable to swallow solid foods for 6 months. She had lost approximately five pounds. The parents and patient recognized that the problem began when the patient witnessed her grandmother choke at the dinner table. The grandmother had no untoward sequelae, but the child was frightened of swallowing solids thereafter. Results of otolaryngological evaluation were normal. We told Susan that she could learn a method to solve the problem herself if she wished. Trance was achieved via the coin induction method and the patient appeared very comfortable while focusing on a favorite place where she could enjoy being happy, comfortable, and safe. We taught her ideomotor signals, and she was asked, while still in trance, if she would like to solve her problem of eating. When her response was immediately positive, we proceeded to ask her to recall a happy meal prior to the frightening event, to remember her favorite foods, how good they tasted, how easy it was to swallow them. When the patient seemed comfortable with this, we suggested she imagine the same menu in a future meal, enjoying eating, tasting, swallowing, knowing she was in control of swallowing, and that she had solved the problem herself. General suggestions were given for relaxation, feeling better than before, and finding it easy to review the exercise at home. The patient went home and ate her first complete dinner in 6 months without difficulty. One-year follow-up revealed no recurrences.

Charlie Y., age 24 months, had a history of chronic ear infections. During many ENT visits, he had been restrained on a mummy board for examination and treatment. Hypnotherapy was requested when his anxiety increased to the point that he began crying as soon as he walked through the clinic door. He was seen for three hypnotherapy sessions during which suggestions for comfort and ease were given as he played with toys and participated in mock ear examinations, alternately taking the role of doctor and patient. Clinic staff agreed to discontinue use of the mummy board. At the end of 3 weeks, his anxiety was markedly reduced and he cooperated easily with subsequent ear examinations. This little boy's mother was a nurse who prompted the referral by insisting that "there had to be a better way." Many parents are not as assertive. We hope to see surgical staff members make increasing use of techniques that minimize anxiety in their young patients. We also hope to see decreasing use of such methods as mummy boards, which are bound to increase anxiety.

UROLOGY

Hinman and Baumann (1976) have reported the use of suggestion and hypnotherapy in seven of eight boys with complications after corrective surgical procedures for dysfunction of the voiding mechanism. Four of these patients improved. It was pointed out that operation or reoperation in five of these children might have been unnecessary if bladder coordination had been established earlier.

These patients had been referred to the urologist because of incontinence, recurrent infections of the urinary tract, or both. Two children had posterior urethral valves, one had an imperforate anus, three had bilateral reflux without demonstrable anatomical abnormality in the lower tract, and two had large bladders with upper tract changes. All patients were diagnosed as having voiding incoordination on a psychological basis. The authors pointed out the hazards of complex urological procedures, such as reimplantation of ureters, if the problem of bladder incoordination is not solved. In the case of these patients, hypnotherapy was associated with achievement of bladder coordination as demonstrated by urodynamic assessment.

CONCLUSIONS

Hypnotherapy can be a useful adjunct in many surgical situations and can often be used as the sole anesthetic for minor surgical procedures. Children who use hypnotherapy successfully can be more cooperative with surgical care, and may experience fewer complications and more rapid recovery.

REFERENCES

Alpert, J. J. Accidental stresses: Stressful accidents. *Pediatric Audio Digest Foundation,* 1975, *21*(2). (Tape)

Andolsek, K., & Novik, B. Procedures in family practice: Use of hypnosis with children. *The Journal of Family Practice,* 1980, *10,* 503–507.

Antitch, J. L. S. The use of hypnosis in pediatric anesthesia. *Journal of the American Society of Psychosomatic Dentistry and Medicine,* 1967, *14,* 70–75.

Bensen,V. B. One hundred cases of post-anesthetic suggestion in the recovery room. *The American Journal of Clinical Hypnosis,* 1971, *14,* 9–15.

Bernick, S. M. Relaxation, suggestion, and hypnosis in dentistry: What the pediatrician should know about children's dentistry. *Clinical Pediatrics,* 1972, *11,* 72–75.

Bernstein, N. R. Management of burned children with the aid of hypnosis. *Journal of Child Psychology and Psychiatry,* 1963, *4,* 93–98.

Bernstein, N. R. Observations on the use of hypnosis with burned children on a pediatric ward. *The International Journal of Clinical and Experimental Hypnosis,* 1965, *13,* 1–10.

Betcher, A. M. Hypnosis as an adjunct in anesthesiology. *New York State Journal of Medicine,* 1960, *60,* 816–822.

Browning, C. W., Quinn, L. H., & Crasilneck, H. B. The use of hypnosis in suppressing amblyopia of children. *The American Journal of Ophthalmology,* 1958, *46,* 53–67.

Cheek, D. B. Unconscious perception of meaningful sounds during surgical anesthesia as revealed under hypnosis. *The American Journal of Clinical Hypnosis,* 1959, *1,* 101–113.

Crasilneck, H. B., & Hall, J. A. *Clinical hypnosis: Principles and applications.* New York: Grune & Stratton, 1975.

Crasilneck, H. B., McCranie, E. J., & Jenkins, M. T. Special indications for hypnosis as a method of anesthesia. *Journal of the American Medical Association,* 1956, *162,* 1606–1608.

Cullen, S. C. Current comment and case reports: Hypno-induction techniques in pediatric anesthesia. *Anesthesiology,* 1958, *19,* 279–281.

Daniels, E. The hypnotic approach in anesthesia for children. *The American Journal of Clinical Hypnosis,* 1962, *4,* 244–248.

Dikel, W., & Olness, K. Self-hypnosis, biofeedback, and voluntary peripheral temperature control in children. *Pediatrics,* 1980, *66,* 335–340.

Edel, J. W. Nosebleed controlled by hypnosis. *The American Journal of Clinical Hypnosis,* 1959, *2,* 89–90.

Erickson, M. H. Pediatric hypnotherapy. *The American Journal of Clinical Hypnosis,* 1958, *1,* 25–29.

Gaal, J. M., Goldsmith, L., & Needs, R. E. The use of hypnosis, as an adjunct to anesthesia, to reduce pre- and post-operative anxiety in children. Paper presented at the annual meeting of the American Society of Clinical Hypnosis, Minneapolis, November 1980.

Gardner, G. G. The use of hypnotherapy in a pediatric setting. In E. Gellert (Ed.), *Psychosocial aspects of pediatric care.* New York: Grune & Stratton, 1978.

Hinman, F., Jr., & Baumann, F. W. Complications of vesicoureteral operations from incoordination of micturition. *The Journal of Urology,* 1976, *116,* 638–643.

Jones, C. W. Hypnosis and spinal fusion by Harrington instrumentation. *The American Journal of Clinical Hypnosis,* 1977, *19,* 155–157.

Kelly, L. J. Hypnosis and children in the emergency department. Paper presented at the annual meeting of the American Society of Clinical Hypnosis, Chicago, October, 1976.

Kroger, W. S., & DeLee, S. T. Use of hypnoanesthesia for caesarean section and hysterectomy. *Journal of the American Medical Association,* 1957, *163,* 442–444.

LaBaw, W. L. Adjunctive trance therapy with severely burned children. *International Journal of Child Psychotherapy,* 1973, *2,* 80–92.

Lewenstein, L. N. Hypnosis as an anesthetic in pediatric ophthalmology. *Anesthesiology,* 1978, *49,* 144–145.

Look, Y. K., Choy, D. C., & Kelly, J. M., Jr. Hypnotherapy in strabismus. *The American Journal of Clinical Hypnosis,* 1965, *7,* 335–341.

Lucas, O. N. Dental extractions in the hemophiliac: Control of the emotional factors by hypnosis. *The American Journal of Clinical Hypnosis,* 1965, *7,* 301–307.

Marmer, M. J. Hypnosis as an adjunct to anesthesia in children. *AMA Journal of Diseases of Children,* 1959, *97,* 314–317.

Mirvish, I. Hypnotherapy for the child with chronic eczema: A case report. *South African Medical Journal,* 1978, *54,* 410–412.

Neiburger, E. J. Waking hypnosis through sensory confusion: 302 cases of dental prophylaxis. *Journal of the American Society of Psychosomatic Dentistry and Medicine,* 1976, *23,* 88–98.

Neiburger, E. J. Child response to suggestion: Study of age, sex, time, and income levels during dental care. *Journal of Dentistry for Children,* 1978, *45,* 396–402.

Olness, K. In-service hypnosis education in a children's hospital. *The American Journal of Clinical Hypnosis,* 1977, *20,* 80–83.

Olness, K., & Gardner, G. G. Some guidelines for uses of hypnotherapy in pediatrics. *Pediatrics*, 1978, *62*, 228–233.

Scott, D. L. Hypnosis as an aid to anesthesia in children. *Anesthesia*, 1969, *24*, 643–644.

Shaw, S. I. A survey of the management of children in hypnodontia. *The American Journal of Clinical Hypnosis*, 1959, *1*, 155–162.

Smith, G. G., Crasilneck, H. B., & Browning, C. W. A follow-up study of suppression amblyopia in children previously subjected to hypnotherapy. *The American Journal of Ophthalmology*, 1961, *52*, 690–693.

Tasini, M. F., & Hackett, T. P. Hypnosis in the treatment of warts in immunodeficient children. *The American Journal of Clinical Hypnosis*, 1977, *19*, 152–154.

Thompson, K. F. A rationale for suggestion in dentistry. *The American Journal of Clinical Hypnosis*, 1963, *5*, 181–186.

Trustman, R., Dubovsky, S., & Titley, R. Auditory perception during general anesthesia —Myth or fact? *The International Journal of Clinical and Experimental Hypnosis*, 1977, *25*, 88–105.

Wakeman, R. J., & Kaplan, J. Z. An experimental study of hypnosis in painful burns. *The American Journal of Clinical Hypnosis*, 1978, *21*, 3–12.

Wangensteen, O. H. New operative techniques in intestinal obstructions. *Wisconsin Medical Journal*, 1962, *62*, 159–169.

Williams, D. T., & Singh, M. Hypnosis as a facilitating therapeutic adjunct in child psychiatry. *Journal of the American Academy of Child Psychiatry*, 1976, *15*, 326–342.

Winkelstein, L. B., & Levinson, J. Fulminating pre-eclampsia with caesarean section performed under hypnosis. *American Journal of Obstetrics and Gynecology*, 1959, *78*, 420–423.

13

Hypnotherapy with the
Terminally Ill Child

Reports of hypnotherapy with terminally ill patients have focused on three areas (1) modification of pain, anxiety, and other symptoms and by-products of the disease and its treatment; (2) modification of the disease process itself; and (3) modification of the patient's ability to respond with mastery in the dying process.

We will review published reports and our own clinical experience with children in all these areas. Then, to illustrate the ways in which hypnotherapy can facilitate mastery, integration, and even creativity in the dying child and his family, we reprint portions of the previously published report of David, a 12-year-old boy who died of leukemia on Christmas day (Gardner, 1976).*

THE USES OF HYPNOTHERAPY WITH DYING CHILDREN

It is virtually impossible to be certain that hypnotherapy per se is the source of positive clinical results. However, especially in cases of dying children, it has often been demonstrated that ordinary forms of

---

*While many of our examples concern children who die of leukemia, it is important to remember that about 50 percent of children with leukemia now achieve full recovery from their disease. The outlook for childhood leukemia has improved considerably since 1960.

reassurance and counseling, medications, and other traditional therapies have failed. Therefore, even in the complete absence of controlled
studies, and usually in the absence of any formal measures of ability
to enter the hypnotic state, we are inclined to believe that hypnotherapy is indeed valuable for many who suffer terminal illness.

Modification of Symptoms and By-Products of the Disease and Treatment

Reports from several centers agree that hypnotherapy can be valuable—sometimes in dramatic ways—for a vast array of physical and
psychological problems that arise in children with terminal illness.

Crasilneck and Hall (1973, 1975) described their work with two
boys, 4 and 8 years old, one with inoperable brain cancer and the
other with leukemia. The specific problems treated included severe
pain, poor tolerance of medical procedures, generalized anxiety, fear
of dying, depression, insomnia, anorexia, and behavioral difficulties.
Each of the boys went into deep hypnosis and responded very well to
direct suggestions for symptom relief after one session. The younger
boy was seen daily the first month, then three times weekly until his
death in the first week of the third month of hypnotherapy. The older
child achieved rapid remission of his leukemia and was to be seen
when necessary for further hypnotherapy. At the time of the report,
this boy was successfully using self-hypnosis for therapeutic procedures.

Anecdotal reports of this kind are now common, as hypnotherapy
becomes widely used with children who have cancer. Recently, three
research studies have reported results for a series of patients, both
adding to our understanding and bringing out some of the complex
issues not yet understood in the area of symptom relief.

LaBaw and his colleagues (1975) utilized adjunctive hypnotherapy, in both group and individual sessions, with 27 pediatric cancer
patients, age 4 to 20 years. In addition to the specific problems treated
by Crasilneck and Hall (1975), this study reported successful modification of nosebleeds and of vomiting associated with chemotherapy.
The results were presented in the form of brief clinical vignettes for 12
of the children, said to be representative of the group as a whole.
Based on these 12 descriptions, we have classified the response to
hypnotherapy as follows—none or minimal: 3; moderate: 3; good: 6.
The authors did not draw conclusions as to which types of symptoms
were most amenable to treatment. In this small group of 12, successful
response to hypnotherapy did not appear to be clearly related to age or
sex, though there was a tendency for girls to respond better than boys
(Table 13-1).

Table 13-1
Response to Hypnotherapy by Sex and Age

Age (years)	Minimal		Moderate		Good	
	M	F	M	F	M	F
5–6	1	–	1	–	–	–
7–8	–	–	–	–	2	–
9–10	1	–	1	1	–	1
11–12	–	–	–	–	–	–
13–14	1	–	–	–	1	–
15–18	–	–	–	–	–	–
19–20	–	–	–	–	–	2
Total	3	0	2	1	3	3

Adapted from LaBaw et al., 1975.

The authors noted that reasons for difficulty in using hypnosis and/or self-hypnosis included excessive dependency needs, extreme anxiety or pain, defensive passivity, and lack of parental support.

J. R. Hilgard and Morgan (1978) reported their use of hypnotherapy for modification of specific problems—chiefly pain and anxiety—in 34 pediatric cancer patients, age 4 to 19 years. Seven other children were offered hypnotherapy but refused this treatment modality. The children's ability to use hypnotherapy for symptom relief was associated with age, score on the Stanford Hypnotic Clinical Scale (SHCS), anxiety level, and the nature of the problem. The data are summarized in Table 13-2.

Olness (1981) taught self-hypnosis for symptom relief to 21 pediatric cancer patients from a group of 25 consecutive referrals; 3 children and 1 set of parents refused this treatment modality. The age range at referral was 3 to 18 years. Symptom relief was defined as a reduction in pain associated with procedures, such as intravenous injections, spinal taps, and bone marrow aspirates, and/or a reduction in anorexia, nausea, or vomiting associated with radiation or chemotherapy. Specific indicators of improvement included reduction in analgesic or antinausea medication.

Of the 21 patients taught self-hypnosis, 12 were referred at the time of initial diagnosis. These 12 all demonstrated substantial symptom relief. Of the nine patients first trained during relapse, seven demonstrated substantial symptom relief. Of the other two, a 3-year-old had only one practice session, and a 4-year-old was referred on the day of his death. Children who practiced most regularly obtained the most consistent relief. Benefits accrued about equally to both younger (5 to 11) and older (12 to 18) children, but the younger chil-

Table 13-2
Response to Hypnotherapy for 34 Pediatric Cancer Patients

| Problem | Age Range (years) | No. of Patients | Degree of Symptom Relief* | |
			Poor or Partial	Substantial or Excellent
Ancillary symptoms†	14–19	10	2(2)	8(2)
Poor tolerance of short procedures‡	9–16	5	1	4
Continuous pain	13–19	3	3(1)	0
Poor tolerance of bone marrow aspirates	4–6	10	10(several)	0
or lumbar punctures§¶	7–13	6	2	4
Totals		34	18	16

Adapted from J. R. Hilgard and Morgan, 1978.

*The numbers in parentheses refer to the number in each group obtaining a low score on the Stanford Hypnotic Clinical Scale. For these subjects, significant symptom relief cannot be attributed to the use of hypnosis and is probably related to anxiety reduction by other means.

†Includes diffuse anxiety reactions, depression, insomnia, nausea, high blood pressure.

‡Includes intravenous injections and bandage changes; does not include bone marrow aspirates and lumbar punctures.

§Data grouped separately for younger and older children.

¶Children in this group manifested the most severe anxiety.

dren achieved symptom control more quickly, in an average of two sessions as compared to four sessions for the older children.

It is difficult to make meaningful comparison of these three studies. In the first two, about half the patients achieved significant symptom relief following hypnotherapy; in Olness's study the success rate was 90 percent. In the LaBaw, et al. study, girls seemed to fare better than boys; the other two studies did not report sex differences. J. R. Hilgard and Morgan found that children 4 to 6 years old responded poorly as compared to older children; Olness found no such difference. J. R. Hilgard and Morgan noted that the younger children had the most severe anxiety about major medical procedures, a finding similar to that of Katz, Kellerman, and Siegel (1980). It is not clear whether Olness treated anxiety in her young patients differently or whether they were less anxious. J. R. Hilgard and Morgan found different success rates according to the nature of the problem; Olness's report does not permit this kind of comparison. Olness stressed the value of regular practice and early referral; the other studies did not comment on these issues. In two studies, the patients were trained from the beginning to use self-hypnotic techniques; J. R. Hilgard and Morgan encouraged self-hypnosis but apparently not to the same extent. Only J. R. Hilgard and Morgan used any formal measure of ability to achieve hypnosis and found two patients whose low scores on the SHCS suggested that their symptom improvement was due to factors other than hypnosis; we do not know how many similar cases were included in the other studies.

In all three studies, we do not know whether or how the results are related to the fact that the patients all suffered from cancer. Would the results be different for children suffering chronic illnesses that are not life-threatening? Or are these data representative of pediatric patients as a whole? In short, we are unable to explain the available data in any truly satisfactory way. Now that three independent studies have demonstrated the possibility of moving from anecdotal reports to studies including a series of patients, we urge researchers to move a step further to controlled clinical trials in which identical research protocols are used simultaneously at several medical centers.

Modification of Disease Process

The idea that physiological and psychological processes are intertwined goes back many centuries. More recently, there have been reports of the association of psychological factors with a variety of children's diseases, including cancer (Greene & Miller, 1958, Jacobs & Charles, 1980). Since these are retrospective studies, the data are very difficult to interpret. For example, Jacobs and Charles (1980) emphasized that their review of life stress events for children with cancer and with other illnesses must be interpreted only as contextual and not as causal. They also noted that a given event, such as parental divorce or change of residence might be very stressful for one child while having little impact on another. Other important variables cited included the availability of social supports and the child's habitual coping skills. None of these factors has been adequately studied.

While we agree with the Jacobs and Charles (1980) conclusion that the role of psychological factors as antecedents of childhood cancer remains a matter of conjecture, we also agree with their conclusion that there is a strong possibility that childhood cancer is a psychobiological phenomenon.

If psychological factors play a role in the development of cancer, then it is conceivable that psychological treatment might also affect the course and ultimate outcome of the disease. Recently, there has been a great deal of interest, especially in the press, in the possibility of using certain imagery techniques—which we would put in the gen-

eral category of self-hypnosis—to affect the course of potentially terminal disease, especially cancer. Basically, the technique consists of
asking a patient to visualize some process in which cancer cells are
destroyed and to focus on images of physical health and general well-
being. The process is both appealing and benign to cancer patients,
and some who have used it have gone on to make a good recovery
from their disease, with the aid of more traditional forms of treatment.
The data consist mainly of anecdotal reports, and there exist no reports
of prospective studies documenting causal relationships between
these imagery techniques and positive therapeutic outcomes. Yet, despite the lack of any supporting scientific data, desperate cancer patients are increasingly asking their physicians for treatment by imagery techniques. These requests come not only from adult patients
but also from pediatric cancer patients and their families.

We respond to requests for imagery therapy in the same way we
respond to requests for other experimental forms of treatment. We tell
our patients the nature of the available data, noting that, while there
is no good evidence that the method can affect the course of cancer,
there is also no good evidence that it cannot do so. We say that the
treatment has no known harmful effects, provided patients continue
with other prescribed treatment such as radiation or chemotherapy.
Further, while the treatment may have no effect on tumor growth, its
use may have benefit in other ways. Patients who focus on positive
ideation may become more hopeful, more motivated to get adequate
nourishment and exercise, and more able to relax and get adequate
rest. In such instances, patients can improve the quality of their lives
even in the face of continued tumor growth.

For these reasons, we have both provided imagery therapy to patients who requested it and who continued to show interest after hearing our cautionary remarks. Some have died; others continue to use
the method with enthusiasm. Until further data are available, we will
continue to use imagery with patients who request it, always in the
context of scientific integrity and modesty.

An example of the imagery method to combat cancer is cited from
Olness's (1980) report of her work with cancer patients. A 13-year-old
boy described his cancer cells as black knights lined up for attack, but
smaller, weaker, and fewer in number than his healthy white blood
cells, depicted as white knights. The white knights continually chop
up the black knights with daggers. The drugs are vicious beasts who
support the white knights in their attack. This patient thinks about
his imagery several times daily and, after 30 months in remission, ex-
presses confidence that he is winning in the fight against his disease.

Another of our patients was a 17-year-old boy who requested imagery therapy 4 years after losing an arm to cancer. He was well for 3

years after diagnosis, and achieved national ranking as a handicapped downhill skier. When he then developed multiple lung metastases, he underwent vigorous chemotherapy; he began imagery therapy several months later. He visualized himself in a downhill slalom race, increasing his feelings of love, safety, strength, health, and competence as he passed each flag on the course. Then he visualized feelings of physical, mental, and spiritual well-being held tight in his hand and absorbed into his entire body. He enthusiastically practiced these and related techniques at least twice daily. His metastases disappeared, but he later suffered another relapse. He died about 1 year after beginning imagery therapy, having survived more than 5 years since initial diagnosis.

Modification of Patient's Ability to Respond with Mastery in the Dying Process

There comes a time in the lives of some terminally ill children when it is clear to them that they will inevitably die as a result of their disease. The possibility and even the probability of dying have been stated directly by several of our young patients. One 4-year-old leukemic boy said to his therapist, "Leukemia is a bad disease and you could die from it. [Die?] Yes, you just lie there and never wake up and you can't do anything any more and then you are just bones." Another 4-year-old boy, who was losing his life-long battle against chronic granulomatous disease, said simply to his mother, "Mommy, I'm going to die."

Although denial is a common and frequently adaptive defense mechanism for children with life-threatening illness, as well as for their families and their doctors (LaBaw et al., 1975), it is also true that most of these children have quite an accurate understanding of their chances for survival. Families and doctors—more often than they would like to admit—are tempted to impose their own need for denial on the child, creating a maladaptive conspiracy of silence in which the child must bear the burden of dying alone. For example, a 12-year-old girl with a recently diagnosed inoperable brain stem tumor told her psychologist that she knew she would eventually die. When asked if she had talked about dying with her parents, she replied, "Oh no, it would upset them too much!"

Gardner (1977) outlined four basic rights of dying children. First is the right to know the truth about the probable outcome of their illness. Actually, since most children have already figured it out for themselves, it would be more accurate to say affirm the truth rather than to imply that these children are learning it for the first time. Second is the right to share thoughts about dying, not just the probability of death, but the many questions that follow. Does it hurt to die? Are your parents with you when they bury you? What do you wear when you get buried? If they bury you down in the ground, how do you get up to heaven? Third is the right to live as full and normal a life as possible, truly to live until they die. Fourth is the right to participate in the process of dying, to have input concerning whether treatment should be continued or stopped, to state a preference for dying in the hospital or at home, and so on. Not all children choose to exercise these rights, but we believe the option of choosing should be available to them.

We have found that hypnotherapy can sometimes facilitate the process in which dying children exercise their rights. The mechanisms are occasionally direct; that is, interviewing the dying child in hypnosis concerning his or her problems. Much more often, hypnotherapy facilitates these goals indirectly. In such cases, the terminally ill child is usually first referred for hypnotherapy for some sort of specific symptomatic relief. A positive transference develops between the child and the therapist. In the context of a safe and trusting alliance, the child becomes more able to exercise his or her rights, usually with full parental support. After achieving initial symptom relief with the aid of hypnotherapy, much of the work toward the larger goals of solving problems rather than enduring them may be done in the waking state, with hypnotherapy used adjunctively as needed. Three case vignettes illustrate these direct and indirect processes.

Markowitz (1980) described to us his hypnotherapeutic work with an intelligent adolescent boy, on the day of his death from leukemia. In a waking interview the previous day, the boy had said he wanted to "write a will." That is, he wanted to state what he would like done with some of his personal belongings, and he wanted to give some advice to his parents concerning how they should deal with their lives after his death. Unfortunately, he went into coma before making the will. The following day, the therapist went to the boy's home, where he lay unconscious, and repeated a hypnotic induction that he had used successfully on earlier occasions. He reminded the boy of his previously stated wish and told him that, if making a will was still important to him, he could become more alert, open his eyes, and dictate his thoughts to the therapist. In 90 seconds, the boy opened his eyes, and he then dictated to the therapist for nearly 2 hours, giving his skis to his father, his guitar to his sister, and so on. He then talked with his family for another 45 minutes, following which he relapsed into coma and died 3 hours later.

Becky S. was a 7-year-old girl in the end stages of cystic fibrosis, who was initially referred to us for hypnotherapy to improve her tolerance of painful medical procedures such as fingersticks and arterial blood gases. She achieved better pain control after one hypnotherapy session and proudly told the therapist the next day that she had pricked her own finger. Some weeks later, during her terminal hospitalization, she complained to the therapist of diffuse anxiety, dizziness, and double vision. Recognizing the symptoms of hypoxia, and noting the results of a recent blood gas evaluation, the therapist asked the ward nurse whether the child could be given higher levels of oxygen. The nurse replied that the child was getting maximal oxygen through the nasal prongs she was using. She could get additional oxygen if she would use an oxygen mask instead of the nasal prongs, but she had refused suggestions from nurses and doctors that she wear a mask, apparently because she was afraid to have her face covered. The therapist returned to Becky's room and offered the same explanation and suggestion previously given by others. Becky immediately accepted the mask. The increased oxygen eliminated her hypoxic symptoms and allowed her to spend the evening cheerfully talking and playing with her family. It seemed that the context of the hypnotherapeutic relationship allowed this child to make more constructive decisions about her own treatment.

Steven T., a 10-year-old boy, also in the end stages of cystic fibrosis, was referred to us for hypnotherapy because of depression and decreased tolerance of medical procedures including postural drainage and intravenous infusions. He would resist and cry, asking the medical staff members why they continued these painful treatments when they knew as well as he did that he was going to die anyway. In the first hypnotherapeutic session, Steven quickly learned self-hypnosis to control pain and to decrease his anxiety about being unable to get enough air during postural drainage treatments that resulted in prolonged and violent coughing. He was also able to clarify that he really did want continued treatment, since he wanted to live as long as possible, and he asked that the nurses ignore his pleas when his frustration resulted in "temper tantrum" behavior. He immediately developed a strong positive alliance with the therapist. His mother concurrently responded well to brief counseling from the therapist and to more extensive therapy from her social worker.

In a later nonhypnotic psychotherapy session, Steven openly discussed his concerns about dying, especially his awareness that vigorous antibiotic therapy was no longer producing significant improvement in his pulmonary status. The therapist introduced a "life and death game" in an effort to modify the boy's increasing obsession with dying. Outlining a "life circle" and a "death circle" on a sheet of white paper, the therapist showed Steven two crayons, red and green, stating that life was to be represented by the color green and death by the color red. She then affirmed that treatment was of decreasing value and sometime soon would be of no value at all. She agreed that some-day the doctors would have no more "life" (treatment) to give Steven and could offer him only a relatively comfortable death, with medications as needed for pain and/or anxiety. She then removed the green crayon, illustrating the problem. Steven said he still wanted life, and he asked for the green crayon so that he could color the life circle green. The therapist reminded him that she had no more green to give him, and she challenged him to create green by himself. Steven quickly saw that his only option at this point in the game was to color the death circle red. As he worked at the task, the therapist encouraged him to look at death, to acknowledge death. Then, using the principle of complimentary colors, the therapist asked Steven to look again at the life circle. It turned green before his eyes.*

Both amazed and amused, Steven saw conceptually as well as graphically, that he could take some responsibility for his own experience, acknowledging death, then setting it aside and creating a more enjoyable life. For example, he proceeded to arrange a prebirthday party for himself in the hospital, instead of continuing to worry that he might not live another month until his 11th birthday. This being successful, he arranged a second prebirthday party when he went to visit relatives. Then, on his actual birthday, he enjoyed still a third party.

In many other ways, Steven created life for himself. Shortly before he died, he made a new contract with hospital staff to the effect that he could refuse postural drainage if he wished and have narcotic medication when he requested it, all knowing that this was now his terminal hospitalization. Supported by his family, he spent his last days relating to them and to the hospital staff members, for many of whom he had become a favorite patient. On the night before he died, he requested and fully enjoyed a special dinner sent in from a local restaurant. For Steven, the initial use of hypnotherapy seemed to facilitate this dying child's ability to exercise all four of his basic rights. To a large extent he shifted his approach to the task of dying from helpless frustration to mastery and control.

Hypnotherapy in the Broadest Context of Experience

Recent developments in holistic medicine are rapidly changing the way we treat children with life-threatening illness. Rather than directing efforts only at the disease process, we now emphasize the need for simultaneous attention to the physical, psychological, and spiritual needs of the patient and the family and the involved community.

As compared with the more narrow area of symptom relief, it is even more difficult to assess the value of hypnotherapy in holistic medicine. We can speculate that hypnotherapy may have an impact on several interrelated areas. For the child: (1) symptom relief; (2) decreased anxiety, depression, passivity, helplessness; (3) enhanced ego functions, especially feelings of safety, trust, hope, autonomy, competence, initiative, humor, reality testing, self-esteem, dignity, and grace; and (4) increased ability to relate positively to others in age-appropriate ways. For the family: (1) decreased feelings of anxiety and impotence; (2) increased ability to relate to the child and to offer comfort and reassurance rather than to engage in defensive withdrawal; (3) increased ability to make constructive use of community resources such as friends and clergy; and (4) increased ability to deal creatively with loss of a child, using the grief process in the service of personal growth. For the community: (1) increased responsiveness to the greater receptivity of the child and the family; and (2) increased awareness of the value of such responsiveness.

Every one of these areas affects all others, each making its own contribution, perhaps including enhancing the child's ability to use hypnotherapy, thus coming full circle in a complex set of causal relationships. While the formal use of hypnotherapy may appear to serve limited functions, it can interact with other resources in the child, the family, and the community to facilitate growth and mastery, thus utilizing emotional upheaval in the service of attaining higher levels of ego integration.

We do not mean to overvalue the role of hypnotherapy, but rather to recognize the whole spectrum of possible actions and reactions in the total experience of a dying child who uses this treatment modality. In the context of perceiving hypnotherapy as one resource among many, each affecting the others in the broadest context of experience, we present a previously published account (Gardner, 1976) of the child David.†

---

*For readers unfamiliar with this phenomenon, a similar effect can be produced by staring for 30 to 60 seconds at a red area on the book jacket and then immediately staring at a blank white area on the inside of the cover.

†Reprinted from the April 1976 *International Journal of Clinical and Experimental Hypnosis*. Copyrighted by the Society for Clinical and Experimental Hypnosis, April, 1976.

The authors would like to express their appreciation to David's parents for their assistance in the preparation of this manuscript and especially for their permission to print photographs of David and his family and to include excerpts of a family tape recording.

The Child David

A Brief History

David was the second of four boys born to intelligent, capable, middle-class parents. The family valued religious commitment and, at the time of David's illness, were members of an Episcopal church. Outgoing and sociable, they frequently spent time both with personal friends and with the father's business associates. The father especially enjoyed the challenge of hiking, backpacking, and skiing—activities that demand and develop physical and mental stamina, independence, and persistence in the face of difficulty. He encouraged the children in these and other rigorous pursuits such as baseball, football, and swimming. The mother, through her qualities of gentleness, tenderness, and obvious pleasure both in sharing laughter and in relieving distress, complemented the father in conveying to the children that sense of security and involvement in living that is the foundation for personal growth. Of course, there were differences of opinion and periods of significant tension and strain, but, more than most, this family found real reward in doing things together. Birthdays and holidays were special family "happenings," so much so that every year each child had two birthday celebrations, a party with his friends and a separate birthday dinner for the family alone.

Up to the age of 11, David was healthy. He often lacked enthusiasm at school, annually causing enough concern that his teacher requested a conference with his parents; yet his schoolwork was satisfactory. He excelled in outdoor activities with family and peers, while at the same time he was able to enjoy himself when alone. A bright child, he shared his parents' good sense of humor and enjoyed playing jokes on people. Though capable of anger, he also expressed love and tenderness to his family, and especially to his dog. He tended not to worry about things and to take life as it came, proud of his past, secure in the present, and not giving a great deal of thought to the future.

Then, soon after his 11th birthday, a routine blood test showed abnormalities that led to hospitalization and to a diagnosis of acute lymphatic leukemia. The parents were stunned, but found hope in the knowledge of many potentially helpful drugs. David reacted characteristically, without much concern, even enjoying the new experiences of his first hospitalization, yet very happy to return home to his family and his dog. Having achieved remission, David perceived his disease primarily as a nuisance and joined his parents in their developing denial that it was really a serious threat. Life routines returned essentially to normal. He completed the school year successfully, went on a family backpacking trip, and pitched his Little League baseball team to a first place win.

The Introduction of Hypnotherapy

In early fall, 10 months after the initial diagnosis, relapses began, and inexorably the periods of remission became progressively shorter. The parents faced the truth all over again, this time more realistically and more painfully. They counseled with their priest and with a few very close friends, trying to make some sense theologically out of their predicament and to begin planning a funeral that could properly reflect their evolving feelings about the meaning of death. Fundamentally, knowing they might not function very well if they had to face the situation alone, they began building a support system, both interpersonally and philosophically. Active planning replaced denial as a coping mechanism.

Though David's outlook remained essentially positive, he too was more often confronted with the devastating consequences of his illness. Soon after he began sixth grade, he was told he could no longer play football. On Halloween, he began to revel in neighborhood fun, but became too tired and returned home after he had visited only three houses. On his 12th birthday, he was again sick and spent much of the day sleeping. In these difficult times, he was frustrated and depressed, sometimes in tears, but he responded well to overtures from others; on Halloween, his little brothers shared their candy with him, and, on his birthday, a high school choral group came to the house to sing him an hour of show tunes. He was also sustained by his own resources, especially his undaunted desire to enjoy living. Important as it was that his family and friends never deserted him, it was more important that he never deserted himself.

Then during a hospitalization in November, David developed vomiting that did not respond to medication. Both for him and his parents, frustration quickly mounted into anxiety and then into depression and despair. It was Michael, a male nurse, who, sharing in the frustration, first discussed the problem with the author, a psychologist experienced in using hypnotherapy with pediatric patients. We agreed that hypnosis might alleviate David's vomiting and, after discussing the situation with the medical staff, proposed the idea to David and to his mother who was staying with him at the time. They both voiced immediate enthusiasm, ready to grasp at anything that might help. David's positive response was further enhanced by his curiosity about hypnosis, which he put in the same category of intrigue as black magic, and his anticipated pleasure in experiencing it. Thus, there were no problems with initial motivation and cooperation.

Selecting induction techniques.   The selection of appropriate induction and deepening techniques was based on several factors. First, since David now feared he had lost control of his disease, it was important to use techniques that would enhance his sense of control and mastery. He needed to feel that hypnosis was not something done to him by some other powerful person but rather a state he could achieve for himself after proper training. Thus, hypnosis was described as analogous to learning to write or ride a bike, and techniques were avoided which involved any sort of gadgetry or emphasis on cues from the hypnotherapist.

Second, the induction techniques needed to be consistent with David's capabilities and interests, especially in the case of visual imagery. Through interviews with David and his mother, the therapist obtained the relevant information, including knowledge about David's enjoyment of new experiences and his love of imaginative activities. For example, his mother described how he and his brother enjoyed creating an imaginary house from pine shrubs on a recent backpacking trip.

Third, since it seemed likely that David would be taught self-hypnosis, the most preferable induction techniques were those he could use himself or with only minimal aid from his mother. Corollary to this, the induction techniques needed to be easily mastered by the mother, since her interest in the method suggested that she could become a hypnotherapeutic ally, assisting her son in hypnosis when the therapist was not available. Parents have been taught to be effective therapists for children's behavior problems (Stabler, Gibson, & Cutting, 1973), and this author has had successful experiences in teaching parents to assist with hypnotherapy.

Based on this initial information, the therapist decided to begin with suggestions for progressive relaxation and guided visual imagery related to David's interests and experiences. The boy was first given some elementary facts about hypnosis (e.g., that it was not the same as black magic and that he would be awake and able to remember what happened) in order to minimize confusion and develop a concept of active partnership in the therapeutic alliance. After this brief teaching session, the induction was carried out as planned, and David went into hypnosis without difficulty.

Early goals.   The immediate goal was, of course, to try to reduce the nausea and vomiting. The therapist first reminded David of his own wish to work on this problem and added her agreement that the vomiting served no useful purpose and therefore should be eliminated. She then asked David to recall specific foods that he particularly enjoyed and to bring these vividly to mind, together with sensations of mild hunger and gustatory pleasure. As he enhanced these images, he was told that these good feelings could fill his entire body and mind more and more, until there was just no room left for the unpleasant feelings which had plagued him. Generally, the idea was to create a positive state that would be antithetical to nausea. As David indicated that he was immersed in the good feelings and the bad ones had disappeared, he was given posthypnotic suggestions that he could maintain the good feelings after returning to the normal waking state, could actually enjoy food and fluids, and could take medication without difficulty. After he was aroused, the therapist remained with him while he ate a small meal. He was both astonished and proud to find that the problem was resolved after this one session.

Toward the larger goal of mastery, the therapist suggested during the hypnotic session that, just as David was now able to achieve physical relaxation and visual imagery when he wished, he could look forward to using this method for other purposes such as pain control, knowing that he had more control over his physical and emotional state than he realized previously. This sense of control could make him more relaxed and less anxious, and then he would be even more able to reach his goals. He was asked to recall earlier experiences of mastery, such as winning at baseball, and then to bring these feelings into the present, with posthypnotic suggestions that they could carry over into the future. Thus, the therapist created the growth cycle that seems so often to be at the root of successful hypnotherapy.

David was indeed pleased with his new skill and readily found that, in addition to achieving control of the nausea, he could respond to hypnotherapy for control of pain and of marked anxiety related to the start of an intravenous infusion. Here the therapist used the same paradigm as for control of nausea, namely creating an antithetical feeling state. David was asked to recall his arm feeling very comfortable, to bring that comfort into the present so thoroughly that there was simply no room for pain.

Extensions of Mastery

Self-hypnosis. It was David himself who asked to learn self-hypnosis so that he could better control problems of nausea, pain, or anxiety that might arise at home. Accordingly, prior to discharge from the hospital, and after careful discussion with him and his mother about the nature and use of hypnosis, David was taught self-hypnosis. He was cautioned regarding abuse by being told that it was so easy to learn hypnotic induction that he could probably hypnotize his friends or other people, but that he should not do this because, though it is easy to learn *how* to hypnotize, it takes special training to learn *when* and *why* to use hypnosis and *what* suggestions to give people. He was reminded that, just as special training is needed to know when and why to use medications, the same is true for hypnosis. He and his mother agreed that he could be responsible in this regard. There were no particular limitations put on his using hypnosis for himself, except to emphasize that it was not to be done "just for fun" and to suggest that he talk with his mother or the therapist before using it for any new problem.

Some interesting difficulties arose at this point which are illustrative of the need to be alert to idiosyncratic responses to hypnosis, to be skilled in a variety of induction methods, and to be ready to modify therapeutic techniques on short notice. The first problem concerned induction in self-hypnosis. Most patients, including children, can readily adapt the induction methods of heterohypnosis to autohypnosis, providing the therapist has not structured the situation otherwise. Thus, in David's case, he was asked simply to close his eyes and allow himself to enter the state of physical relaxation now familiar to him, while focusing his attention on pleasant visual imagery. As he began to respond, he became curiously anxious. When asked what troubled him, he said that he could achieve the relaxation and imagery but was worried because, without any comments from the therapist, he didn't know whether or not he was "really in hypnosis." That is, he wanted some sort of clear external cue that hypnosis had been achieved, and did not feel comfortable or confident having to rely solely on his experiential state. It was easy enough to give him the needed cue by adding reverse arm levitation to the induction procedure. He was asked to raise one arm and then to notice how it would begin to feel heavy and drift downward as he relaxed. He was told that the arm would drift lower and lower and that, when it reached his lap or the bed or chair, he could be sure he was in hypnosis. David accepted this suggestion without question, and used this technique successfully up until 3 days before his death.

The second problem that arose in teaching David self-hypnosis concerned anxiety when he was asked to do something in self-hypnosis that he had not done in any previous heterohypnosis session, namely to talk. He had never been required to give any verbal response, since simple motor responses such as nodding or shaking his head were sufficient for communication around the problems at hand. Now, however, it seemed desirable to demonstrate to him and his mother that he could respond to her verbally or initiate verbalization while in hypnosis, should the need arise. When this was first proposed, David expressed his fear that he would "come out of hypnosis and wake up" if he talked. Despite reassurance, he maintained this anxiety during the hypnotic induction and avoided the problem of having to talk by soon drifting off to sleep. The therapist took the opportunity to note to the mother this example of ego control in the hypnotic state, with David finding a way to avoid the feared unwanted self-arousal that would have impaired his confidence that he could use hypnosis alone. The therapist also used this incident to demonstrate to the mother that, if David were to fall asleep while using hypnosis, it was quite easy to awaken him gently, just as one might awaken any sleeping child. Once David was awake, the therapist provided further reassurance and explanation. Following this, David again induced self-hypnosis and, this time, gave appropriate verbal responses to questions and commands from his mother as well as from the therapist. It is important to note here that the therapist did not respond to the unexpected events with anxiety, but turned the situation into an opportunity for teaching and further development of skills. If hypnosis has been initially presented as a technique which may have to be modified to fit individual needs, then it is not a disaster when problems of this sort occur.

The third problem in teaching David self-hypnosis was related to his mother. Both she and the therapist agreed that it might be useful for her to experience a hypnotic induction herself, since she wanted to know "what it feels like" and since first-hand knowledge of the state might enhance her effectiveness in helping David use hypnosis. When this was suggested, David expressed interest in seeing his mother in hypnosis. She was willing, and it was convenient to have her go into hypnosis in David's room since the therapist's office was in another part of the hospital, and only a brief experience of induction and dehypnotization was anticipated. The mother went into hypnosis without difficulty, but soon became spontaneously alert, commenting briefly that she felt a bit silly. She later told the therapist, "Really I was getting so relaxed and my defenses were breaking down; I was near tears and I didn't want to cry in front of David." It seems that sharing the hypnotic experience with her dying child brought out feelings of sadness and anticipatory grief that she did not want David to have to bear in addition to his already heavy burden. More than the other two problems, in retrospect it seems this one could have been anticipated. It would have been better to have insisted on David not being present when his mother experienced hypnosis. Then, perhaps she could have made constructive use of the emergence of her feelings of grief.

In spite of these difficulties, both David and his mother gained confidence that he could use hypnosis himself and that she could assist him as needed. As with induction, the method of dehypnotization was simple, merely counting silently to five. David never abused the privilege of learning self-hypnosis. With characteristic responsibility and humor, he later told the therapist that he had resisted the temptation to talk in detail about hypnosis to his friends, but he confessed that he had tried to hypnotize his dog.

The eagle dream.   In chronic and terminal illness, one sees extended hope and relief when the patient and the family learn that hypnosis can be useful not only for the treatment of painful or negative experiences, but also for enhancement of positive experiences such as safety and joy. This idea was introduced to David by suggesting that he might have a pleasant hypnotic dream that he could repeat as often as he liked. He dreamed that he was an eagle who enjoyed flying from one safe and peaceful place to another; whenever anything disturbed him, he could simply fly off to another, even safer and happier place. At home, when David was in distress, he successfully combined reverse hand levitation with the eagle dream to achieve quietness and calm enjoyment, sometimes at his own initiation and sometimes following his mother's suggesting, "David, just find your peaceful place." Family friends, who were unaware of what was happening, were astonished at the rapidity and ease with which he could shift from a negative to a positive feeling state.

For David and his family it became more possible to tolerate gradual physical deterioration and to avert the threat of psychological disintegration by learning to achieve a feeling of emotional ease and dignity. The sense of threat gradually gave way to a sense of challenge and then to task accomplishment and general mastery. That is, David expressed and at the same time enhanced his growing trust in himself and turned his attention to solving problems rather than enduring them. The therapist took this opportunity to remind him and his mother that they could consider using hypnosis for new problems as they arose, feeling free to contact the therapist for consultation and assistance as needed.

An example of contraindication.   On Thanksgiving Day, just before being discharged from the hospital, David suddenly asked a doctor if having leukemia meant that he was going to die. To his horror he learned that he would die "in a month at the least and a year at the most." Despite his size, he sat in his mother's lap and wept bitterly

in the car driving home; then, as if to indicate his beginning acceptance, he began parceling out his belongings, emphasizing that he
wanted his dog "to be for the whole family." By the time he got home,
less than an hour later, he had somehow regained his sense of trust,
hope, and integrity. He shared the news with his older brother, again
with tears, though only briefly, and then told a few friends who immediately came to the house. After talking about his problems, they
resumed normal activities, as if to say there was no great reason for
concern or for deviating from their usual habit of enjoying life and
taking things as they came. The hospital staff reported the incident to
the therapist by telephone, but by the time she telephoned the family,
everything was under control and no special intervention was needed.

   During the next couple of weeks, when David did not talk any
more about his impending death, both his family and his doctors
wondered if he had questions or ideas he wanted to share but was
reluctant to do so. It was hard to believe that he had either denied the
truth, which had been put to him so plainly, or integrated it successfully into his general life style. At the next outpatient visit, his mother
asked if it might be valuable to question him about these issues in a
hypnotic session and then to create amnesia for the session so that he
would not be upset by the content of the interview. She was told that
it is extremly difficult to predict how a person will react to this type of
hypnotic interview, and that it is especially difficult to be sure of obtaining amnesia. Therefore the plan was abandoned, not only because
of the uncertainty of success, but also because we did not want to take
the risk of having a distressing hypnotic experience interfere with
David's successful use of hypnosis in other areas.

   Since a hypnotic approach seemed contraindicated in this instance, the mother asked for other ideas and accepted the suggestion
that we ask David quite straightforwardly if he had any questions
about his illness or about death. She feared that she might upset him
if she herself wept during the interview, but she overcame her fear
when reminded that we had solved difficult problems before and
could surely trust in our resourcefulness now. We agreed to terminate
the interview by observing David's response and following his lead.
In response to questions, David said calmly that he knew he was
going to die but was not worried and had no questions. Like many
dying children, his only stated concern was that he did not want his
parents to be sad or upset because of him. Though assured that he
could bring up the subject at any time in the future, he never raised
it again.

   An example of creative use of hypnosis.   Glad to have a treatment
technique that was both painless and portable, David and his family

went to visit relatives in Texas in mid-December. The therapist taught David to go into hypnosis by telephone, demonstrating this with him during a clinic visit. Putting a hypnotic induction on tape was considered, but not carried out since, with David's condition now likely to change in unknown ways almost from day to day, there was little chance that suggestions on prerecorded tape would be useful.

Once in Texas, David developed a ravenous appetite associated with high-dose steroids which had recently been prescribed. When it got to the point that he woke two or three times a night to have his mother fix eggs and toast, they decided to try hypnotherapy for appetite control. David was assisted by his uncle, who is a psychotherapist, and, after one session, his appetite returned to normal levels.

After a week, David was again in relapse. His parents conferred with their doctor and agreed to return home, not to attempt further treatment, and to keep David as comfortable as possible so that he might die in dignity and peace.

The Last Three Days

Early Saturday, December 23, David entered the hospital for the last time. He had vomited blood several times during the night, and neither he nor his parents had had much sleep. He had recurring sharp pain in his leg, which he could no longer control with hypnosis. He was admitted to a private room and intravenous morphine was begun. Though in such poor condition, David once again spontaneously raised his arm and lowered himself into hypnotic comfort before the needle was put into his vein. Even the therapist now marvelled at this continuing ability to maintain some degree of control of experience.

In the hallway, both parents wept. The father was angered that there seemed to be no way to hold off this inexorable march toward death until David had had one last Christmas. The mother feared that she would "fall apart" and be unable to support David now, when he most needed her. The therapist decided to stay to try to help the family regain touch with their inner resources so that they could once again express the courage and love and tenderness that had sustained them before. The father went home to arrange for the other three children to be with grandparents. David and his mother slept. By afternoon, the parents were refreshed and David was comfortable, sleeping most of the time.

On December 24, when David's condition was relatively stable and when he seemed comfortable in spite of labored breathing, the decision was made to reduce the morphine, which seemed to be controlling his pain and anxiety but only at the expense of his ability to maintain ego functions. It was hoped that a smaller amount of morphine combined with hypnotic suggestions might control the pain and still allow him to be more alert and to spend maximal time relating to his family. Likewise, if he was more alert, his parents could be more active in comforting him, caring for his needs, and sharing conversation, thus again averting passive submission and impotence.

True to himself, David maintained his capacity for trust and hope. Once when his leg hurt, he responded readily to a suggestion that he could "just let the pain go," but he said he feared it might come back. When reassured that he could "just let it go again," he immediately relaxed; further episodes of the leg pain were infrequent and brief. That afternoon he unexpectedly became fully alert and began spontaneously reminiscing about pleasant experiences of the past. Wishing to preserve this precious experience, his mother asked that this conversation be tape recorded. The therapist found a tape recorder and granted the request. In the evening, his older brother brought his Christmas presents, but David was sleepy and showed little interest. Friends and hospital staff brought food and wine, and someone remarked that a new family began to be created, united by some mysterious sense of sharing, freedom, and warmth, enhanced by David's attitude of calm as he began his final approach toward death. Christmas Eve was quiet.

On Christmas Day, again without warning, David became alert and now asked to see his presents. He opened several, making his usual wisecracks, and then gave gifts to his father and mother. He tired easily, and his breathing became increasingly labored. His father helped him to a more comfortable position in bed while his mother spoke softly to him, repeating simple phrases remarkably similar to the rhythm and language of hypnotherapy. Since the tape recorder had been running, this, too, was recorded, an excerpt of which follows:

That's a boy. Find your quiet place and just rest now. There David. There Davey, there Davey, just rest honey. Just rest. Just rest honey. Just rest honey. Just rest. That's a boy. It's all right honey. Just relax. Just rest. Just relax honey. Just rest. That's a boy, honey. That's a boy. Just rest honey. That's a boy. We'll open more presents later, honey. There now. There now, there now, there now. There now. There Davey, just relax, just relax. There. Just relax honey. That's a boy. That's a boy, find your quiet place. Just relax. That's a boy. Okay honey, okay just relax honey. Just rest, just find your peaceful place and rest. Just find your peaceful place and rest. Mommy and Daddy are right here and we're going to keep you good and safe. It's okay honey. It's okay.

Joined by a close family friend, the therapist, and Michael the nurse, both parents continued to comfort their son. Later, on that Christmas afternoon, David died.

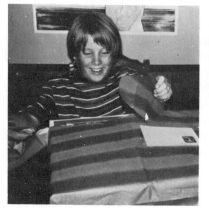

1. *Eleventh birthday party.*

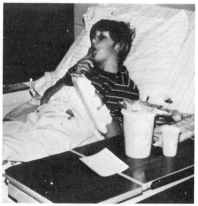

2. *First hospitalization.*

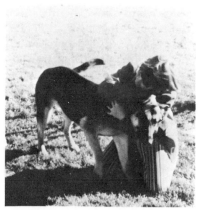

3. *First return home.*

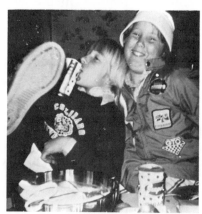

4. *Clowning with a friend.*

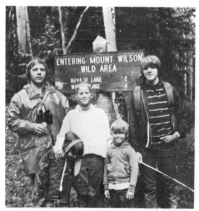

5. *Family backpacking trip.*

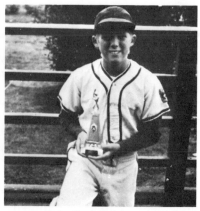

6. *Baseball victory.*

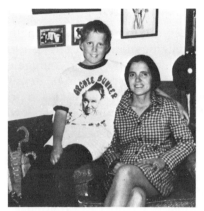

7. *David and his mother.*

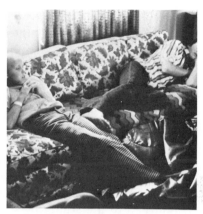

8. *The last Thanksgiving.*

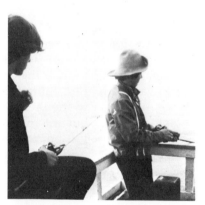

9. *Fishing, a week before death.*

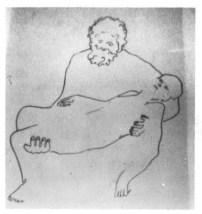

10. *Sketch of Michael holding David after death.*

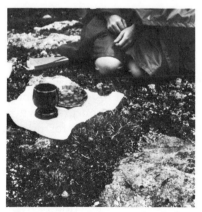

11. *Outdoor Mass before scattering of ashes.*

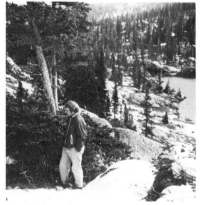

12. *Father at the scattering site a month later.*

Hypnotherapy in the Grieving Process

David's parents had many sources of strength to sustain them through the next months, especially religious faith and strong ties to the community and to the church, in addition to inner courage and creative acceptance. Family and friends participated in a Requiem Mass. In the summer when the snow melted in the mountains, a priest and a few friends hiked with the family to an alpine lake. Following the Eucharist, they scattered David's ashes amidst the pine shrubs where earlier he had joined his brother in imaginative games.

The parents and children each found their individual ways of expressing their grief and integrating David's death into a concept of meaningful life. The children talked with friends and family. The parents returned to the scattering site in early October to experience the beauty of the first snowfall. A family friend drew a sketch of Michael holding David after death, when told that this scene had reminded the therapist of the Michelangelo Pietà in Rome.

The mother, having experienced hypnosis before, now used it again to enhance her capacity for full expression of her feelings, to enjoy fresh and vivid memories of David, to find meaning in her loss, and to allow opportunity for further personal development in the context of her son's death. She said, "Dying was the hardest thing Dave ever had to do, and he did it well." Once, in a letter to the therapist, she wrote, "David is so real to me—not externally but internally—bound up in all that I cherish and wonder at and reflect on, that his reality is very present, very real, very full of meaning. And so I rejoice, mainly, that God should so bless me as to make meaning out of chaos."

CONCLUSIONS

While hypnotherapy seems to be valuable for many children with life-threatening illness and for their families, there are instances in which it is of limited value or none at all. Some children and parents simply refuse this treatment modality. Other children eagerly embark on learning hypnotic skills only to fail, for known and unknown reasons. Still other children respond well to hypnotherapy for one purpose but not for another, or respond well at one time and poorly at another. We still have a great deal to learn about potential uses of hypnotherapy with dying children. How do we help them maximize their use of hypnotic talent? What are the limits of the possible uses of hypnotherapy? How can we best facilitate the interaction of hypnotherapy with many other forms of medical, surgical, and psychological treatment?

Child health professionals who utilize hypnotherapy with dying children must also consider issues related to their own involvement. The hypnotherapeutic relationship is characterized by more intense emotional responses, not only in the patient but also in the therapist. When working with dying children, the hypnotherapist must be able to deal with his or her own reactions to loss and with the emotional stress of personal involvement, combining human caring with professional objectivity in such a way that the end result is positive not only for the child and the family but for the therapist as well.

REFERENCES

Crasilneck, H. B., & Hall, J. A. Clinical hypnosis in problems of pain. *The American Journal of Clinical Hypnosis*, 1973, *15*, 153–161.

Crasilneck, H. B., & Hall, J. A. *Clinical hypnosis: Principles and applications.* New York: Grune & Stratton, 1975.

Gardner, G. G. Childhood, death, and human dignity: Hypnotherapy for David. *The International Journal of Clinical and Experimental Hypnosis*, 1976, *24*, 122–139.

Gardner, G. G. The rights of dying children: Some personal reflections. *The Psychotherapy Bulletin*, 1977, *10*, 20–23.

Greene, W. A., Jr., & Miller, G. Psychological factors and reticuloendothelial disease. IV. Observations on a group of children and adolescents with leukemias: An interpretation of disease development in terms of mother–child unit. *Psychosomatic Medicine*, 1958, *10*, 124–144.

Hilgard, J. R., & Morgan, A. H. Treatment of anxiety and pain in childhood cancer through hypnosis. In F. H. Frankel & H. S. Zamansky (Eds.), *Hypnosis at its bicentennial: Selected papers.* New York: Plenum Press, 1978.

Jacobs, T. J., & Charles, E. Life events and the occurrence of cancer in children. *Psychosomatic Medicine*, 1980, *42*, 11–24.

Katz, E. R., Kellerman, J., & Siegel, S. E. Behavioral distress in children with cancer undergoing medical procedures: Developmental considerations. *Journal of Consulting and Clinical Psychology*, 1980, *48*, 356–365.

LaBaw, W., Holton, C., Tewell, K., & Eccles, D. The use of self-hypnosis by children with cancer. *The American Journal of Clinical Hypnosis*, 1975, *17*, 233–238.

Markowitz, D. M. Personal communication, August, 1980.

Olness, K. Imagery (self-hypnosis) as adjunct therapy in childhood cancer: Clinical experience with 25 patients. *American Journal of Pediatric Hematology/Oncology*, 1981, *3*, 313–321.

Stabler, B., Gibson, F. W., Jr., & Cutting, D. S. Parents as therapists: An innovative community-based model. *Professional Psychology*, 1973, *4*, 397–402.

14

Looking to the Future

We have brought together a variety of ideas concerning hypnotic responsiveness in childhood and the use of hypnotherapy in childhood disorders. In our attempt to integrate clinical observations with research studies, we have found that most have significant methodological shortcomings. The weight of evidence suggests that most children are responsive to hypnosis and that hypnotherapy can often be useful in their treatment. At the same time, the data are usually not compelling and often raise more questions than they answer. There is a great deal of work still to be done.

We now present issues of research methodology, pointing out some technical considerations that should enhance the value of future research. Finally, specific problem areas in which we expect future research to provide clarification are addressed.

More so than in earlier chapters, we engage in speculation in the hope that our ideas may stimulate creative thought and action in our colleagues. We stretch our own imaginations!

RESEARCH METHODOLOGY

While we cannot attempt a full discussion of methodological issues in child hypnosis research, we would like to mention several problems that come up again and again in the studies previously cited. For a thorough review of technical aspects of hypnosis research, we refer the reader to the excellent book edited by Fromm and Shor,

Hypnosis: Developments in Research and New Perspectives (1979); almost every chapter contains ideas that are relevant to child hypnosis research.

Hypnotic Responsiveness

We hope the Children's Hypnotic Susceptibility Scale (London, 1963) will be revised. Some items should be changed or deleted. Other items could be added, especially with a view toward studying hypnotic responsiveness in very young children. The standardization sample should include children from a wide range of social and cultural backgrounds.

We anticipate reports of normative data for the Stanford Hypnotic Clinical Scale: Child (Morgan & J. R. Hilgard, 1979), providing more information both on normal populations and on special groups of children.

We hope that studies with both of these scales will further clarify the relationship between age and hypnotic responsiveness, including delineation of moderating variables. We look for more sophisticated research on other correlates of hypnotic responsiveness, especially the role of imaginative skills. Sheehan (1979) reviewed the literature on adult hypnosis and the process of imagination. This is an area of study that is more complex than it first appears.

There has been almost no research on the role of imagination in childhood hypnotic responsiveness. We strongly urge our colleagues to make advances in this area, for we strongly believe that imagination is the key factor underlying the benefits of child hypnotherapy.

Clinical Research

While descriptive case studies will always have their place, we anticipate fewer reports of this type that do little more than repeat information that is already widely disseminated, for example, that hypnotherapy seems to be helpful for asthmatic children. We look for an increase in valuable reports describing the results of hypnotherapy with a series of cases of children allowing better assessment of the merits of hypnotherapy for childhood problems. These studies should provide evidence that the children actually are responsive to hypnosis. Proper control groups should be utilized so that it is reasonable to conclude that positive results are due to hypnosis and not to other factors, such as attention or task motivation. By the same token, measures of hypnotic responsiveness should also be used to ascertain that so-called nonhypnotic control groups do not include children who go into hypnosis without any formal induction.

Where possible, the data should be analyzed by persons who do not know which children had hypnotherapy and which did not; otherwise experimenter bias makes the results difficult to interpret.

Researchers in clinical applications of hypnotherapy with children must carefully consider their choice of statistical maneuvers before completing study designs. They should be encouraged and challenged by Feinstein's (1977) following statement:

> One of the most pernicious scientific delusions now prevalent in the world of medical research is the idea that concepts of random sampling can be readily applied to clinical populations. The idea is completely vitiated by the use of patients as the material of clinical investigations because a patient—unlike a rat—chooses the investigator rather than vice versa. The statistical literature contains many precise instructions for tests that quantify the operations of chance but almost no instructions for the judgment needed to make decisions of science. [p. 23]*

In all research studies, both negative and positive results should be reported, and there should be special attention to communicating effectively in oral presentations and in published reports. We recommend review of three papers on effective communication with colleagues in the field of hypnosis (Frankel, 1981; Fromm, 1981; Orne, 1981).

In short, if colleagues interested in child hypnosis and hypnotherapy are more careful both in doing research and in reporting it, there will be fewer instances in which there is more heat than light.

TOPICS FOR FUTURE RESEARCH

Consciousness and Imagination

We have taken the position that hypnosis is an altered state of consciousness and that hypnotherapy is a treatment modality, distinct from other forms of medical and psychological therapy, that has unique benefits for many child patients. It is possible that we are wrong on both these points. If we are right, we would hope to be able to increase our level of confidence through research in several areas: the nature of consciousness in general; the nature of altered states of consciousness, how these are best achieved, and how they vary in

---

*From *Clinical Biostatistics* by A. R. Feinstein, St. Louis: Mosby, 1977. With permission.

terms of potential value; the nature of imagination and how imagery skills may be fostered and preserved.

Future research concerning child applications of hypnotherapy must take into account why childhood imagery skills peak and subsequently fade as the child moves into adulthood. Imagery is intrinsic to child hypnotherapy; it is also part of child development, play patterns, creativity, and adult achievements.

Plato, in *The Republic,* was keenly aware of the tremendous influence of imaginative involvement on child development. He argued, for example, that children should be exposed to certain kinds of literature, drama, and music while other kinds should be suppressed. Otherwise children would learn inappropriate values and behave as adults in ways which would be harmful to themselves and to society. Plato may have been right; we certainly hear similar arguments today, especially with respect to children's television programming.

It is one thing to restrict the focus of a child's imagination; it is something else to devalue imagination generally. While many people would agree with the former but not the latter, our society seems to be producing just the reverse situation. Bronowski (1974) wrote: "All great civilizations have failed in one regard. They have limited the freedom of imagination of their young."* This idea is not new. William Blake, writing in 1788, lamented the loss of childhood imagination to the repressive forces of reason, and expressed hope that "the real man, the Imagination" would be found again (Kazin, 1974, p. 83).

We all think we know what imagination is, and yet scientists are still trying to define it. There are many questions. Is imagination essentially a single process or is it a set of discrete skills? Why does it persist in some people and drop out in others? Why do some people use it adaptively and others maladaptively? Since it appears to be of great value in dealing with certain potentially devastating situations, such as when one is a hostage or a prisoner of war, why don't we make a greater effort to teach people to preserve it, to use it for relatively minor problems as well as for major ones? Who should be the teachers and how should they teach?

How is imagination related to eidetic imagery, a skill seen in some children but only rarely in adults (Haber, 1980)? How is it related to extrasensory perception, another skill that has been reported to be available to some children (Peterson, 1975; Schwarz, 1970)?

If imaginative skills facilitate hypnotic responsiveness, might it also be true that experience with hypnosis fosters the development

---

*From *The Ascent of Man* by Jacob Bronowski, Boston: Little, Brown, 1974. With permission.

and preservation of imaginative skills? Should all children be taught self-hypnosis? Are children who are familiar with self-hypnosis better able to adapt to life's challenges and to develop their own assets? Frankel (1976) has described hypnosis as a coping mechanism especially useful in the treatment of certain clinical disorders, such as phobias, where the development of the problems seems to be associated with high hypnotic responsiveness. If this is true, might not hypnotic skills be used to prevent certain problems and to minimize the impact of others?

Links between Mental and Physiological Processes

John Wheeler, Professor of Physics at Princeton, has written, "Today no mystery more attracts the minds of pioneers from the field of molecular biology than the mechanism of brain action. Many workers . . . feel that the decisive step forward is waiting for an idea . . . we can believe that it will somehow touch the tie between mind and matter" (1974, p. 690).

It is not beyond our wildest dreams that physics and chemistry may provide the tools needed to explain hypnosis just as they provided tools to enable the use of oil and electricity. If molecules arrange into images that result in Nobel-prize-winning discoveries in chemistry, might they not also arrange into images that result in changed behavior and symptom relief? For example, we now know that children's thought processes are associated with deliberate changes in temperature of their finger tips. How? Might we one day explain this phenomenon at a molecular level?

Every adult human body contains 100 trillion cells. These fundamental components of living things were first discovered in the 17th century. Since then, we have learned much about what happens inside cells but very little about how it happens. Researchers ponder why genes in individual cells switch themselves on and off and perform differently in varying circumstances. For example, why does messenger ribonucleic acid (m-RNA) not always transmit the complete messages that it carries from deoxyribonucleic acid (DNA)? The whole issue of regulation of the function of the 100 trillion cells is a mystery at this time. There is no clear explanation for how microtubules carry instructions between cell nuclei and surfaces. It is possible that some of the regulation of cell behavior comes from messages that begin with thought and mental images. Tracing transmission to the cell, to the m-RNA, to the microtubules and using that knowledge to alleviate the human condition must be the task of the remainder of the 20th century and the 21st.

Both clinical observations of responses to hypnotherapy and experimental laboratory work in hypnosis may provide a suitable launching pad for the inevitable understanding of these mechanisms. E. R. Hilgard's (1977) work on the nature of consciousness is a step in this direction. Studies of hypnotic amnesia are also relevant. Would it be useful to do research on the mechanisms of hypnotic amnesia or pain control in children? Might we learn more about the interaction between mind and body?

A growing body of data finds no relationship between physiological processes and the presence or absence of hypnosis (Sarbin & Slagle, 1979). Have we missed something here?

An even larger body of data (e.g., Sarbin & Slagle, 1979) suggests that mental processes occurring in hypnosis are related to somatic effects. A recent study (MacDonald, Hogan, & Olness, 1981) assessed the ability of children to change voluntarily brain stem auditory evoked potentials with and without hypnosis. This pilot study measured tracings at 85 and 65 decibels for the left ear for 10 children, ages 7 to 11, and repeated these tracings after giving the verbal suggestion that the sound intensity was much less. One group of children had previous experience in self-hypnosis; the other did not. Both groups showed significant prolongation of interwave latencies after verbal suggestion alone. Following this, one group listened to a hypnosis tape and the measurements were repeated. The hypnosis group demonstrated greater reduction in brain stem auditory evoked potentials than did the control group. The three children most clinically responsive to the use of self-hypnosis demonstrated the most notable prolongation of interwave latencies in response to suggestion both before and after the self-hypnosis tape.

How do these changes occur? There are many theories but no real answers. No one is, at this time, close to tracing the impulse associated with a thought or feeling through to its translation into bronchospasm, blood pressure elevation, or increased peristalsis. What is the role in hypnotherapy of biological rhythms, already known to be associated with variations in drug response? Are hypnotic suggestions more effective at certain times than at others? Should we be scheduling hypnotherapy to fit children's biological rhythms and not to fit arbitrary office hours? Do certain drugs minimize the results of hypnotherapy? Do others enhance it?

Role of the Hypnotherapist in Hypnotherapy

It seems logical that mental processes—including affect, imagery, and expectations—of hypnotherapists are related to treatment outcomes. For example, some studies (e.g., Rutter, 1980) have found a relationship between teacher expectations and student performance, independent of IQ levels. Many people have had the experience of feeling worse if a friend or neighbor says, "You don't look well. Are you sick?" What happens when a hypnotherapist anticipates a poor treatment outcome? What are the cues by which such an expectation gets communicated to a patient? The "hanging crepe phenomenon" (Siegler, 1975), common in the medical profession, should be studied with regard to hypnotherapy.

What about biological rhythms, moods, and other variables in hypnotherapists? It is possible that we will develop objective measures of these variables that will enable us to decide that we should not work with children at certain times.

Do some child hypnotherapists work more successfully with their patients than others? Which people are most suited to be child hypnotherapists and which least? Should we discourage certain people from becoming child hypnotherapists? Should we be more selective in whom we accept for training in this field?

How and to what extent should child hypnotherapists communicate their own imagery to patients? How should we foster and direct our own imaginative processes so as to be of maximal help to our patients?

Role of the Child in Hypnotherapy

We hope that, in future years, a more prescriptive approach to hypnotherapy will be seen. More than many people now recognize, the design of a hypnotherapeutic approach for a particular child patient must take into account such factors as age; developmental level; verbal and imaginal fluency; activity level and other temperamental variables; personality factors such as motivation; internal–external locus of control; mechanisms of coping and defense; needs and conflicts; anxiety level and the manner of its expression; physical strengths and disabilities. We must consider the child's role in the family, the school, and other social settings that have direct or indirect influences on treatment. We may find it important to measure a child's variations in handling of neurohumoral mediators such as enkephalins, serotonin, and catecholamines, before titering doses of hypnotherapy.

We already have some data suggesting that children respond differently to different kinds of hypnotic inductions. It is also likely that children respond differently to different kinds and amounts of hypnotherapeutic suggestions. Which children benefit most from direct suggestion? Which do better with more indirect, symbolic approaches? Which children need special emphasis on self-hypnosis? Which require more therapist contact? Which children do best with which therapists? Which children benefit most from treatment in groups and which from individual sessions?

When a child wants to master a problem, at what specific points is hypnotherapy likely to be helpful? For example, in a child with maladaptive anxiety regarding learning and performance, should we employ hypnotherapy before learning begins, during initial learning, during review of learned material, before performance, during performance, or at several of these points?

How can we predict these variations in response so that treatment programs can be designed more effectively and carried out with minimal cost of time and money?

ART AND SCIENCE

As answers to these questions and to others not yet raised are learned, we will become better able to employ child hypnotherapy in the scientific context of prescriptive treatment. The application of approaches found to have particular value will be expanded. Useless approaches will be eliminated. We will learn how best to combine hypnotherapy with other treatment modalities. We will question basic assumptions and define new problems.

Hypnotherapy will always involve art as well as science. Intuition and hunches will continue to be important. But we hope that scientific developments will lead to more creative and effective use of intuition.

Most of all, we hope that our synthesis of available observations and information will provide inspiration, clues, and nuggets for those who wish to expand the frontier of child hypnosis and hypnotherapy. The future involves a lot of hard work. It also contains the potential for excitement and satisfaction as we use our own skills to find better ways of allowing children to develop their potential to the fullest, to be all that they really are.

> *Piping down the valleys wild*
> *Piping songs of pleasant glee*
> *On a cloud I saw a child.*
> *And he laughing said to me.*
>
> *Pipe a song about a lamb;*
> *So I piped with merry chear,*
> *Piper pipe that song again—*
> *So I piped, he wept to hear.*
>
> [William Blake, 1788/1977]

REFERENCES

Blake, W. Songs of innocence and experience. In Ostriker, A. (Ed.), *William Blake: The complete poems.* New York: Penguin Books, 1977. (Originally published, 1788.)

Bronowski, J. *The ascent of man.* Boston: Little, Brown, 1974.

Feinstein, A. R. *Clinical biostatistics.* St. Louis: Mosby, 1977.

Frankel, F. H. *Hypnosis: Trance as a coping mechanism.* New York: Plenum, 1976.

Frankel, F. H. Reporting hypnosis in the medical context: A brief communication. *The International Journal of Clinical and Experimental Hypnosis,* 1981, *29,* 10–14.

Fromm, E. How to write a clinical paper: A brief communication. *The International Journal of Clinical and Experimental Hypnosis,* 1981, *29,* 5–9.

Fromm, E., & Shor, R. E. (Eds.). *Hypnosis: Developments in research and new perspectives* (2nd ed.). New York: Aldine, 1979.

Haber, R. N. Eidetic images are not just imaginary. *Psychology Today,* 1980, *14,* 72–82.

Hilgard, E. R. *Divided consciousness: Multiple controls in human thought and action.* New York: John Wiley & Sons, 1977.

Kazin, A. (Ed.). *The portable Blake.* New York: Viking Press, 1974.

London, P. *Children's Hypnotic Susceptibility Scale.* Palo Alto, Calif.: Consulting Psychologists Press, 1963.

McDonald, J., Hogan, M., & Olness, K. Self-hypnosis and voluntary control of brain-stem auditory evoked potentials in children. *Proceedings of the Ambulatory Pediatric Association,* 1981.

Morgan, A. H., & Hilgard, J. R. The Stanford Hypnotic Clinical Scale for Children. *The American Journal of Clinical Hypnosis,* 1979, *21,* 148–155.

Orne, M. T. The why and how of a contribution to the literature: A brief communication. *The International Journal of Clinical and Experimental Hypnosis,* 1981, *29,* 1–4.

Peterson, J. W. Extrasensory abilities of children: An ignored reality? *Learning,* 1975, *4,* 10–14.

Rutter, M. School influences on children's behavior and development. *Pediatrics,* 1980, *65,* 208–220.

Sarbin, T. R., & Slagle, R. W. Hypnosis and psychophysiological outcomes. In E. Fromm & R. E. Shor (Eds.), *Hypnosis: Developments in research and new perspectives* (2nd ed.). New York: Aldine, 1979.

Schwarz, B. E. *Parent–child telepathy: A study of the telepathy of everyday life.* New York: Garrett-Helix, 1970.

Sheehan, P. W. Hypnosis and the process of imagination. In E. Fromm & R. E. Shor (Eds.), *Hypnosis: Developments in research and new perspectives* (2nd ed.). New York: Aldine, 1979.

Siegler, M. Pascal's wager and the hanging of crepe. *The New England Journal of Medicine,* 1975, *293,* 853–857.

Wheeler, J. A. The universe as home for man. *American Scientist,* 1974, *62,* 683–691.

Appendix A

Children's Hypnotic Susceptibility Scale

Perry London, Ph.D.

GENERAL INSTRUCTIONS

The ability of experimenters or practitioners to make effective use of the Children's Hypnotic Susceptibility Scale depends more on the ease with which they establish effective relationships with children than upon any experience they may have had in the use of hypnosis. The scale has been constructed as an individual psychological test for children which incorporates sufficient flexibility within its standard procedures to approximate the experiences contained in many conventional clinical hypnosis sessions. Examiners who have training and experience both in the administration of individual psychological tests such as the Stanford-Binet or Wechsler Intelligence Scale for Children and in the use of hypnotic techniques are thus ideally prepared to administer the Children's Hypnotic Susceptibility Scale. But neither of these skills is adequate substitute for a sensitive appreciation of the needs and concerns with which children of all ages may approach an

Reprinted from *The Children's Hypnotic Susceptibility Scale* by P. London, Palo Alto, Ca.: Consulting Psychologists Press, Inc., 1963. Copyright © 1962 by Perry London. With permission.

unfamiliar situation like a test, or a readiness to respond helpfully to the sometimes subtle communications of discomfiture or embarrassment that children may convey by word or gesture in the course of testing. It is as nearly impossible to overstate the importance of getting and keeping good rapport in testing children as it is to overstate the importance of adhering to standard test procedures. Serious or persistent violation of either rule will invalidate the test results.

In training personnel to administer the Children's Scale, we have encountered two characteristic misconceptions on the part of novice examiners which tend to interfere with their performance:

1. Some examiners attempt to induce very profound trances at the expense of standard procedure.
2. Some examiners adhere to the procedure with almost senseless rigidity, disregarding significant features of a child's behavior.

1. The purpose of the Children's Scale, like that of the Stanford Hypnotic Susceptibility Scale from which it derives, is to discover the extent to which a child will respond to hypnotic suggestions which are made in an entirely standard way and which permit a standard means for evaluating responses. The Children's Scale is thus a test of *typical* performance rather than one of *maximum* performance. Used properly, it should give reliable information about how susceptible a child is to attempts at hypnotic induction under certain typical conditions, *not* how susceptible he is to the application of a maximum effort at induction. Maximum effort with children may indeed produce a very deceptive test result, for young children in particular are likely to sense a coercive urgency in the examiner's voice or manner and, accustomed to responding with docility to the wishes of adult authority, may produce those responses which they think are being demanded of them without in fact being hypnotized. The text of the scale itself contains sufficient repetitive and insistent wordings in appropriate places to permit examiners to conscientiously attempt induction without either improving or adding to the wording or communicating it with undue vehemence.

2. Children, like living organisms in general and human beings in particular, are highly variable in ways that cannot always be predicted in advance. The variations in the text of the scale, such as alternate wordings or procedures, are attempts to provide the examiner with suitable standard responses to the many situations for which it *is* possible to predict much variation among different children. In general, alternative wordings have been designed with the intent of protecting children against a disappointing feeling of failure, a feeling of humiliation at being patronized, or a feeling that they are being sub-

jected to an absurd and senseless experience. The entire Older Form (ages 13 years, 0 months to 16 years, 11 months) differs from the Younger Form only with respect to some wordings which have been "upgraded" because of complaints from adolescent subjects in our laboratory that some of the language was infantile.

But not all exigencies of response can be foreseen or treated within the regular scale instructions. While competent administration requires careful advance study and knowledge of the scale, and close adherence to it, it also may require occasional ingenuity or at least a degree of common sense not included in writing.

Many young children, for example, do not like to leave their eyes closed for any length of time. If they pop open, the examiner should calmly interrupt himself long enough to instruct the child to close his eyes again and keep them closed. While this differs from the prescribed routine somewhat, it is much less serious than the disturbance of procedure which may otherwise occur. The Eye Catalepsy item (No. 10), for example, cannot be administered at all if the child's eyes are open when it is begun!

Another situation which requires slight divergence from the written instructions is that in which literal adherence becomes absurd. On the Taste Hallucination item (No. 17), for example, an occasional child will put the stick in his mouth as per instructions, respond affirmatively to the question, "Is it good?" and then, to the question, "What does it taste like; what flavor?" will say, "It tastes like wood!" Now the standard instruction assumes that the response will have been "grape" or "orange" or some such, and continues, "Oh, _____. Well, go ahead and lick it all up." Such a procedure is absurd in this case, and it is more reasonable to assume that the "wood" response is a cue for the examiner to switch to the standard script for handling *negative* responses to this item, which reads, "That's all right. . . . Sometimes it is kind of hard to taste things."

The possibilities for such surprises as the foregoing are very many, and it is no more possible to specify all the good and bad ways of handling them than to identify all the forms they may take. Perhaps a good rule of thumb might be to think of the entire test situation as a kind of game between examiner and child in which the examiner makes a serious but good-natured attempt to hypnotize the child, relying for his procedures and wordings on a prepared script. Since the child does not know the script and may not, in any case, wish to be bound by it, his responses may occasionally force the examiner to depart from it. In such cases, the examiner should respond in a courteous, reasonable way that departs from his script as little as possible and that permits him to return to it as soon as possible.

Physical Arrangements

Our laboratory arrangements have been generally similar to those used in the standardization of the Stanford Hypnotic Susceptibility Scale, i.e., we have hypnotized children seated in an easy chair in a small room furnished like an office. The hypnotist is seated at a type-writer table near the child and on his left, so that the table, etc. are just outside the line of vision. Floor lamps are the main source of light. In our laboratory, the child sits half facing a large mirror which is, in fact, a one-way vision screen through which he may be observed by parents and examiners. When seated, he cannot see in the mirror, however, without actually turning his head to the side.

While an easy chair is not necessary, it is important to use a chair with arms for administering the scale, as the Eye Closure item (No. 2) requires that the child's elbow be supported for several minutes. Floor lamps are generally preferable to overhead lighting as they give off less glare. Excessive noise and drafts from fans or windows should be avoided as undesirable distractions. Undisturbed and pleasant sur-roundings are obviously most conducive to a relaxed and enjoyable experience.

Test Materials

In addition to the text of the scale, some easily obtained materials are needed:

1. Stopwatch, timer, or watch with sweep-second hand. Many items are timed.
2. Chevreul pendulum, or other bright metal or glass object sus-pended from one-foot chain; used for Eye Closure (No. 2) and Arm Lowering (No. 3) items.
3. A pin, sharp stylus, or well-sharpened hard lead pencil; used for Anesthesia (No. 16).
4. Tongue depressors; used for Cold Hallucination (No. 15), Anes-thesia (No. 16), and Taste Hallucination (No. 17).
5. A small bottle with a screw cap, containing a very mildly offensive liquid; used for Smell Hallucination (No. 18). We have successfully experimented with a number of odoriferous materials for this item. The most suitable, an insect skin repellant, is no longer manufactured. Other satisfactory compounds include tincture of Valerian and *dilute* household ammonia. The general principle which has guided our use of a smelly substance has been that it should be mild enough so that slight inhalation would produce no reaction or could easily be misinterpreted as pleasant, while

strong inhalation should reveal it as distinctly unpleasant to most people without being startling to them.
6. Writing pencils and a pad of 8½ × 11 inch unlined paper. Used for Regression (No. 20).

Preparing Subjects

In our laboratory, parents were asked to prepare their children for the test session by explaining the nature of the experiment in language appropriate to the age and understanding of the child. We have found that remarks such as those contained in the Establishing Rapport section of the scale are quite suitable for this purpose. It is probably more important for children to receive advance preparation when they are to be hypnotized for scientific purposes than when the scale is to be used clinically, as they may otherwise find the former situation bewildering. We have routinely prepared the parents themselves, in the course of arranging appointments by telephone, by describing several scale items to them and suggesting specific information which could be usefully communicated to the children. Telephoning appointment schedules offers a particularly good opportunity for answering parents' questions and clarifying misconceptions or allaying concerns they may have about hypnosis.

Test Procedure

Several minutes should be devoted to putting the subject at ease before beginning the scale proper with item 1, Postural Sway. The Preliminary Tests and Establishing Rapport sections are intended to orient the subject towards the test situation and familiarize him with the examiner. They can be suitably conducted in the examination room with the subject seated in the examining chair and the experimenter beside him, and they should be conducted in a relaxed, unhurried manner, leading naturally into the first item. The items are then administered consecutively.

The scale has been divided into two parts in order to provide a breather for the participants and to allow the experimenter to abbreviate the proceeding, should he wish to do so, without embarrassing himself or the subject. Termination may be advisable if a child has been generally unresponsive to Part I. The twelve items of Part I parallel the Stanford Hypnotic Susceptibility Scale, and require about 20 minutes for administration. Part II contains 10 items which require about 30 additional minutes for administration and is dependent upon

Part I in the sense that it begins with the reinduction of hypnosis by a posthypnotic signal issued at the end of Part I.

In composing items, we made some attempt to provide continuity from one item to another. In Part I, items 2 and 3 (Eye Closure and Hand Lowering) are connected by references to the Chevreul Pendulum, and item 4 (Arm Immobilization) is further associated with item 3 by reference to the feeling of heaviness which had previously been suggested for that arm. In Part II, item 15 (Cold Hallucination) begins with a reference to the television set of item 14, and item 18 (Smell Hallucination) ends with a similar reference. Items 15 (Cold), 16 (Anesthesia), and 17 (Taste Hallucination) are all administered as a unit which centers around the image of a cold popsicle, and item 18 (Smell) begins with a reference to the popsicle's lack of odor.

The purpose of these continuities is to facilitate the smooth administration of the Scale with minimum risk of boring children or trying their patience. Though the great majority of children remain fascinated throughout the proceedings, and quite unaware of the passage of time, the complete Scale administration often requires a full hour, which may particularly tax very young children as well as those older children who are relatively unsusceptible. Connected items are not meant to be dependent upon one another, however; they are all scored independently, and the administration of any one is not contingent on the child's having responded favorably to the previous suggestion. Provision is made within the standard script, moreover, for omitting or altering such references to earlier items as would be incongruous with the observed performance.

Recording and Scoring Responses

Each item of the Children's Scale may be scored either in terms of a simple dichotomy of pass (+) or fail (−) or along a 4-point continuum (0–1–2–3) which provides a somewhat more refined index of the child's responses. The dichotomous scoring is intended to be comparable to that employed on the Stanford Hypnotic Susceptibility Scale, though the criteria for each item were developed independently on a pilot sample of children. It is recommended that examiners regularly record performances on 4-point continuum, however, since this can readily be collapsed to dichotomous scoring if desired, whereas dichotomous scores cannot be expanded to 4-point scores. In either case, a high (2 or 3) or pass (+) score indicates that a child responded to a particular suggestion in a fashion consistent with what might be expected from a hypnotized person, while a low (0 or 1) or fail (−) score represents inadequate compliance with suggestion.* Since the 22 items of the Scale sample a very wide variety of common hypnotic phenomena, it is felt that a reasonable approximation of a child's hypnotic susceptibility is obtained simply by summing his favorable responses. Total susceptibility score, therefore, is the sum of scores for the individual items. When dichotomous scoring is used, pass (+) items are scored 1 and fail (−) items are scored 0.

A scoring key is provided for the entire Scale, but the user must carefully note that it is sometimes exemplary rather than comprehensive and precise, particularly with respect to evaluating responses in Part II. Most items of Part II, like item 12 (Amnesia) of Part I, must be judged more in terms of verbalizations that the child does or does not make than in terms of any very concrete set of overt behaviors. Even when a suggested sequence involves a combination of motor and verbal responses, as in the case of most Part II items, the verbal part of the response must generally be given priority for judging success or failure so long as the motor response does not clearly contradict it. If a child says he smells perfume, for example, when we suggest that he do so, we must accept his report as valid no matter what else he does, provided only that he not contort his face in disgust, hold his nostrils closed, etc. A certain amount of experience in administering and scoring the Scale is necessary before one can feel confident in diverging from the literal dicta of the key, but the very high interscorer and retest reliabilities obtained in our experiments from relatively inexperienced examiners make it clear that this can be done without violence to the test norms.†

Those items whose performance depends on relatively simple motor responses can be scored with confidence immediately upon completion, but this is not always the case with items requiring much verbalization, especially considering that what constitute good verbal

---

*The scoring system described here measures only one aspect of compliance to hypnotic suggestions, i.e., motor or verbal behaviors which are overtly like those of a hypnotized person. They take no account of the fact that a subject can easily perform these acts without in fact being hypnotized, or that two subjects giving the same overt responses may be experiencing radically different feelings. A series of studies is currently in progress for assessing the relationship between a subject's overt behavior and his subjective involvement in the hypnotic experience, but adequate means for assessing the latter and satisfactorily quantifying it for use as part of the Scale's scoring procedure have not been sufficiently demonstrated at this time (1962). A report of preliminary work in this direction is contained in "Hypnosis in Children: An Experimental Approach" by P. London, International Journal of Clinical and Experimental Hypnosis, 1962, 10, 79–91.

†P. London. Hypnosis in Children: An Experimental Approach. International Journal of Clinical and Experimental Hypnosis, 1962, 10, p. 84.

responses will vary somewhat depending on the age and intelligence of the child. Since the latter must be kept in mind when the item is scored, and reasonable allowance made for the different expectations one may have of the verbal skills of a 5-year-old and an adolescent, *verbatim recording* of items such as 12 (Amnesia) and 21 (Dream) is indispensable. It may also be very helpful to record appropriate details of verbalizations to items like 14 (Television Hallucination), 17 (Taste Hallucination), 19 (Rabbit Hallucination), and 20 (Age Regression). In general, the examiner should record all those comments and remarks of the child which can make anecdotal contributions to an understanding of the dynamics of his behavior as well as those which are required to score his performance. A sample form for recording scores and observations of the child's performance is presented on pp. 332–339.

Normative Data

At this writing (1962), the present form of the Children's Hypnotic Susceptibility Scale has been administered in standard fashion to over 250 children of both sexes within the age range for which the test was developed; data collection is still in process. Information from pilot studies clearly indicates that the scale is sufficiently reliable to warrant publication. Norms will be reported at the earliest possible date. By making the Scale available at this time, we hope to encourage other investigators of hypnosis in children to employ standard procedures for their investigations and to facilitate the comparison of results obtained in investigations conducted at many different laboratories.

YOUNGER FORM (AGES 5–12), PART I

Preliminary Tests

The following form of the Goodenough Draw-A-Man-Test is routinely administered prior to the scale, since it is particularly useful for judging the effectiveness of the Age Regression item of the scale.*

Note: *The text for the Younger Form contains both italicized and nonitalicized material. The sentences in italic type are instructions to the experimenter (E). Those in roman type are verbal instructions to the subject (S). Alternate wordings for instructions to older children (ages 8–12) are enclosed in square brackets.*

*Although the Goodenough test is primarily designed for estimating the intelligence of young children, we have limited its use in our studies of the Children's Scale to assessing Age Regression and have preferred to rely on the Vocabulary Subtest of the Wechsler Intelligence Scale for Children for a relatively rapid and valid estimate of intelligence.

To start off, I'd like you to take this pencil and put your name on the top of this paper. *Hand child pencil and a single sheet of typewriter-size blank paper. Note dominant hand.*

That's fine. Now, draw a picture of a man. *Cue, if necessary:* Draw the whole man, draw all of him. *If child objects, insist gently, or in the case of a girl, suggest picture of a lady.*

Establishing Rapport (Ages 5–7)

After drawings are completed, E makes the following remarks, which should be memorized or paraphrased.

You must be wondering what we're going to do here. Well, we're going to play a kind of game. It is called hypnotism, and I'll tell you how it works. Have you ever heard about hypnotism? *Note remarks.* I'm going to ask you to think of some different things and to do some things, and we will see how good an imagination you have. It is fun to do, and you have probably never done anything just like the things I'm going to tell you about. So let's see how good you can be at this.

After a while, I'll tell you to get very comfortable and relaxed, just like you were all ready to go to sleep, and then I want you to try not to think about anything but what I tell you. As I tell you to do different things, you will want to do them, and they will happen very easily.

When I do this with other boys and girls, it often makes them feel very good and happy. All I want you to do is to listen very carefully to me and just see what happens. It should be fun for you, so pay close attention, and we'll start right now.

Establishing Rapport (Ages 8–12)

You must be wondering just what we are going to do here. Well, this is an experiment in science, and it is about hypnotism. Do you know what that is? *Record child's impressions and previous experiences.* What we are going to do is this: I am going to ask you to think about some different things which I will describe and to do some things, and we will see how good your imagination is. You probably have never before done anything exactly like this, so pay very close attention to what I say, and let's see how well you can do this. You will find that it is fun to do.

Ask for questions. Avoid direct answers to questions asking for details of the hypnotic procedure.

Would you like me to tell you why we are doing this experiment? Well, hypnosis is something that doctors use a lot nowadays to help sick people with their troubles. By coming here today and doing these things with me, you are helping science learn more about it, and that will make it possible for us to give more help to people who are sick or troubled.

All I want you to do is listen very carefully to me and just see what happens. I think you will enjoy it a lot—so pay close attention, and let's start now.

1. Postural Sway

To start off, I want you to see what it's like to think real hard of [concentrate on] the things I tell you about and try to do them.

1.   So stand up right here with your back to me and I'll show you something. First, stand very straight, with your feet together and your hands at your sides. That's fine. Now just close your eyes, that's it— and with your eyes closed, I want you to see a picture of yourself [imagine yourself] on a swing. You've been on a swing before, and you know just what it feels like to go back and forth on one. If you think real hard about that picture, then soon you will really start to swing yourself. When the swing goes up and back, you can feel yourself bending with it, and when it goes forward, you just bend again with it. Let me show you how it will be.

Grasp S by the shoulders and push gently forward and backward several times to set in motion. Once swaying starts, take a position which will break child's fall in either forward or backward direction. Do not touch child until after a definite loss of balance has occurred.

2.   As you think about that, you really will bend back and forth, back and forth. You'll go back and forth so much that you'll finally tip over backwards—and when that happens, just let yourself tip backwards, and I'll catch you so you won't fall down.

3.   Think about being on a swing, going back and forth, back and forth—that's fine, you're really starting to swing, more and more, swinging and swinging, back and forth, a little more backwards everytime, swinging, swinging, more and more, further and further. . . .

4.   You're swinging further and further backwards, swinging and swaying, going backwards, going backwards, going backwards, . . . you're going, going . . . falling back, falling back, all the way backwards, all the way backwards . . . tipping over, tipping over, tipping over . . . TIP OVER!

If fall occurs

If no fall occurs

That's fine. Now you see how thinking about being on a swing makes you feel like you really are on one. Now we're going to do that again, only this time I want you to think even harder about it until you really go all the way over backwards. Think about being on a swing, and . . .
Repeat paragraphs 2, 3, and 4. If S still fails, induce a voluntary fall.

That's fine. Now you see how thinking about doing something makes you feel like you really are doing it.

Seat S in the chair again and record the score.

2. Eye Closure

Use Chevreul pendulum. Take it out of case, hold it by the end of the chain, and swing it in front of child.

1.   Look at this ball on the chain, _____. See the way it swings when I hold it like this. Even if I hold the chain very still, the ball keeps on swinging all the time. Here, you try it now. Hold your arm like this and hold the end of the chain. *Take left arm, prop elbow on chair arm, with forearm at right angles to upper arm, and place end of chain in hand so ball swings freely. Have S lean back in chair if it can be done comfortably.* Now, look at [concentrate on] the ball very hard and see if you can keep it from moving. Pay close attention to it, and hold your arm very still, so it won't move at all. Keep right on looking at the ball all the time, and while you do, just keep on listening to me. Don't pay attention to anything else but the way the ball looks and the things that I say to you. Don't pay attention to anything but the ball and the sound of my voice.

The remainder of this section should be read quite slowly in an even tone. If eyes close at any time, finish the sentence and turn to the corresponding paragraph of 2A, continuing through the end of the section.

2.   To play this game [To be hypnotized], all you need to do is keep looking at the ball and listening to my voice. And while you do that, you will start to feel very nice, and warm, and comfortable—and

you will even get a little bit sleepy. Pretty soon your eyes will get tired, and you will feel like closing them. When that happens, just let it happen. It will be all right. The ball may look a little bit funny sometimes; it might get hard to see it very clearly. And your eyes will get so tired they will just feel like closing all by themselves. When that happens, just let them close, and you can go on looking at the ball in your mind even with your eyes closed.

3. It feels so nice to just sit there and relax and listen to my voice. . . . It feels very warm and good and pleasant, like it feels when you have been playing real hard on a hot day and just flop down on the grass to rest in the shade. . . . It is such a nice tired feeling, it makes you feel all good inside. . . . You feel so nice all over, and your eyes are getting so heavy. . . . They feel like somebody is just pushing them slowly shut, like they can't help closing all by themselves, closing all by themselves.

4. You start to feel so drowsy and sleepy, so nice and tired and sleepy, like you are all relaxed and want to sleep, all warm and comfortable. . . . You feel so good and so nice. . . . It is so pleasant to listen to my voice and to pay attention just to my voice and not to listen to anything else. . . . It makes you feel so quiet and good and drowsy and sleepy to listen to my voice . . . very drowsy, very sleepy . . . sleepy, sleepy, sleepy.

5. Your eyes are getting heavy, so very heavy. You feel tired and good, very good, and there is such a nice feeling of being warm and sleepy all over. You are tired and drowsy. Tired and sleepy. Sleepy. Sleepy. Just listen to my voice. Don't pay attention to anything else but my voice. Your eyelids are very heavy, and they are feeling heavier and heavier, just like something was pressing them shut. Your eyes are tired and blinking, blinking, blinking . . . closing, closing . . . closing.

If eyes have not closed voluntarily within 10 seconds after this point, item has been failed.

> *If eyes have not yet closed*
> Soon your eyes would close by themselves, but you don't need to wait any longer. You have been listening carefully to me and paying attention to the ball. Now you are comfortable and drowsy, and you may just let your eyes close. *If no response:* That's it, now close them.

As soon as eyes close: Now just leave your eyes closed until I tell you to open them or to wake up, and keep right on like you were still looking at the little ball only with your eyes closed.

Record score.

2A. Eye Closure

This item is for those who close their eyes before completion of item 2, paragraph 5. As soon as eyes close, terminate sentence appropriately, then:

1a.   You feel very relaxed and good, tired and drowsy, but you are going to get even more tired and drowsy. Your eyes are closed now. Just leave your eyes closed until I tell you to open them or to wake up, and keep right on like you were still looking at the little ball, only with your eyes closed.

Resume reading at the appropriate place and continue the Scale. Should eyes reopen, instruct S to close them.

2a.   And while you do that, keep on listening to my voice, and soon you will start to feel very nice, and warm, and comfortable—and you will even get more sleepy, so that sometimes my voice will sound like it is part of a dream. That will be all right. You will still be able to hear me and pay attention to the things I say, even though it may feel like you are dreaming. Whatever happens, just let it happen and go on getting more and more sleepy, more and more drowsy, while you keep on listening to my voice and watching the picture of the little ball in your mind, even with your eyes closed.

3a.   It feels so nice to just sit there and relax and listen to my voice. . . . It feels very warm and good and pleasant, like it feels when you have been playing real hard on a hot day and just flop down on the grass to rest in the shade. . . . It is such a nice tired feeling, it makes you feel all good inside. . . . You feel so nice all over, and you are getting very sleepy. . . . You are going more and more deeply asleep, into a soft pleasant sleep where this good feeling grows better and better.

4a.   You are feeling so drowsy and sleepy, so nice and tired and sleepy, like you are all relaxed and want to sleep, all warm and comfortable. . . . You feel so good and so nice. . . . It is so pleasant to listen to my voice and to pay attention just to my voice and not to listen to anything else. . . . It makes you feel so quiet and drowsy and sleepy to listen to my voice . . . very drowsy, very sleepy . . . sleepy, sleepy, sleepy.

5a.   You feel as if you are in a nice bed, very nice and soft. You feel tired and good, very good, and there is such a nice feeling of being warm and sleepy all over. You are tired and drowsy. Tired and

sleepy. Sleepy. Sleepy. Just listen to my voice. Don't pay attention to
anything else but my voice. My voice sounds like it is coming to you
in a dream, and listening to it puts you in a deep, deep, sleep. But
you will always keep on hearing my voice no matter how sleepy you
feel you are.

6 and 6a.   You feel nice and drowsy and sleepy while you keep
on listening to my voice. Just keep listening to what I am saying. Soon
you will be fast asleep, but you will still hear what I say. And don't
wake up until I tell you to. I'm going to count from one to ten, and
every time I count you will get more and more sleepy, but you will
still be able to do all the things I ask you to do. *Stroke forehead lightly.*
One . . . two . . . deep asleep, deeper and deeper . . . three . . .
four . . . more and more asleep . . . five . . . six . . . seven . . . fast
asleep, feeling warm and good . . . eight. . . . Just keep listening to
me and the things I tell you to think of . . . nine . . . ten . . . DEEP
ASLEEP! Do not wake up until I tell you to. Stay deep asleep and
listen to the things I talk about.

3.   Hand Lowering (Left)

*If hand has already dropped, raise arm into position again, saying, Lift
up your arm again.*

Now that you're so comfortable and drowsy, you start to notice
something interesting happen. While you hold the chain with the ball
at the end of it, it starts to get heavy. And it gets heavier and heavier,
so that you want to drop the ball. It is getting much too heavy to hold
on to. *Put hand under ball to catch it.* It just is getting so heavy it's too
heavy to hold, you can just let it go. It's much too heavy to hold onto,
and you can just let it go.

If chain is not released soon, gently take it from child's hand.

And now your arm is getting heavy, too, just like something was
pulling it down. It starts going down, a little bit down, more and more
down . . . further and further . . . so heavy . . . so very heavy.
. . . It just goes down all by itself, all by itself, further and further
down, till it comes to rest all by itself. *Wait 10 seconds.*

If hand doesn't lower

That's fine. Now you can put
your arm down all the way. You
saw how hard it was to hold it
up. Now just let it lie there, so
heavy.

When all the way down

That's good. . . . Now just let
your hand lie there and rest, but
it still feels heavy to you.

Record score.

4. Arm Immobilization (Left)

And now I want you to keep paying attention to this arm some
more—*stroke child's left arm*—because it feels very heavy now . . .
heavier and heavier. . . . It feels just like it is being pressed against
the arm of the chair, it's so heavy. . . . And it keeps pressing against
the chair, so very heavy, that it feels like you can't lift it. Maybe it's
just too heavy to lift now, maybe that is just too hard to do now that
it's so heavy. Why don't you see how heavy it is? . . . Just try to lift
your hand up, just try. *Wait 7 seconds.*

If hand does not lift	*If hand lifts*
	That's fine. . . . You can put your arm back down again. You see how hard it was for you to lift it—much harder than it usually is. Now you can just relax again and feel nice and sleepy some more.
That's fine. . . . Stop trying. . . . Your hand and arm don't feel heavy any more. You can lift it now. . . . Go ahead and lift it up a little. Now just relax again and feel all nice and sleepy.	

Record score.

5. Finger Lock

Now let's do something else. Put your fingers together, lock them
together. *Take child's hands and position correctly.* That's it. Now press
your hands tightly together. Make them get tighter and tighter . . .
very tight. . . . Make them so tight that you can't take them apart.
Lock them together, tightly together, very tight. Now just try to take
them apart when they are locked up so tight together, just try. . . .
Wait 5 seconds.

If not taken apart   *If taken apart*

All right, now just relax your
hands again. See how hard it was
to pull them apart? But they
aren't tight any more now. You
can just relax again, very
comfortably, very deeply.

Stop trying now. . . . They'll
come apart right away, they
won't stay tight together any
more. That's it, take them apart
and just relax.

Record score.

6. Arm Rigidity (Right)

Now hold this arm straight out—*take child's right arm*—and the
fingers straight out too. That's it, your arm straight out. *Stroke once
down entire arm.* Now think about your arm getting very stiff and
straight, very, very stiff. . . . Think about it like you were a tree and
your arm was a branch of the tree, very straight and very stiff and
strong, so it couldn't bend no matter how hard it got pushed . . . as
stiff and strong as a branch of a tree, very straight and stiff . . . so
stiff that you can't bend it. . . . That's right. . . . Now see if you have
made it stiff enough. . . . Try and bend it. . . . Try. . . . *Wait 5
seconds.*

If arm does not bend   *If arm bends*

That's all right. See how hard it
was for you to bend your arm?
But it isn't stiff any more. You
can just put it back the way it was
and relax. That's right, just relax.

There, that's enough now. . . .
Just relax. . . . Don't try to bend
your arm any more and don't
make it like a tree branch any
more. . . . It isn't stiff now, and
you can just let it go back on your
lap—*or the chair arm, whichever is
appropriate.*

Record score.

7. Hands Together

Now put your hands out in front of you just like you were going to start clapping. Here, I'll show you how. *Place child's hands about a foot apart, palms inward.* That's right. Now I want you to imagine that there is a big rubber band around your hands, a big rubber band stretched out around your hands. . . . And it is pulling them together, pulling them together. . . . And when you think about that, your hands will start coming together just like a rubber band was around them . . . pulling them together, closer and closer . . . slowly at first, but they come closer together, closer . . . moving . . . moving . . . closer and closer. . . . *Wait 5 seconds.*

If hands have touched	*If hands have not touched*
	That's fine. They've come very close together. Let me show you how near they are to touching. *Move S's hands together fairly rapidly.* That's fine. Now just let them relax on your lap—*or chair arm*—and get very comfortable again.
That's fine. All right, now just let your hands relax and get very comfortable again.	

Record score.

8. Verbal Inhibition (Name)

You feel very good and relaxed now, very comfortable and warm and sleepy and drowsy. And when you're all sleepy like that, all you want to do is just sit back and listen. . . . You don't feel like doing anything else. . . . You don't even want to talk, just listen quietly to my voice. . . . It is just too much trouble to talk. . . . So if I asked you now to tell me your name, you probably couldn't even do it. . . . It would just be too much trouble because it is so nice just to listen and not do anything else. . . . Just try now to tell me your name and see how hard it is. . . . Just try. *Wait 10 seconds.*

If name spoken

There, you did it. . . . It was a lot of trouble, but you did it anyway even though it was harder than it

If name not spoken

>   usually is. That's fine. . . . Now
>   just relax.

Don't try anymore. . . . That's it.
. . . Stop trying. . . . You can
say your name now easily. . . .
Say it, go ahead. . . . Good. . . .
Now just get all sleepy and
relaxed again.

>   *Record score.*

9. Auditory Hallucination (Fly)

You have been listening very well to me, paying close attention. You haven't been listening to anything but my voice, but now I want you to listen to another thing. There has been a fly buzzing around you, going buzzzzzz the way flies do. You can hear it now as it flies right around your left hand. *Touch hand.* It's landing right on your hand. . . . Maybe it tickles a little. . . . There it flies away again. . . . You hear it buzz. . . . It's back on your hand tickling. . . . You don't like that old fly. . . . You'd like to get rid of it. . . . Go ahead, brush it off. . . . Get rid of it if it bothers you. . . . *Wait 10 seconds.*

There it's gone now. . . . That's good. . . . It doesn't bother you now. . . . It's all gone and disappeared. . . . Now relax, and feel all comfortable again.

>   *If no response*
>   The fly is gone now, so you won't
>   hear it. Now relax and feel all
>   comfortable again.
>   *Record score.*

10. Eye Catalepsy

You have had your eyes closed for a long time while you stayed comfortable and sleepy. By now, your eyes are very tightly closed, tightly shut. . . . If you tried to open them now, they probably would feel just like they were stuck together with glue . . . tightly glued shut. . . . Maybe, pretty soon, you'd like to try to open your eyes even though they feel so heavy and so completely, so tightly glued shut. Go ahead. . . . Try to open your eyes. *Wait 10 seconds.*

If eyes remain shut	*If eyes open*
	That's fine. You see how hard it was to try and open your eyes. But now you can shut them again and you can relax and be comfortable again.
Now relax. . . . Stop trying to open your eyes. They feel all right again, they aren't stuck, but just keep them closed and get all comfortable again.	

Record score.

Conclusion Part I
Introduction Part II

At this point, the experimenter has the alternatives of either introducing the second part of the Scale or terminating the entire proceeding. Except for experimental purposes, it may be unwise to continue with Part II unless the child has passed five or more items in Part I and/or shown considerable clinical indications of having experienced hypnosis.

If test is to be continued	*If test is to be terminated*
	Now, in just a little while, after you have relaxed a little bit longer, I am going to wake you up very slowly and we will end this session. When we do, you will feel like you have just finished a nice sleep, and then . . . *Conclude with items 11 and 12.*
Now we are going to do some things that are different from the ones we've been doing. I'm going to show you some things that are really interesting—and you're really going to have a good time with them. But before we start that . . .	

11.   Posthypnotic Suggestion (and Amnesia)

I want you to forget all about the things that we've been doing and not to pay attention to them anymore. In a minute, I am going to count backwards from ten to one, and you are going to wake up a little bit at a time. When I say five, your eyes will open, and when I get to one, you will be wide awake. You'll feel real good, just like you had a nice sleep, and you won't remember all the things we did because it will be too much trouble. Later on, I'll tell you that you CAN remember everything, and THEN YOU WILL REMEMBER.

Now when I say one, you'll be wide awake, and you'll stand right up and stretch your arms out wide, but you won't remember that I said to.

If test is to be continued	*If test is to be terminated*
	Ready now, ten—nine—eight—seven—six—five—four—three—two—one.
Then we'll talk a while, and after that, I'll clap my hands two times—when you hear me clap, you'll get all sleepy and drowsy again and your eyes will close, and then we'll start doing some more things. Ready now, ten—nine—eight—seven—six—five—four—three—two—one.	
If eyes open	*If eyes remain closed*
	Wake up! Wide awake! How do you feel?
How do you feel? Wide awake?	

Wait 10 seconds. If child does not stand: Now stand up and stretch so you'll be wide awake. That's fine. Now sit down again. I want to ask you some questions.

Record score.

12. Amnesia

Now, please tell me all about the different things that we've been doing, and what's been happening since you came in here.

Record verbatim. When child stops reporting: That's fine. Now listen to me very carefully—NOW YOU CAN REMEMBER EVERYTHING. Anything else now . . . that's fine.

Part I Ends Here

YOUNGER FORM, PART II

13. Posthypnotic Suggestion (Reinduction)

Clap hands twice sharply. Wait 10 seconds.

If eyes close	*If eyes do not close*
	Now just let your eyes close again, and let them stay closed till I tell you to open them or I tell you to wake up.
That's it. . . . Now just leave your eyes closed until I tell you to open them or to wake up.	

Record score.

After eyes are closed: You can remember now how you felt before when you were like this . . . all sleepy and comfortable, kind of drowsy and relaxed . . . feeling all good inside, nice and warm and comfortable and pleasant. It gives you such a good feeling to just sit there and listen quietly to my voice . . . to pay attention only to what I am saying and not to listen to anything else. . . . It makes you feel all quiet and kind of tired . . . and a little bit sleepy, and drowsy. . . .

Just keep listening to my voice and to what I am saying. . . . Pretty soon it will put you fast asleep, but you'll still hear what I say. . . . And later on, we'll talk to each other, and you'll be able to stay fast asleep but talk to me at the same time. . . . It will be very easy for you to do, to just stay all relaxed and sleepy but to talk to me when I ask you to. I'm going to count from one to ten, and every time I count you will get more and more sleepy, but you will still be able to do all the things I ask you to do. One . . . two . . . deep asleep, deeper and deeper . . . three . . . four . . . more and more asleep . . . five . . . six . . . seven . . . fast asleep, feeling warm and good . . . eight . . . nine . . . ten . . . DEEP ASLEEP! And stay deep asleep, all relaxed and comfortable, all the time that we do these different things.

14. Visual and Auditory Hallucination (Television)

Tell me, do you ever watch TV? What shows do you like best? *If S does not specify some program, suggest Disneyland, Huckleberry Hound, or any popular network children's program.* Oh, ＿＿! Well, that's fine.

Now, if you could watch any program you chose, which one would you like to see right now? Well, you CAN see it if you really want to, and I'll tell you how. When I count to three, I want you to see a TV set standing right in front of you. Then, when I tell you, you can turn it on and then you can watch _____ (*name of program*). Ready? one—two—three. Look at the set now. Do you see it?

If yes	*If no*
	That's all right—sometimes it takes a while to catch on to how to do this. So just wait a little while, and I think you'll start to see it pretty soon. *Wait 5 seconds.* There, are you starting to see the TV set now?
Why don't you turn it on? They're going to show _____. Is it on? Do you see it now? Is the picture clear? (Why don't you fix it?)	*If yes*
	If still no
	All right. I'm going to count to three again, and when I reach three, you're going to remember some program of _____ that you've seen before. And it will be so clear, that you'll even see and hear the whole program, and the music and everything. Okay now, one—two—three. Do you remember?
What's happening? Can you hear the program? Is it loud enough? Tell me about it. . . . All right, now you can watch the rest of the program while I do some other things.	*If yes*
	If still no
	That's okay. We'll find some other things you can do now. Just forget all about the TV. There isn't any there. Just relax and keep listening to my voice.

Record score.

If child responded positively to TV: Now I bet you like to eat a little snack when you're watching TV.

15. Cold Hallucination

Do you like popsicles? *If no, try ice cream bars.* What flavor do you like? Well, you can have a nice icy cold _____ flavored popsicle right now. Now you think real hard about what a popsicle is like, so cold and hard, and I'm going to put one in your hand, only it will be up-side down so the icy part will be in your hand. When you hold it a little while, your hand will start to feel cold. Later on, I'll tell you that you can eat the popsicle . . . okay?

Place tongue depressor in hand, close child's palm around it. Observe temperature of back of hand.

There now, do you feel how cold and hard the popsicle is? Pretty soon, it will feel so cold that it will make your hand get cold too. As you hold it longer, your hand will feel colder and colder. It may get so cold that you cannot hold on to it any more. Does it feel cold now? *Feel hand and note any apparent temperature change.*

If yes	*If no*
	Well, you just hold it a little bit longer. You know how cold ice in your hand feels, don't you? Well, this feels just like ice—so hard and cold. Does your hand feel very cold now?
Fine. It's going to get so cold that pretty soon it will feel numb. It will be cold as ice and then it will . . .	

If still no

Well, after holding it so long, some people never feel COLD . . . because their hand just starts to get NUMB from holding it, and then they do . . .

16. Anesthesia

not feel anything. Your hand is going to get very numb, just like when it goes to sleep. It won't be able to feel anything at all, it will be so numb. *Make continuous circular motion with finger on hand in area between thumb and forefinger.* Even if something sharp pressed your hand, or stuck it or cut it, you wouldn't feel it. It won't hurt or feel anything at all. Your hand is becoming more and more numb. It can't feel anything at all, no matter what.

Stick child's hand gently but firmly with pin. There now, did you feel anything?

If yes	*If no*
	Press again, harder: Do you feel anything now? All right, now you'll start to get some feeling back in your hand. Pretty soon it will stop feeling numb and will feel just like it usually does.
What did it feel like? It didn't really hurt, did it? *Press again, more gently:* Do you feel anything now? All right, now your hand will stop feeling numb, and it will feel just like it usually does.	

Now, is it starting to feel all right again? Good. Now it should be just like it was before it got numb. It isn't numb any more.

Record score for items 15 and 16.

17.   Taste Hallucination

If still holding stick	*If not holding stick*
	Now that your hand isn't numb anymore, you can have the popsicle back. It's still icy cold like before, and . . .
Now that your hand isn't numb anymore, you should still be able to feel the icy cold of your popsicle.	

In just a few seconds, you can eat it. Imagine how good it is going to taste, cold and sweet. And the more you suck it, the better it will taste. Now you can put the popsicle in your mouth. Go ahead and lick it now. *Make sure child places end of stick in mouth.* Can you taste it?

If yes

If no

That's okay. Sometimes it takes a few seconds before you can really taste it. Think of how good and sweet and cold it is. . . . Can you begin to taste it now?

Is it good? What does it taste like; what flavor? Oh, _____. Well go ahead and lick it all up. *Wait 10 seconds.* Now you're almost through with the popsicle. There now, you've finished it. Can you still feel the sweet taste in your mouth? Now that the popsicle is gone, the taste will all go away. . . . All right, now it's gone.

If yes

If still no

That's all right. . . . Sometimes it is kind of hard to taste things that are very cold. Here I'll take the popsicle back and you can forget all about it.

If child saw TV

Now just relax again and keep real nice and comfortable and sleepy. You were watching TV a little while ago, but now the program's over and the TV is all gone.

Record score.

18. Smell Hallucination (Perfume)

Now (that you are through with your popsicle), I want you to think about some other things. You know, popsicles are cold and sweet, but they hardly have any smell. But a lot of other things have a real strong smell—and there are some real good smells, like when your mom is baking a cake or when you smell burning leaves. And you know how your mother has a lot of sweet smelling things that she likes to use when she gets all dressed up, like perfume and powder. Doesn't she like to use perfume? Well, you know how sweet that smells.

Now I'm going to give you a bottle of perfume. *Place bottle in child's hand.* I'm going to take off the cap, and in a minute you'll start to smell the perfume. It may smell only a little bit at first, but it will get stronger and stronger until you can smell it very well. Do you smell it yet?

If yes	*If no*
	Well, it usually takes a little while for the smell to reach you. *If appropriate:* Put the bottle right under your nose, and in a few seconds it will get stronger and you'll be able to smell it more. Can you smell it?
Good. Can you tell it's perfume? Put the bottle right under your nose. Now it will start to get even stronger, and you will smell it even more. Does it smell closer and sweeter? All right. Now in a minute you won't be able to smell it anymore. I'll take the bottle away and it will get weaker. *Remove bottle.* It will get weaker and weaker like it was farther away . . . so weak that you can't smell it at all. You will forget all about the perfume and feel good and comfortable and relaxed.	

If still no

That's all right. Some people find it harder to smell perfume than others, and some kinds are not very strong anyway. So we'll just forget about it. *Take bottle away.* There isn't any perfume now, so you cannot smell it anymore. Just forget all about it and feel good and comfortable and relaxed.

Record score.

19. Visual Hallucination (Rabbit)

When I next clap my hands like this—*demonstrate with mild but audible clap*—you will see a table in front of you, and you will notice a small bunny rabbit sitting on it. . . . You will want very much to pick it up and hold it. . . . *Clap hands.* There. See the rabbit?

| *If yes* | *If no* |

If no

Well, wait a minute, and think real hard about what a bunny rabbit is like—*pause 5 seconds*—and maybe you will. I'm going to clap again now, and then you may see it. *Clap.* Do you see it now?

If yes

What is it doing? It's not big is it? . . . Would you like to hold it? You can if you want but be very gentle with him because he is a very young rabbit . . . just a baby. . . . Hold him tight because he will wiggle and squirm a lot at first and will be hard to hold. . . . Go ahead, pick him up and pet him. . . . Don't let him get away or fall. . . . Kind of cute, isn't he? . . . Isn't his fur soft? Feel how warm it is. . . . What color is the bunny? What color are his eyes? . . . It looks like he is about ready to go to sleep. . . . Why don't we just let him stay on your lap? . . . Just forget about him for a while. . . . He won't fall off. Just forget about the bunny on your lap.

If still no

Well, that's all right. Some people see this and others don't. You can just forget about the rabbit now. That's not important, so forget all about it.

Record score.

20. Regression (Age)

Now we are going to do something a little different. You should still be nice and comfortable and relaxed, just listening to my voice. Pretty soon I'm going to put a pencil in your hand. When I do, you will stay just as quiet and drowsy and relaxed as you are now, but your eyes will come open. Here is the pencil. *If necessary, cue:* Open your eyes now but stay deeply relaxed.

Now put your name at the top of this paper. *Hand a blank 8½ ×11 inch paper to child on a pad firm enough to support writing in his lap.* That's fine. Now draw a picture of a man. *Cue if necessary:* Draw the whole man, draw all of him.

All right, now let your eyes close again . . . and something very interesting is going to happen. . . . You are going to start to get smaller. I want you to think about being younger and smaller, think real hard about the time when you were only 5 years old. *If child is under 8, say 4 years old.* And in a little while, you are going to start to feel like you are growing younger and smaller, till you will be only 5 years old.

Then you will feel just as good and happy as could be, but you will feel younger. . . . I will count to five, and when I count, you get younger and smaller until I get to five. Pretty soon you'll be a little boy (girl) again, and then you will be able to do things like you used to do. *Count slowly.* One—two—three—you're getting younger—four—five. There you are.

- How old are you now?
- What is your best friend's name?
- How much is two and two?
- How much is six and five?
- What games do you like to play best?

That's fine. Can you write your name?

If yes	*If no*
	Well, that's all right. But I bet you can draw, and . . .
Good. Open your eyes and put your name on this paper. . . . That's fine. And . . .	

Now, I would like you to draw a picture of a man. Draw it right on this paper. *If necessary, cue:* Draw the whole man, draw all of him.

Good. Now let your eyes close again. That's right. *Pause 5 seconds.* Now, you will forget all about being 5, and you'll start to grow up again till you are _____ years old. That's right. Now you're growing up, getting bigger, getting bigger. . . . How old are you now? Oh, ____! That's fine.

Score for items 20, 21, and 22 can be recorded after the session on the basis of E's verbatim records of child's responses.

21. Dream

Now I am going to let you relax for a little while longer and get comfortable just like you do when you go to bed at night. In a minute I will stop talking and then you are going to have a dream, just like when you sleep . . . a nice happy dream. You can sleep and dream about anything you want to. Just let any happy dream come into your mind. Now you are falling asleep, deeper and deeper asleep. . . . Soon you will be deeply, soundly asleep. . . . As soon as I stop talking you will begin to dream. When I speak to you again, you will finish your dream, and you will listen to me just as you have been doing. If your dream ends before I talk to you again, you will stay pleasantly and deeply asleep. Now just sleep and have your dream. *Wait 30 seconds.* The dream is over now, but you can remember it very well and clearly. Now I want you to tell me about your dream, right from the beginning. Tell me all about it.

Record verbatim.

That's fine. Just forget about the dream now.

22. Awakening and Posthypnotic Suggestion

In just a minute, we are going to end this game [experiment]. I will count backwards from ten to one, and you will slowly wake up while I count. When I get to one, your eyes will open and you will be wide awake. Then you will remember the little bunny rabbit in your lap, and you'll look down and see it in your lap, sound asleep. . . . Soon it will wake up, and it will ask you what your name is. You tell it. . . . And then you will forget about the bunny, and he will be all gone.

After you wake up, you will feel real good and happy all the rest of the day. All right, here we go: ten—nine—eight—seven—six—five—four—three—two—one. All wide awake? *If not:* Wake up, wide awake now. *Wait until child has had time to respond spontaneously to rabbit suggestion.* How do you feel?

Record verbatim.

Inquiry: Tell me about the things we've been doing, _____. *If child shows amnesia, ask for details of what happened before beginning test.*

OLDER FORM (AGES 13–16), PART I

The Older Form of the Children's Hypnotic Susceptibility Scale is written primarily for adolescents. It is identical in order of item presentation, general item content, and scoring standards with the form for younger children.

It differs from the Younger Form only in that we have paid careful attention to preserving the dignity of adolescent subjects. Whenever possible, we have tried to avoid using language which was considered patronizing, humiliating, or babyish by pilot teenaged subjects.

Preliminary Tests

The following form of the Goodenough Draw-A-Man Test is routinely administered prior to the scale, since it is particularly useful for judging the effectiveness of the Age Regression item of the scale.*

To start off, I'd like you to sign your name at the top of this page. *Hand S pencil and a single sheet of typewriter-size blank paper. Note dominant hand.*

That's fine. Now, I would like you to use this same paper to give me a sample of your drawing, just like you gave me a sample of your signature. Draw a picture of a man. *Cue if necessary:* Draw the whole man, draw all of him. *If S objects, insist gently, e.g.:* It doesn't need to be fancy or elaborate, just fairly complete, *or* Either sex is all right.

Establishing Rapport (Ages 13–16)

After drawings are completed, E makes the following remarks which should be memorized or paraphrased.

You already know, of course, that we are going to do a scientific experiment here on the subject of hypnosis. But before we do, I thought we would talk a while so that I could tell you some things about it and find out what you already know about it. Have you ever had any experience with hypnosis, such as being hypnotized or watching someone else be hypnotized?

Note: *The text for the Older Form contains both italicized and nonitalicized material. The sentences in italic type are instructions to the experimenter (E). Those in roman type are verbal instructions to the subject (S).*

**Although the Goodenough test is primarily designed for estimating the intelligence of young children, we have limited its use in our studies of the Children's Scale to assessing Age Regression and have preferred to rely on the Vocabulary Subtest of the Wechsler Intelligence Scale for Children (WISC) for a relatively rapid and valid estimate of intelligence. The Goodenough test cannot, moreover, be suitably employed for estimating the intelligence of adolescents, whereas the WISC Vocabulary Subtest can be used for this purpose.*

Note information and previous experiences, as well as subject's impressions of hypnosis.

What we are going to do here is simply this: I am going to ask you to concentrate on different things which I suggest to you to imagine and do, and we will find out how good your imagination is. We are not going to do anything that would be embarrassing for you, though, nothing to make you feel stupid, and we will not pry at all into your private and personal affairs. I think you will find that this is an interesting and enjoyable experience, so I hope you will pay close attention to the things I say.

Ask for questions. Avoid direct answers to questions which ask for details of the hypnotic procedure.

Would you like me to tell you something about why we are doing these experiments? Well, hypnosis is being used widely in different kinds of medicine nowadays to help people with many different kinds of illnesses and other troubles—by coming here today, and doing these things with me, you're helping science to learn more about it, which will eventually make it possible for us to apply it more helpfully to people who are sick or troubled.

All I want you to do throughout this session is listen very carefully to me and let yourself just see what happens. I think you will enjoy it a lot—so pay close attention, and let's start in now.

1. Postural Sway

To begin, I want you to see what it feels like to concentrate on my suggestions and respond to them when you are not hypnotized.

1.   Please stand up right here with your back to me. First, stand straight, with your feet together and your hands at your sides. That's fine. Now just close your eyes, that's it—and with your eyes closed, I am going to ask you to think of an experience you have had in the past. I want you to imagine yourself on a swing. You've been on a swing before, and you know just what it feels like to go back and forth on one. When you were younger, you used to like to swing. When the swing goes up and back, you can feel yourself bending with it, and when it goes forward, you just bend again with it. Let me show you how it will be.

Grasp S by the shoulders, push gently forward and backward several times to set in motion. Once swaying starts, take a position which will break subject's fall in either forward or backward direction. Do not touch subject till after a definite loss of balance has occurred.

2.   As you think about that, you really will bend back and forth, back and forth. You'll go back and forth so much that you'll finally tip

over backwards—and when that happens, just let yourself go over. I am right here, and I'll catch you so you won't fall down.

3.   Think about being on a swing, going back and forth, back and forth—that's fine, you're really starting to swing, more and more swinging and swinging, back and forth, a little more backwards every time, swinging, swinging, more and more, further and further. . . .

4.   You're swinging further and further backwards, swinging and swaying, going backwards, going backwards . . . you're going, going . . . falling back, falling back, all the way backwards, all the way backwards . . . falling over, tipping over, falling, falling . . . FALL!

If fall occurs   *If no fall occurs*

That's fine. Now you see how thinking about an experience can make you feel like you really are having it. Now we're going to do that again, only this time, I want you to think even harder about it until you really do go all the way over backwards. Think about being on a swing, and . . .
Repeat paragraphs 2, 3, and 4. If S still fails, induce a voluntary fall.

That's fine. Now you see how thinking about something makes you feel like you really are doing it.

Seat S in the chair again and record the score.

2.   Eye Closure

Use Chevreul pendulum. Take it out of case, hold it by the end of the chain, and swing it in front of child.

1.   Look at this ball and chain, _____. Notice the way it swings when I hold it like this. Even if I hold the chain quite still, the ball stays in motion, it keeps on swinging all the time. Here, you try it now. Hold your arm like this and take the end of the chain. *Take left arm, prop elbow on chair arm, with forearm at right angles to upper arm, and place end of chain in hand so ball swings freely. Have S slump down in chair if it can be done comfortably.* Now, concentrate on the ball very hard and see if you can keep it from moving. Pay close attention to it, and hold your arm very still, so it won't move at all. Keep right on looking at the ball all the time, and as you do, just keep on listening

to me. Don't pay attention to anything else but the way the ball looks and the things I say to you. Don't pay attention to anything but the ball and the sound of my voice, and you will gradually enter a hypnotic state.

The remainder of this section should be read quite slowly in an even tone. If eyes close at any time, finish the sentence and turn to the corresponding paragraph of 2A, continuing through the end of the section.

2.   To find out what it's like to be hypnotized, all you need to do is keep looking at the ball and listening to my voice. And while you do that, you will start to feel very nice, a little warm, and very comfortable—and you will even get a little bit drowsy. In a short time, your eyes will get tired, and you will feel like closing them. When that happens, just let it happen. It will be all right. The ball may look a little strange sometimes, a little blurred, so that it is hard to see it clearly. That's all right. And your eyes will get so tired they will just feel like closing as if by themselves. When that happens, just let it happen, and you can go on imagining the ball in your mind with your eyes closed.

3.   It feels so nice to just sit there and relax and listen to my voice. . . . It feels warm and good and pleasant, like it feels sometimes when you have been playing or working hard on a hot day and lie down on the grass to rest in the shade. . . . It is such a nice tired feeling, it makes you feel so good and relaxed. . . . You feel so nice all over, and your eyes are getting so heavy. . . . They feel like somebody is just pushing them slowly shut, like they can't help closing all by themselves, closing all by themselves.

4.   You start to feel drowsy and sleepy, so nice and tired and sleepy, like you are all relaxed and want to sleep, all warm and comfortable. . . . You feel so good, so nice. . . . It is so pleasant to listen to my voice and to pay attention just to my voice and not listen to anything else. . . . It makes you feel so quiet and good and drowsy and sleepy to listen to my voice . . . very drowsy, very sleepy . . . sleepy, sleepy, sleepy.

5.   Your eyes are getting heavy, so very heavy. You feel tired and good, very good, and there is such a nice feeling of being warm and sleepy all over. You are tired and drowsy. Tired and sleepy. Sleepy. Sleepy. Just listen to my voice. Don't pay attention to anything else but my voice. Your eyelids are very heavy, and they are feeling heavier and heavier, just like something was pressing them shut. Your eyes are tired and blinking, blinking, blinking . . . closing, closing, closing.

If eyes have not closed voluntarily within 10 seconds after this point, item has been failed.

If eyes have not yet closed

Soon your eyes would close by
themselves, but you don't need to
wait any longer. You have been
listening carefully to me and
paying attention to the ball. Now
you are comfortable and drowsy,
and you may just let your eyes
close. *If no response:* That's it,
now close them.

As soon as eyes close: Now just leave your eyes closed until I tell
you to open them or to wake up, and keep right on like you were still
looking at the little ball only with your eyes closed.

Record score.

Go to paragraph 6, page 315.

2A.   Eye Closure

*This item is for those who close eyes before completion of item 2, para-
graph 5. As soon as eyes close, terminate sentence appropriately, then:*

1a.   You feel very relaxed and good, tired and drowsy, but you
are going to get even more tired and drowsy. Your eyes are closed
now. Just leave your eyes closed until I tell you to open them or to
wake up, and keep right on looking mentally at the little ball, but with
your eyes closed.

*Resume reading at the appropriate place and continue the Scale.
Should eyes reopen, instruct subject to close them.*

2a.   And while you do that, keep on listening to my voice, and
soon you will start to feel very nice, a little warm, and very comfortable—and you will even get more sleepy, so that sometimes my voice
will sound like it is part of a dream. That will be all right. You will
still be able to hear me and pay attention to the things I say, even
though it may feel like you are dreaming. Whatever happens, just let
it happen and go on getting more and more sleepy, more and more
drowsy, while you keep on listening to my voice and watching the
picture of the little ball in your mind, with your eyes closed.

3a.   It feels so nice to just sit there and relax and listen to my
voice. . . . . It feels warm and good and pleasant, like it feels sometimes when you have been playing or working real hard on a hot day
and lie down on the grass to rest in the shade. . . . . It is such a nice
tired feeling, it makes you feel so good and relaxed. . . . . You feel so
nice all over, and you are getting so very sleepy. . . . . You are going

more and more deeply asleep, into a soft pleasant sleep where this good feeling grows better and better.

4a.   You are feeling so drowsy and sleepy, so nice and tired and sleepy, like you are all relaxed and want to sleep, all warm and comfortable. . . . You feel so good, so nice. . . . It is so pleasant to listen to my voice and to pay attention just to my voice and not listen to anything else. . . . It makes you feel so quiet and drowsy and sleepy to listen to my voice . . . very drowsy, very sleepy . . . sleepy, sleepy, sleepy.

5a.   You feel as if you are in a nice bed, very nice and soft. You feel tired and good, very good, and there is such a pleasant feeling of being warm and sleepy all over. You are tired and drowsy. Tired and sleepy. Sleepy. Sleepy. Just listen to my voice. Don't pay attention to anything else but my voice. My voice sounds like it is coming to you in a dream, and listening to it puts you in a deep, deep, sleep. But you will always keep on hearing my voice no matter how sleepy you feel you are.

6 and 6a.   You feel nice and drowsy and sleepy while you keep on listening to my voice. Just keep listening to what I am saying. Soon you will be fast asleep, but you will still hear what I say. And don't wake up until I tell you to. I'm going to count from one to ten, and every time I count you will get more and more deeply asleep, but you will still be able to hear me and to do all the things I ask you to do. *Stroke forehead lightly.* One . . . two . . . deep asleep, deeper and deeper . . . three . . . four . . . more and more asleep . . . five . . . six . . . seven . . . fast asleep, feeling warm and good . . . eight. . . . Just keep listening to me and the things I tell you to think of . . . nine . . . ten . . . DEEP ASLEEP! Do not wake up until I tell you to. Stay deep asleep and listen to the things I talk about.

3.   Hand Lowering (Left)

If hand has already dropped, raise arm into position again, saying, Lift up your arm again.

Now that you're so comfortable and drowsy, you start to notice something interesting happen. While you hold the chain with the ball at the end of it, it starts to get heavy. And it gets heavier and heavier, so heavy that you want to drop the ball. It is getting much too heavy to hold on to. *Put hand under ball to catch it.* It just is getting so heavy it's too heavy to hold, and you can just let it go. It's much too heavy to hold onto, and you can just let it go.

If chain is not released soon, gently take it from child's hand.

And now your arm is getting heavy, too, as if something was

pulling it down. It starts going down, a little bit down, more and more down . . . further and further . . . so heavy . . . so very heavy. . . . It just goes down all by itself, all by itself, further and further down, till it comes to rest all by itself. *Wait 10 seconds.*

When all the way down	*If hand doesn't lower*
	That's fine. Now you can relax your arm like it was before, let it relax down. You noticed how hard it was to hold it up, how heavy it felt. Now just let it lie there, so heavy.
That's good. . . . Now just let your hand lie there and rest, but notice that it still feels heavy to you.	

Record score.

4. Arm Immobilization (Left)

And now I want you to keep paying attention to this arm some more, because it feels very heavy now. *Stroke S's left arm.* As I stroke your arm, you will feel it being pressed down in the chair . . . heavier and heavier. . . . It feels just like it is being pressed against the arm of the chair, it's so heavy. . . . And it keeps pressing against the chair, so very heavy, that it feels like you can't lift it. Maybe it's just too heavy to lift now, perhaps that is just too hard to do now that it's so heavy. Why don't you see how heavy it is? . . . Just try to lift your hand up, just try. *Wait 7 seconds.*

If hand does not lift	*If hand lifts*
	That's fine. . . . Now you can let your arm relax back down again. You saw how hard it was for you to lift it—much harder than it usually is. Now you can just relax again and feel nice and sleepy some more.
That's fine. . . . Stop trying. . . . Your hand and arm don't feel heavy anymore. You can lift it now. . . . Go ahead and lift it up	

a little. That's fine. Now just relax
again, and feel all nice and
sleepy.

Record score.

5. Finger Lock

Now let's do something else. Put your fingers together, lock them
together. *Take the child's hands and position correctly.* That's it. Now
press your hands tightly together, lock them tighter and tighter together . . . very tight. . . . Lock them so tightly that you cannot take
them apart. Lock them together, tightly together, very tight. Now just
try to take them apart when they are locked up so tight together, just
try. . . . *Wait 5 seconds.*

If not taken apart	*If taken apart*
	All right, now just let your hands relax again. You saw how hard it was to separate them. But they aren't tight any more now. You can just relax again, very comfortably, very deeply.
Stop trying now. . . . They'll come apart right away, they won't stay locked together any more. That's it, let them separate and just relax.	

Record score.

6. Arm Rigidity (Right)

Now hold this arm straight out—*take S's right arm*—and the fingers straight out too. That's it, your arm straight out. *Stroke once down
entire arm.* Now imagine that your arm is getting very stiff and
straight, very, very stiff. . . . Think about your arm as if it were in a
splint. Your arm is splinted, held very straight and stiff within a tight
splint so that it could not bend no matter what . . . stiff and strong in
a tight splint, very straight and stiff . . . so stiff that you can't bend
it. . . . That's right. . . . Now see how stiff it is, see if you have made
it stiff enough. . . . Try and bend it. . . . Try. . . . *Wait 5 seconds.*

If arm does not bend	*If arm bends*
	That's all right. You saw how hard it was for you to bend your arm. But it isn't stiff any more. You can just put it back the way it was and relax. That's right, just relax.
There, that's enough now. . . . Just relax. . . . Don't try to bend your arm any more and don't leave it in a splint any more. . . . It isn't stiff now, and you can just let it relax back onto your lap—*or the chair arm, whichever is appropriate.*	

Record score.

7. Hands Together

Now put your hands out in front of you just like you were about to start clapping. Here, I'll show you. *Place S's hands about a foot apart, palms inward.* That's right. Now I want you to imagine that there is a big elastic band around your hands, a big elastic band stretched out around your hands. . . . And it is pulling them together, pulling them together. . . . And as you think about that, your hands will start coming together, just as if an elastic band was stretched around them . . . pulling them together, closer and closer . . . slowly at first, but they come closer together, closer . . . moving . . . moving . . . closer . . . closer and closer. . . . *Wait 5 seconds.*

If hands have touched	*If hands have not touched*
	That's fine. They've come very close together. Let me show you how near they are to touching. *Move S's hands together fairly rapidly.* That's fine. Now just let them relax on your lap—*or chair arm*—and get very comfortable again.
That's fine. All right, now just let your hands relax, and get very comfortable again.	

Record score.

8. Verbal Inhibition (Name)

You feel very good and relaxed now, very comfortable and warm and sleepy and drowsy. And when you feel so sleepy and drowsy, all you want to do is just sit back and listen. . . . You don't feel like doing anything else. . . . You don't even want to talk, but just to listen quietly to my voice. . . . It is just too much trouble to talk. . . . So if I asked you now to tell me your name you probably couldn't even do it. . . . It would just be too much trouble because it is so pleasant just to listen and not do anything else. . . . Just try now to tell me your name and see how hard it is. . . . Just try. *Wait 10 seconds.*

If name not spoken	*If name spoken*
	There, you did it. . . . It took a lot of effort, but you did it anyway, even though I'm sure you noticed it was harder than it usually is. That's fine. . . . Now just relax.
Don't try anymore. . . . That's it. . . . Stop trying. . . . You can say your name easily now. . . . Say it, go ahead. . . . Good. . . . Now just get all sleepy and relaxed again.	

Record score.

9. Auditory Hallucination (Fly)

You have been listening very well to me, paying close attention. You haven't been listening to anything but my voice, but now I want you to listen to another thing. There has been a fly buzzing around you, going buzzzzzz the way flies do. You can hear it now as it flies right around your left hand. *Touch hand.* Now it's landing right on your hand. . . . Maybe it tickles a bit. . . . There it flies away again. . . . You can hear it buzz. . . . It's back on your hand tickling. . . . You don't care for that fly. . . . You'd like to get rid of it. . . . Go ahead, brush it off. . . . Get rid of it if it bothers you. . . . *Wait 10 seconds.*

There, it's gone now. . . . That's good. . . . It doesn't bother you now. . . . It's gone, disappeared. . . . Now relax, and feel all comfortable again.

If no response

The fly is gone now, so you can't
hear it. Now relax and feel all
comfortable again.

Record score.

10.   Eye Catalepsy

You have had your eyes closed for a long time while you stayed
comfortable and sleepy. By now, your eyes are very tightly closed,
tightly shut. . . . If you tried to open them now, they probably would
feel just like they were stuck together with glue . . . tightly glued
shut. . . . Maybe, pretty soon, you'd like to try to open your eyes
even though they feel so heavy and so completely, so tightly glued
shut. Go ahead. . . . Try to open your eyes. *Wait 10 seconds.*

If eyes remain shut	*If eyes open*
	That's fine. Now close your eyes again. You saw how hard it was to open your eyes. But now you can leave them shut and you can relax and be comfortable again.
Now relax. . . . Stop trying to open your eyes. They feel all right again, they aren't stuck, but just leave them closed and get all comfortable again.	

Record score.

Conclusion Part I
Introduction Part II

*At this point, the experimenter has the alternatives of either introduc-
ing the second part of the Scale or terminating the entire proceeding. Except for experimental purposes, it may be unwise to continue with Part II
unless the subject has passed five or more items in Part I and/or shown
considerable clinical indications of having experienced hypnosis.*

If test is to be terminated

Now, in just a few moments,
after you have relaxed a little
while longer, I am going to wake
you up very slowly and we will
finish this experiment. When we

If test is to be continued

do, you will feel as if you have just finished a pleasant nap and then . . .

Now we are about to do some things that are different from the kind we have been doing. I'm going to show you some new things that I think you will find very interesting—and that you will enjoy very much. But before we start that . . .

11. Posthypnotic Suggestion (and Amnesia)

I want you to forget all about the things that we have been doing and not to pay attention to them anymore. In a minute, I am going to count backwards from ten to one, and you are going to wake up slowly as I count. When I say five, your eyes will open, and when I get to one, you will be wide awake. You'll feel real good, just like you had a pleasant sleep, and you won't remember all the things we did because it will be too much trouble to do so. Later on, I'll tell you that you CAN remember everything, and THEN YOU WILL REMEMBER.

Now when I say one, you'll be wide awake, and you'll stand right up and stretch your arms out wide, but you won't remember that I said to.

If test is to be continued

If test is to be terminated

Ready now, ten—nine—eight—seven—six—five—four—three—two—one.

Then we'll talk a while, and after that, I'll clap my hands two times—when you hear me clap, you'll get all sleepy and drowsy again and your eyes will close, and then we'll start doing some more things. Ready now, ten—nine—eight—seven—six—five—four—three—two—one.

If eyes remain closed

Wake up! Wide awake! How do you feel? Are you wide awake?

If eyes open
How do you feel? Are you wide
awake?

Wait 10 seconds.

If subject stands	*If subject does not stand*
	Now stand up and stretch so you'll be wide awake. That's fine. Now sit down again. I want to ask you some questions.

*or stretches or otherwise responds
positively, imitate his movement in
such a way as to prevent him from
being embarassed by his own
response. Do not make such a
movement, however, unless his
response is unmistakable.*

Record score.

12.   Amnesia

Now please tell me all about the different things that we have
been doing, and what has happened since we came in here.

Record verbatim.

When subject stops reporting: That's fine. Now listen to me very
carefully—NOW YOU CAN REMEMBER EVERYTHING. Anything
else now? . . . That's fine.

Part I Ends Here

OLDER FORM, PART II

13.   Posthypnotic Suggestion (Reinduction)

Clap hands twice sharply. Wait 10 seconds.

If eyes close	*If eyes do not close*
	Now just let your eyes close again, and let them stay closed till I tell you to open them or to wake up.
That's it. . . . Now just leave your eyes closed until I tell you to open them or to wake up.	

Record score.

After eyes are closed: You can remember now how you felt before when you were like this . . . sleepy and comfortable, kind of drowsy and relaxed . . . feeling all good inside, pleasant and warm and comfortable. It gives you such a good feeling to just sit there drowsily and listen quietly to my voice . . . to pay attention only to what I am saying and not to listen to anything else. . . . It makes you feel all quiet and sort of tired . . . and a little bit sleepy, drowsy and sleepy. . . .

Just keep on listening to my voice and to what I am saying. . . . Soon it will send you deeply asleep, but you will still hear what I say. . . . And later on, we will talk to each other, and you will be able to stay deep asleep and yet talk to me at the same time. . . . It will be very easy for you to do, to just stay deeply relaxed and sleepy but to talk to me when I ask you to. Now I am going to count from one to ten, and with each count you will get more and more sleepy, but you will still be able to hear me and to do all the things I ask you to do. One . . . two . . . deep asleep, deeper and deeper . . . three . . . four . . . more and more asleep . . . five . . . six . . . seven . . . fast asleep, feeling warm and good . . . eight . . . nine . . . ten . . . DEEP ASLEEP! And stay deep asleep, all relaxed and comfortable, all the time that we do these different things.

14. Visual and Auditory Hallucination (Television)

Tell me, do you ever watch TV? What shows do you like best? *If S does not specify some program, suggest Route 66, American Bandstand, Huckleberry Hound, or any popular network (children's) program.* Oh, _____! Well, that's fine.

Now if you could watch any program you chose, which one would you like to see right now? Well, you CAN see it if you really want to, and I'll tell you how. When I count to three, I want you to see a TV set standing right in front of you. Then, when I tell you, you can turn it on and then you can watch _____ *(name of program)*. Ready? one—two—three. Look at the set now. Do you see it?

If no

That's all right—sometimes it takes a while to catch on to how to do this. So just wait a little while and I think you'll start to see it pretty soon. *Wait 5 seconds.* There, are you starting to see the TV set now?

If yes

Why don't you turn it on?   *If yes*
They're going to show _____. Is it
on? Do you see it now? Is the
picture clear? (Why don't you fix
it?)

                                              If still no
                                     All right. I'm going to count to
                                     three again, and when I reach
                                     three you're going to remember
                                     some program of _____ that
                                     you've seen before. And it will be
                                     so clear, that you'll even see and
                                     hear the whole program, and the
                                     music and everything. Okay.
                                     Now, one—two—three. Do you
                                     remember?

What's happening, can you hear   *If yes*
the program? Is it loud enough?
Tell me about it. . . . All right,
now you can watch the rest of the
program while I do some other
things.

                                              If still no
                                     That's all right. Different people
                                     have different experiences, and
                                     some have this one and some
                                     have others. We'll find some
                                     other things you can do now. Just
                                     forget all about the TV. There
                                     isn't any there. Just relax and
                                     keep listening to my voice.

                              Record score.

  If child responded positively to TV: Now I bet you like to eat a little
snack when you're watching TV.

15.   Cold Hallucination

  Do you like popsicles? *If no, try ice cream bars.* What flavor do you
like? Well, you can have a nice icy cold _____ flavored popsicle right
now. Now you think real hard about what a popsicle is like, so cold

and hard, and I'm going to put one in your hand, only it will be up-
side down so the icy part will be in your hand. When you hold it a
little while, your hand will start to feel cold. Later on, I'll tell you that
you can eat the popsicle . . . okay?

*Place tongue depressor in hand, close S's palm around it. Observe tem-
perature of back of hand.*

There now, do you feel how cold and hard the popsicle is? Pretty
soon, it will feel so cold that it will make your hand get cold too. As
you hold it longer, your hand will feel colder and colder. It may get so
cold that you cannot hold on to it any more. Does it feel cold now?
Feel hand and note any apparent temperature change.

If yes	*If no*
	Well, you just hold it a little bit longer. You know how cold ice in your hand feels, don't you? Well, this feels just like ice—so hard and cold. Does your hand feel very cold now?
Fine. It's going to get so cold that pretty soon it will feel numb. It will be cold as ice and then it will . . .	

                                        If still no
                                Well, after holding it so long,
                                some people never feel COLD
                                . . . because their hand just
                                starts to get NUMB from holding
                                it, and then they do . . .

16. Anesthesia

not feel anything. Your hand is going to get very numb, just like
when it goes to sleep. It won't be able to feel anything at all, it will be
so numb. *Make continuous circular motion with finger on hand in area
between thumb and forefinger.* Even if something sharp pressed your
hand, or stuck it or cut it, you wouldn't feel it. It won't hurt or feel
anything at all. Your hand is becoming more and more numb. It can't
feel anything at all, no matter what.

Stick child's hand gently but firmly with pin. There now, did you
feel anything?

<table>
<tr><td>If yes</td><td>If no</td></tr>
</table>

If yes

If no

Press again, harder: Do you feel
anything now? All right, now
you'll start to get some feeling
back in your hand. Pretty soon it
will stop feeling numb and will
feel just like it normally does.

What did it feel like? It didn't
really hurt, did it? *Press again,
more gently:* Do you feel anything
now? All right, now your hand
will stop feeling numb, and it
will feel just like it normally does.

Now, is it starting to feel all right again? Good. Now it should be
just like it was before it got numb. It isn't numb any more.
Record scores for items 15 and 16.

17.   Taste Hallucination

If still holding stick

If not holding stick

Now that your hand isn't numb
anymore, you can have the
popsicle back. It still feels icy cold
like before, and . . .

Now that your hand isn't numb
anymore, you should still be able
to feel the icy cold of your
popsicle.

In just a few seconds, you can eat it. Imagine how good it is going
to taste, cold and sweet. And the more you suck it, the better it will
taste. Now you can put the popsicle in your mouth. Go ahead and lick
it now. *Make sure S places end of stick in mouth.* Can you taste it?

If yes

If no

That's okay. Sometimes it takes a
few seconds before you can really
taste it. Think of how good and
sweet and cold it is. . . . Can you
begin to taste it now?

Is it good? What does it taste like;
what flavor? Oh, _____. Well go

If yes

ahead and lick it all up. *Wait 10 seconds.* Now you're almost through with the popsicle. There now, you've finished it. Can you still feel the sweet taste in your mouth? Now that the popsicle is gone, the taste will disappear. . . . All right, now it's gone.

If still no

That's all right. . . . Sometimes it is kind of hard to taste things that are very cold. Here I'll take the popsicle back and you can forget all about it. *Remove stick.*

If S saw TV

Now just relax again and keep real nice and comfortable and sleepy. You were watching TV a little while ago, but now the program's over, and the TV is all gone.

Record score.

18. Smell Hallucination (Perfume)

Now (that you are through with your popsicle), I want you to think about some other things. You know popsicles are cold and sweet, but they hardly have any smell. But a lot of other things have a very strong smell—and there are some real good smells, like when your mom is baking a cake, or when you smell burning leaves. And you know how your mother has a lot of sweet smelling things that she likes to use when she gets all dressed up, like perfume and powder. Doesn't she like to use perfume? Well, you know how sweet that smells.

Now I'm going to give you a bottle of perfume. *Place bottle in child's hand.* I'm going to take off the cap, and in a minute you'll start to smell the perfume. It may smell only a little bit at first, but it will get stronger and stronger until you can smell it very well. Do you smell it yet?

<table>
<tr><td>If yes</td><td>If no</td></tr>
</table>

If no

Well, it usually takes a little while for the smell to reach you. *If appropriate:* Put the bottle right under your nose, and in a few seconds it will get stronger and you'll be able to smell it more. Can you smell it?

Good. Can you tell it's perfume? Put the bottle right under your nose. Now it will get even stronger, and you will smell it even more. Does it smell closer and sweeter? All right. Now in a minute you won't be able to smell it anymore. I'll take the bottle away and it will get weaker. *Remove bottle.* It will get weaker and weaker like it was farther away . . . so weak that you can't smell it at all. You will forget all about the perfume and feel good and comfortable and relaxed.

If still no

That's all right. Some people find it harder to smell perfume than others, and some kinds are not very strong anyway. So we'll just forget about it. *Take bottle away.* There isn't any perfume now, so you cannot smell it anymore. Just forget all about it and feel good and comfortable and relaxed.

Record score.

19. Visual Hallucination (Rabbit)

When I next clap my hands like this—*demonstrate with mild but audible clap*—you will see a table in front of you, and you will notice a small bunny rabbit sitting on it. . . . You will want very much to pick it up and hold it. . . . *Clap hands.* There. See the rabbit?

If yes

If no

Well, wait a minute, and think real hard about what a bunny rabbit is like—*pause 5 seconds*—and now maybe you will. I'm going to clap again now, and then you may see it. *Clap* Do you see it now?

What is it doing? It's not very big, is it? . . . Would you like to hold it? You can if you want, but be very gentle with him because he is a very young rabbit . . . just a baby. . . . Hold him tight because he will wiggle and squirm a lot at first and will be hard to hold. . . . Go ahead, pick him up and pet him. . . . Don't let him get away or fall. . . . Kind of cute, isn't he? . . . Isn't his fur soft? Feel how warm it is. . . . What color is the bunny? What color are his eyes? . . . It looks like he is about ready to go to sleep. . . . Why don't we just let him stay on your lap? . . . Just forget about him for a while. . . . He won't fall off. Just forget about the bunny on your lap.

If still no

Well, that's all right. Some people see this and others don't. You can just forget about the rabbit now. That's not important, so forget all about it.

Record score.

20. Regression (Age)

Now we are going to do something a little different. You should still be very comfortable and relaxed, just listening to my voice. Pretty soon I'm going to put a pencil in your hand. When I do, you will remain just as quiet and drowsy and deeply relaxed as you are now, but your eyes will open. Here is the pencil. *If necessary, cue:* Open your eyes now but stay deeply relaxed.

Now sign your name at the top of this page. *Hand a blank 8 ½ × 11 inch paper to S on a pad firm enough to support writing in his lap.* That's fine. Now draw a picture of a man. *Cue if necessary:* Draw the whole man, draw all of him.

All right, now let your eyes close again . . . and something very interesting is going to happen. . . . You are going to start to feel yourself getting smaller. I want you to think about being younger and smaller, think about the time when you were only 5 years old. And in a little while, as you concentrate on this, you are going to start to feel as if you are growing younger and smaller, till you will feel yourself to be only 5 years old.

You will feel happy and delighted, a happy little child. . . . I will count slowly to five, and as I count, you feel yourself be a little boy (girl) again, and then you will be able to do things like you used to do. *Count slowly.* One—two—three—you're getting younger—four —five. There you are.

- • How old are you now?
- • What is your best friend's name?
- • How much is two and two?
- • How much is six and five?
- • What games do you like to play best?

That's fine. Can you write your name?

If yes	*If no*
	Well, that's all right. But I bet you can draw, and . . .
Good. Open your eyes and put your name on this paper. . . . That's fine. And . . .	

Now, I would like you to draw a picture of a man. Draw it right on this paper. *If necessary, cue:* Draw the whole man, draw all of him.

Good. Now close your eyes again. That's right. *Pause 5 seconds.* Now, you will forget all about being 5, and you will start to grow up again till you are _____ years old. That's right. Now you are growing up, getting bigger, getting bigger. . . . There . . . how old are you now? Oh, _____! That's fine.

Score for items 20, 21, and 22 can be recorded after the session on the basis of E's verbatim records of subject's responses.

21. Dream

Now I am going to let you relax for a little while longer and get comfortable just as you do when you go to bed at night. In a minute I will stop talking and then you are going to have a dream, just as when you sleep at night . . . a nice happy dream. You can sleep and dream about anything you want to. Just let any pleasant dream come into your mind. Now you are falling asleep, deeper and deeper asleep. . . . Soon you will be deeply, soundly asleep. . . . As soon as I stop talking, you will begin to dream. When I speak to you again, you will finish your dream, and you will listen to me just as you have been doing. If your dream ends before I talk to you again, you will stay pleasantly and deeply asleep. Now just sleep and have your dream. *Wait 30 seconds.* The dream is over now, but you can remember it very well and clearly. Now I want you to tell me about your dream, right from the beginning. Tell me all about it.

Record verbatim.

That's fine. Just forget about the dream now.

22. Awakening and Posthypnotic Suggestion

In just a minute, we are going to finish this experiment. I will count backwards from ten to one, and you will slowly wake up as I count. When I reach one, your eyes will open and you will be wide awake. Then you will remember the little bunny rabbit in your lap, and you will look down and see it in your lap, sound asleep. . . . Soon it will wake up, and it will ask you your name. You tell it. . . . And then you will immediately forget about the bunny and have no thoughts about him.

After you wake up, you will feel very pleasant and happy and energetic for the rest of the day. All right, here we go: ten—nine—eight—seven—six—five—four—three—two—one. Wide awake? *If not:* Wake up, wide awake now. *Wait till subject has had time to respond spontaneously to rabbit suggestion.* How do you feel?

Record verbatim.

Inquiry: Tell me about the things we've been doing, _____. *If child shows amnesia, ask for details of what happened before beginning of test.*

Children's Hypnotic Susceptibility Scale
Scoring and Observation Form

Child's name _____   Session no. _____

	Year	Month	Day	
Date	____	____	____	Hypnotist _____
Birthdate	____	____	____	Observer _____
Age	____	____	____	Score _____

Using (check one):
_____ four-point scale
_____ +/− scale

Standard scoring procedures call for a four-point scale, and it is recommended that performances be recorded in this manner. Those who prefer a simple pass (+) versus fail (−) dichotomy may later reduce scores to such a scale by counting 0 and 1 scores as fail (−) and 2 and 3 scores as pass (+). Try to record time in the left-hand margin, but remember that observations of behavior are more important than precise time records. In the blank space under each item, make special note of the child's apparent subjective reaction to the experience, e.g., Is he particularly sluggish? alert? sober? amused? How hard does he seem to be trying on the challenge items? Do some of his responses appear to be "unconsciously" determined, e.g., Does response to posthypnotic suggestion seem natural and unstudied or merely compliant? Check the appropriate response in each item and enter its number on line at right.

PART I

Time

1. Postural Sway   Score
Score only on first attempt, i.e., on basis of performance during initial reading of paragraphs 2, 3, and 4.
____ ____ (3) Falls.   ____
____ ____ (2) Loses balance and recovers without falling.
____ ____ (1) Sways but does not lose balance.
____ ____ (0) Little or no swaying, no loss of balance.

2. Eye Closure
____ ____ (3) Eyes close and remain closed before examiner completes paragraph 5.   ____
____ (2) Eyes close within 10 seconds after completion of paragraph 5 or close before time limit but occasionally reopen briefly.
____ (1) Becomes drowsy, but eyes do not close within limit.
____ (0) No marked drowsiness, and only closes eyes when specifically told to do so.

3. Hand Lowering (Left)

(3) Hand rises less than 1 inch from chair by time limit or, with slow, effortful movement, up to 3 inches.

(2) Hand rises from 1 to 3 inches by time limit or, with slow, effortful movement, up to 4 inches.

(1) Hand rises from 3 to 6 inches, relatively easy, smooth, rapid movement.

(0) Hand rises more than 6 inches, relatively easy, smooth, or rapid motion.

4. Arm Immobilization (Left)

(3) Hand lowers to resting position within time limit.

(2) Hand moves through 30-degree arc or more, but does not lower to rest.

(1) Hand lowers through less than 30-degree arc.

(0) Hand does not move noticeably.

5. Finger Lock

(3) Incomplete separation of fingers by the time limit despite some effort to unlock them.

(2) Incomplete separation of fingers, but no effort made to separate them.

(1) Separation within time limit but only after considerable effort.

(0) Separation within time limit with little difficulty.

6. Arm Rigidity (Right)

(3) Arm bends less than 2 inches at elbow despite effort to bend it.

(2) Arm bends less than 2 inches, but little effort made to bend it.

(1) Arm bends more than 2 inches but only after considerable effort.

(0) Arm bends more than 2 inches with little difficulty.

Time | 7. **Hands Together** | Score
_____ _____   (3) Hands move together and touch within _____
              time limit.

_____   (2) Hands move to within 2 inches of each other.

_____   (1) Hands move to within less than 2 inches of each other or in opposite direction, within time.

_____   (0) Hands do not move noticeably.

8. Verbal Inhibition (Name)

_____ _____   (3) Name not spoken despite effort to speak. _____

_____   (2) Name not spoken, but little effort made to speak.

_____   (1) Name spoken within time limit but only after considerable effort.

_____   (0) Name spoken within time limit with little difficulty.

9. Auditory Hallucination (Fly)

_____ _____   (3) Any appropriate movement, grimacing, acknowledgment of effect, and apparent irritation. _____

_____   (2) Appropriate movement, etc. but no apparent irritation.

_____   (1) Small and irrelevant muscle responses.

_____   (0) No noticeable response.

10. Eye Catalepsy

_____ _____   (3) Eyes remain closed despite effort to open them. _____

_____   (2) Eyes remain closed, but little effort manifested.

_____   (1) Eyes open within the time limit after considerable effort.

_____   (0) Eyes open easily.

11. Posthypnotic Suggestion (Standing Up)

_____ _____   (3) Stands up and stretches. _____

_____   (2) Remains seated and stretches or stands but does not stretch.

_____   (1) Irrelevant movements, e.g., yawning.

_____   (0) No apparent response.

Time   **12. Amnesia**   Score

(3) Three or fewer items recalled with apparent difficulty and/or confusion.

(2) Three or fewer items recalled with relative ease.

(1) More than three items recalled but with difficulty and/or confusion.

(0) More than three items recalled but with relative ease.

PART II

13. Posthypnotic Suggestion (Reinduction)

(3) Closes eyes within time limit and apparently relaxes body.

(2) Closes eyes without apparent body relaxation, or eyes remain open but become glazed and apparently puzzled.

(1) Partial response indicating clap has had some meaning, but no sign of eye closure, dazedness, or body relaxation.

(0) No significant response, and only closes eyes when specifically instructed.

14. Visual and Auditory Hallucination (Television)

(3) Substantially completes suggested sequence, e.g., sees TV set, turns it on, sees picture clearly, describes scene meaningfully.

(2) Completes significant portion of sequence with some failure, e.g., sees TV set, turns it on, but cannot see the picture clearly or describe the program well.

(1) Fails most of sequence, e.g., sees TV set, but does not turn it on, etc.

(0) No apparent response, e.g., does not see TV set.

15. Cold Hallucination

——— ——— (3) Apparent blanching of skin, temperature change, or goose bumps and/or appropriate motor responses, e.g., juggling or dropping stick. ———

——— (2) Appropriate verbal response of cold sensation but no motor or other changes.

——— (1) Repeated indecision ("I'm not sure if it feels cold") without nonverbal positive indicators.

——— (0) No cold response of any kind.

16. Anesthesia
On first trial:

——— ——— (1) Feels point but no pain. ———

——— (0) Feels pain and/or withdraws hand.
Any other response, give second trial.
On second trial:

——— (3) Does not feel anything.

——— (2) Indicates awareness of stimulus but cannot clearly describe it.

——— (1) Feels point but no pain.

——— (0) Feels pain and/or withdraws hand.

17. Taste Hallucination

——— ——— (3) Substantially completes suggested sequence, e.g., takes stick into mouth, makes licking movements, describes appropriate taste sensation. ———

——— (2) Completes significant portion of sequence with some inadequacies, e.g., experiences only very slight or vague taste sensations.

——— (1) Completes sequence but denies effect, e.g., "It tastes like wood."

——— (0) No sequence.

18. Smell Hallucination (Perfume)

——— ——— (3) Affirms and describes odor of perfume. ———

——— (2) Affirms odor of perfume but does not elaborate or describe it.

——— (1) Smells something but not sure it smells like perfume.

——— (0) Smells nothing or smells bad odor.

Time		**19. Visual Hallucination (Rabbit)**	Score

19. Visual Hallucination (Rabbit)   Score

(3) Substantially completes suggested sequence, e.g., picks up rabbit, cuddles, describes it.

(2) Completes significant portion of sequence with some inadequacies, e.g., sees rabbit and describes it but does not pick it up.

(1) Not sure he sees rabbit and performs most of sequence vaguely or inappropriately.

(0) Does not see rabbit.

20. Age Regression

General sequence involves three parts: (a) verbalizations that are not inconsistent with the role of a younger child, (b) changes in writing own name, and (c) changes in figure drawing. For name writing, changing from writing to printing is the most general expectation, though not required. For both (b) and (c), performance changes must be in the direction of sloppier and/or simpler drawing and writing, particularly relative to the prehypnotic performance.

(3) Completes sequence appropriately, i.e., no negations on questions and apparent changes downward on both name and drawings. Regressed drawing cannot be *better* than hypnotic drawing, but it need not be worse so long as hypnotic drawing is simpler, etc. than prehypnotic drawing.

(2) Qualifies on either name or drawing or both regardless of responses to questions.

(1) Neither name nor drawing show regression but no negation on questions.

(0) No changes on either name or drawing and negative responses to questions.

21. Dream

(3) Reports spontaneously and without appearance of concocting story as he goes, and/or some elaboration *or* emotionality (giving the appearance of impact on the child).

(2) Perfunctory report or lack of emotionality but does not appear to be composing the story during the report.

(1) Same as (2) but appears to be composing.

(0) No response or negation.

Time	**22. Awakening and Posthypnotic Suggestion**	Score
_____ _____	(3) Substantially completes suggested sequence, e.g., awakens, looks down at rabbit, recites name.	_____
_____	(2) Completes significant portion of sequence with some inadequacies, e.g., looks down but says, "He can't ask my name, rabbits don't talk."	
_____	(1) Fails most of sequence, e.g., "I'm supposed to tell him my name, but there isn't any rabbit there."	
_____	(0) No apparent response, e.g., neither looks down nor tells name.	

TOTAL SCORE _____

NOTE: These scores reflect the overt behavior (OB) of the child (see Chapter 3). Additional scoring procedures and detailed normative data are included in "Norms of Hypnotic Susceptibility in Children" by P. London and L. M. Cooper, *Developmental Psychology*, 1969, *1*, 113–124.

The mean overt behavior scores and standard deviations for children in the standardization sample, by 1-year age groups, are given below. Age is determined to the nearest birthday (e.g., children who are 4 years, 7 months through 5 years, 6 months are called 5-year-olds).

Age	Mean	Standard Deviation
5	33.50	12.23
6	37.45	14.45
7	40.25	14.67
8	44.90	11.01
9	45.30	18.53
10	49.90	11.19
11	48.55	12.97
12	46.10	14.19
13	43.95	14.96
14	48.35	14.15
15	38.45	16.33
16	44.70	17.86

From "Norms of Hypnotic Susceptibility in Children" by P. London and L. M. Cooper, *Developmental Psychology*, 1969, *1*, 113–124. Copyright 1969 by American Psychological Association. Reprinted by permission of the publisher and authors.

Appendix B

Stanford Hypnotic Clinical Scale for Children

Arlene Morgan, Ph.D.
Josephine R. Hilgard, M.D., Ph.D.

MODIFIED FORM (AGES 4–8)

This form may be substituted for the child who cannot relax and does not like to close his eyes. Typically this will be the very young child (under 6 years of age, and occasionally 7 or 8 years) or the extremely anxious child. This form is similar to the standard version except for the active fantasy induction, a few changes in the wording of tests, and the omission of a posthypnotic suggestion.

Induction

If Standard Form is used first, improvise transition.

I'd like to talk with you about how a person can use his imagination to do or feel different kinds of things. Do you know what I mean by imagination? *If necessary, explain:* Do you know what it's like to pretend things . . . to "make-believe?" Do you ever pretend things or make-believe that you are someone else?

Reprinted from Stanford Hypnotic Clinical Scale for Children *by A. Morgan and J. R. Hilgard,* The American Journal of Clinical Hypnosis, *1979, 21, 155–169. With permission.*

Note: *Detailed normative data for this scale are not yet available. Preliminary data are presented in Figure 3-3 (Chapter 3, p. 27).*

Note: *The text for the Modified Form contains both italicized and nonitalicized material. The sentences in italic type are instructions to the hypnotist. Those in roman type are verbal instructions to the child.*

When you can do anything you want to do, what do you do? That is, what are the things you like to do more than anything else in the world? *Probe for interests, e.g., swimming, hiking, playing on the slide and merry-go-round (playground), having a picnic, etc. Select a favorite activity and engage child in thinking about it. The picnic described here is an illustration.*

Okay, let's do that right now.* Let's imagine [pretend] that we are on a picnic, and there's a big picnic basket right in front of us. What does the basket look like to you? How big is it? . . . I'm going to spread this bright yellow tablecloth on the grass here. . . . Why don't you take something out of the basket now? Tell me about it. . . . That's fine. . . . What else is in the basket? *Continue until a convincing fantasy is developed, or child shows total lack of involvement.*

You know, you can do lots of interesting things by thinking about it this way. It's like imagining [pretending] something so strongly that it seems almost real. How real did it seem to you? Good. Now let's try imagining some other things, okay?

1. Hand Lowering

Please hold your right [left] arm† straight out in front of you, with the palm up. *Assist if necessary.* Imagine that you are holding something heavy in your hand, like a heavy rock. Something very heavy. Shape your fingers around the heavy rock in your hand. What does it feel like? . . . That's good. . . . Now think about your arm and hand feeling more and more heavy, as if the rock were pushing down . . . more and more down . . . and as it gets heavier and heavier, the hand and arm begin to move down . . . down . . . heavier and heavier . . . moving . . . down, down, down . . . moving . . . moving . . . more and more down . . . heavier and heavier. . . . *Wait 10 seconds; note extent of movement.* That's fine. Now you can stop imagining there is a rock in your hand, and let your hand relax. . . . It is not heavy any more. . . .

Score + if hand lowers at least 6 inches at end of 10 seconds.

2. Arm Rigidity

Now please hold your left [right] arm straight out and the fingers straight out, too. . . . That's right, your arm straight out in front of

---

*It is not necessary for the child to close his eyes. If closing eyes appears desirable give child a choice: Some children find it easier to imagine with their eyes closed: You may close your eyes if you wish to, but keep them open if you'd rather.

†Either arm may be used for items 1 and 2; if, for example, one arm is immobilized, use other arm for both items.

you, fingers straight out, too. . . . Think about making your arm very
stiff and straight, very, very stiff. . . . Think about it as if you were a
tree, and your arm is a strong branch of the tree, very straight and
very strong, like the branch of a tree . . . so stiff that you can't bend
it. . . . That's right. . . . Now see how stiff your arm is. . . . Try to
bend it. . . . Try. . . . *Wait 10 seconds.* That's fine. . . . Now your
arm is no longer like a branch of a tree. It is not stiff any longer. . . .
Just let it relax again. . . .

   Score + if arm has bent less than 2 inches at end of 10 seconds.

3 and 4. Visual and Auditory Hallucination (TV)

   What is your favorite TV program? *For the occasional child who
does not watch TV, substitute favorite movie and modify the instructions
appropriately. Record response.* You can watch that program right now
if you want to, and I'll tell you how. When I count to three, you will
see a TV in front of you, and you can watch (*name of program*). . . .
Ready? One . . . two . . . three . . . do you see it?

If yes	*If no*
	That's all right. . . . Sometimes it takes a little while to catch on how to do this. . . .
Is the picture clear? . . . Is it black and white, or is it in color? What's happening? Can you hear the program? . . . Is it loud enough? What are you hearing? . . . *Finally:* Now the program is ending. . . . The TV is disappearing. . . . It's gone now . . . very good.	
	If eyes are open
	Why don't you close your eyes for a moment and try to see it in your mind. . . . Sometimes it's easier to imagine things like this with your eyes closed. . . . *Continue:* Just wait a little while, and I think you'll start to see it pretty soon. *Wait 5 seconds.* There, what do you see now?

What are you hearing? *If sees or
hears, question as above.*

If still no
That's okay. Just forget all about
the TV. . . . We'll do something
else. . . .

*Visual: Score + if child sees a program with sufficient detail to be
comparable to actual viewing.*
*Auditory: Score + if child reports hearing words, sound effects, music,
etc.*

5. Dream

Do you ever dream at night when you are asleep? *If puzzled, explain that a dream is like seeing things going on even when you are asleep.*
I'd like you now to think about how you feel when you are just ready
to go to sleep at night, and imagine that you are about to have a
dream. . . . Just let a dream come into your mind . . . a dream just
like the dreams that you have when you are asleep. . . . *If eyes are
open:* Maybe you'd like to close your eyes while you do this. *Continue:*
When I stop talking, in just a moment, you will have a dream, a very
pleasant dream, just like when you are asleep at night. . . . Now a
dream is coming into your mind. . . . *Wait 20 seconds.*

The dream is over now, and I'd like you to tell me about it. *Record
verbatim, probing as necessary for thoughts or images.* That's fine. You
can forget about the dream now. . . . That's all for the dream. . . .

*Score + if child has an experience comparable to a dream, with some
action.*

6. Age Regression

Now I'd like you to think back to some very special time when
you were younger than you are now . . . some time that you had a lot
of fun . . . a special trip, perhaps, or a birthday party. Can you think
of such a time? What was it? *Record target event.* All right . . . now
I'd like you to think about that time. . . . Think about being back
there again. . . . In a little while you are going to feel just like you
did on that day when (*specify target event*). I am going to count to five,
and at the count of five, you will be right back there again . . . one
. . . two . . . three . . . four . . . five. . . . You are now there. . . .
Tell me about it. . . . Where are you? . . . What are you doing? . . .

How old are you? . . . What are you wearing? . . . *Continue as appropriate and record responses.*

That's fine. . . . Now you can stop thinking about that day and come right back to this day, in this room, with everything just as it was. Tell me how it seemed to be back at (*target event*). . . . Was it like being there, or did you just think about it? *How real was it?* That's fine. . . .

Score + if child gives appropriate answers to questions and reports some experience of being there.

Termination

Well, you've done very well today. What was the most fun of the things I asked you to do? Is there anything else you'd like to talk about? . . . If there isn't, then we're all through.

Stanford Hypnotic Clinical Scale for Children
Modified Form (Ages 4–8)
Scoring Form

Name _____   Date _____   Total score _____

Age _____   Hypnotist _____

SUMMARY OF SCORES
(details on the pages that follow)

		Score (+ or −)
1.	**Hand Lowering**	(1) _____
2.	**Arm Rigidity**	(2) _____
3.	**TV—Visual**	(3) _____
4.	**TV—Auditory**	(4) _____
5.	**Dream**	(5) _____
6.	**Age Regression**	(6) _____
	TOTAL SCORE	_____

Comments:

1. **Hand Lowering** Score

   Describe movement:

   Score + if arm and hand lowers at least 6 inches
   by end of 10 seconds. (1) _____

2. **Arm Rigidity**

   Describe movement:

   Score + if arm bends less than 2 inches by end
   of 10 seconds. (2) _____

3 and 4. **Visual and Auditory Hallucination (TV)**

   Program preferred:

   (3) Visual
   Do you see it?
   Is picture clear?
   Is it black and white or color?
   What's happening? (detail of action)

   Score + if child reports seeing a picture
   comparable to actual viewing. (3) _____

   (4) Auditory
   Can you hear it?
   Is it loud enough?
   Sound reported (words, sound effects,
   music, etc.):

   Score + if child reports hearing some sound
   clearly. (4) _____

5. **Dream**
   Verbatim account of dream:

   Score + if child has an experience comparable to
   a dream, with some action. This does not
   include vague, fleeting thoughts or feelings
   without accompanying imagery. (5) _____

6. **Age Regression**
   Target event:
   Where are you?
   What are you doing?

   How old are you?
   What are you wearing?
   How did it seem to be back there?

   Was it like being there, or did you just think
   about it?

   Other:

   Score + if child gives appropriate responses and
   reports some experience of being there. (6) _____

                                    TOTAL SCORE   _____

STANDARD FORM (AGES 6–16)

Discussion of preconceived ideas that child and/or parent may have about hypnosis should precede administration of the scale. Be sure the meaning of the word "relax" is understood. If necessary, explain it in terms of "letting go" as when the hypnotist holds the child's wrist and lets it drop gently, or "feeling loose like a rag doll."

Induction

I'm going to help you learn some interesting things about imagination today. Most people say that it's fun [fascinating]. I will ask you to think of some different things, and we will see how your imagination works. Some people find it easier to imagine some things than other things. We want to find what is most interesting to you. Listen very carefully to me, and let's see what happens. Just be comfortable in the chair [bed], and let's imagine some things now. Please close your eyes so you can imagine these things better. . . . Now I'd like you to picture yourself floating in a warm pool of water. . . . What is it like? . . . And now can you picture yourself floating on a nice soft cloud in the air? . . . What is that like? . . .

That's fine—just open your eyes. . . . Now I'd like to show you how you can feel completely relaxed and comfortable, because that makes it easier to imagine things, too. . . . I'm going to draw a little face on my thumbnail.* . . . Here it is. . . . *Hypnotist draws face on own thumbnail with red felt pen.* Let's put one on your thumb. Do you want to do it or shall I? *Hypnotist or child does so.* That's a good face! Now please hold your hand up in front of you like this—*assist child so that hand is in front, thumbnail facing him, with elbow not resting on anything*—and look at the little face [thumbnail] as you listen to my voice. Just keep watching the little face [thumbnail], try to think only about the things I talk about, and let your body relax completely. . . . Let your whole body feel loose and limp and relaxed. . . . Relax completely . . . just let all the muscles in your body relax . . . relax

---

Note: *The text for the Standard Form contains both italicized and nonitalicized material. The sentences in italic type are instructions to the hypnotist. Those in roman type are verbal instructions to the child.*

If drawing a face on thumbnail seems awkward for the older child, eliminate it and have him simply stare at the thumbnail. Substitute "thumbnail" for "little face" as indicated.

completely. . . . Be as relaxed as you were while you were imagining that you were floating in the pool of water, or floating on a cloud. . . . Feel your body becoming more and more relaxed . . . more and more relaxed. . . . Your eyelids, too, are relaxing. They are starting to feel heavy. As you keep watching the face [thumbnail], your eyes feel heavier and heavier. . . . Your eyes are starting to blink a little, and that's a very good sign. That means you're relaxing really well. Just keep watching the face [thumbnail], your eyes feel heavier and heavier. . . . Your eyes are starting to blink a little, and that's a very good sign. That means you're relaxing really well. Just keep watching the face [thumbnail] and listening to my voice. . . . Already your eyelids feel heavy. Very soon they will feel so heavy that they will begin to close by themselves. . . . Let them close whenever they feel like it. And when they close, let them stay closed. . . . Even now, and your whole body is feeling so nice, so comfortable, completely relaxed. . . .

If child shows convincing evidence at any time of inability to relax, or unwillingness to let eyes close or remain closed, go to Modified Form.

Now I'm going to count from one to ten, and you will find your body becoming even more relaxed. . . . You will continue to relax as you listen to the counting . . . one . . . more and more relaxed, such a good feeling . . . two . . . three . . . more and more relaxed all the time, feeling so good . . . four . . . five . . . six . . . even more relaxed . . . and your eyes are feeling heavier, heavier. . . . It feels so good just to let go and relax completely . . . seven . . . eight . . . nine . . . VERY relaxed now . . . ten. . . .

If child is still holding hand up: Just let your hand relax completely, too. . . . Let it relax comfortably on your lap [the bed]. . . . That's fine. . . .

If eyes have not closed: Now please let your eyes close, and just relax completely. Just let your eyes close and keep them closed while you listen to me. . . .

For all children: And now as we go on, it will be very easy for you to listen to me because you are so relaxed and comfortable. If you can keep your eyes closed, you can imagine some things better, so why don't you let them stay closed. You'll be able to stay relaxed and talk to me when I ask you to. . . . You are feeling very good. . . . Just keep listening to what I tell you and think about the things I suggest. Then let happen whatever you find is happening. . . . Just let things happen by themselves. . . .

If eyes open at any time, request child gently to close them: Because imagination is easier that way.

1.   Hand Lowering

Please hold your right [left] arm* straight out in front of you, with
the palm up. *Assist if necessary.* Imagine that you are holding something heavy in your hand, like a heavy rock. Something very heavy.
Shape your fingers around the heavy rock in your hand. What does it
feel like? . . . That's good. . . . Now think about your arm and hand
feeling heavier and heavier, as if the rock were pushing down . . .
more and more down . . . and as it gets heavier and heavier, the
hand and arm begin to move down . . . down . . . heavier and heavier . . . moving . . . down, down, down . . . moving . . . moving
. . . more and more down . . . heavier and heavier. . . . *Wait 10 seconds; note extent of movement.* That's fine. Now you can stop imagining
there is a rock in your hand, and let your hand relax. . . . It is not
heavy anymore. . . .

Score + if hand lowers at least 6 inches at end of 10 seconds.

2.   Arm Rigidity

Now please hold your left [right] arm straight out, and the fingers
straight out, too. . . . That's right, your arm straight out in front of
you, fingers straight out, too. . . . Think about making your arm very
stiff and straight, very, very stiff. . . . Think about it as if you were a
tree and your arm is a strong branch of the tree, very straight and very
strong, like the branch of a tree . . . so stiff that you can't bend it.
. . . That's right. . . . Now see how stiff your arm is. . . . Try to
bend it. . . . Try. . . . *Wait 10 seconds.* That's fine. . . . Now your
arm is no longer like a branch of a tree. It is not stiff any longer. . . .
Just let it relax again. . . .

Score + if arm has bent less than 2 inches at end of 10 seconds.

3 and 4.   Visual and Auditory Hallucination (TV)

It is easier to imagine what I am going to ask you to do if you
keep your eyes closed.

What is your favorite TV program? *For the occasional child who
does not watch TV, substitute favorite movie and modify the instructions
appropriately. Record response.*

You can watch that program right now if you want to, and I'll tell
you how. When I count to three, you will see a TV in front of you,

---

*Either arm may be used for items 1 and 2; if, for example, one arm is immobilized, use
other arm for both items.*

and you can watch (*name of program*). . . . Ready? One . . . two . . . three . . . do you see it?

<table>
<tr><td align="center">If yes</td><td align="center">If no</td></tr>
</table>

If yes

If no

That's all right. . . . Sometimes it takes a little while to catch on to how to do this. . . . Just wait a little while, and I think you'll start to see it pretty soon. *Wait 5 seconds.* There, what do you see now? What are you hearing? *If sees or hears, question as above.*

Is the picture clear? . . . Is it black and white, or is it in color? What's happening? Can you hear the program? . . . Is it loud enough? What are you hearing? . . . *Finally:* Now the program is ending. . . . The TV is disappearing. . . . It's gone now . . . very good.

If still no

That's okay. Just forget all about the TV. . . . We'll do something else. . . . Just relax and keep listening to my voice. . . .

Visual: Score + if child sees a program with sufficient detail to be comparable to actual viewing.

Auditory: Score + if child reports hearing words, sound effects, music, etc.

5. Dream

Do you dream at night when you are asleep? *If puzzled, explain that a dream is like seeing things going on even when you are asleep.* I'd like you to think about how you feel when you are just ready to go to sleep at night, and imagine that you are about to have a dream. . . . Just let a dream come into your mind, a dream just like the dreams that you have when you are asleep. . . . When I stop talking, in just a moment, you will have a dream, a very pleasant dream, just like the dreams you have when you are asleep at night. . . . Now a dream is coming into your mind. . . . *Wait 20 seconds.*

The dream is over now, and I'd like you to tell me about it. *Record verbatim, probing as necessary for thoughts or images.* That's fine. You can forget about the dream now, and just relax. . . . Just relax completely and let your whole body feel good. . . .

Score + if child has an experience comparable to a dream, with some action.

6. Age Regression

Now I'd like you to think back to some very special time when you were younger than you are now. Some time that happened last year, or maybe when you were even younger than that . . . a special trip, perhaps, or a birthday party. Can you think of such a time? What was it? *Record target event.* All right . . . now I'd like you to think about that time. . . . Think about being younger and smaller. . . . In a little while, you are going to feel just like you did on that day when (*specify target event*). I am going to count to five and at the count of five you will be right back there again . . . one . . . two . . . three . . . four . . . five. . . . You are now there. . . . Tell me about it. . . . Where are you? What are you doing? How old are you? . . . Look at yourself and tell me what you're wearing. *Continue as appropriate and record responses.*

That's fine. . . . Now you can stop thinking about that day and come right back to today, in this room, with everything just as it is. Tell me how it seemed to be back at (*target event*). . . . Was it like being there, or did you just think about it? *How real was it?* Did you feel smaller? . . . That's fine. Just relax completely again now. . . .

Score + if child gives appropriate answers to questions and reports some experience of being there.

7. Posthypnotic Response

That's it . . . very relaxed . . . feeling so good, so comfortable . . . so relaxed. . . . In a moment I will ask you to take a deep breath and open your eyes and feel wide awake, so we can talk a little about the things we have done today. . . . However, while we are talking, I will clap my hands two times, like this—*demonstrate.* When you hear me clap, you will immediately close your eyes and go right back to feeling just the way you do now . . . completely relaxed. . . . You'll be surprised at how easy it is to let your eyes close, and let your whole body relax completely again, when you hear the handclap . . . relaxed and comfortable, just as you are now. . . . All right, then . . . now take a deep breath and open your eyes. . . . That's fine. . . . Maybe you'd like to stretch just a little so you'll feel alert. . . . You've done very well at imagining these things. . . . Which of the things that I asked you to think about was the most fun? *After approximately 20 seconds, clap hands. Note response.*

Score + if child closes eyes and exhibits characteristics of relaxation.

Do you feel relaxed? Do you feel as relaxed as you did before, before I asked you to open your eyes? . . . That's fine. Now I'm going to count from five to one, and when I get to one, you will open your eyes and feel wide awake again, and you will know that our imagining things together is over for today. Okay, then . . . five . . . four . . . three . . . two . . . one . . . very good. How do you feel now? Let's talk a little about the other things we did today. *Remind child of specific items so that he recalls all suggestions.* Now I'm going to clap my hands again, and this time it will not make you drowsy and relaxed. *Clap hands, record response, and be sure that child is fully alert.*

Termination

You've done very well today. What was the most fun of the things I asked you to do? Is there anything else you'd like to talk about? . . . If there isn't, then we're all through.

Stanford Hypnotic Clinical Scale for Children
Standard Form (Ages 6–16)
Scoring Form

Name _____   Date _____   Total score _____

Age _____   Hypnotist _____

SUMMARY OF SCORES
(details on the pages that follow)

		Score (+ or −)
1.	**Hand Lowering**	(1) _____
2.	**Arm Rigidity**	(2) _____
3.	**TV—Visual**	(3) _____
4.	**TV—Auditory**	(4) _____
5.	**Dream**	(5) _____
6.	**Age Regression**	(6) _____
7.	**Posthypnotic Response**	(7) _____
	TOTAL SCORE	_____

Comments:

1. **Hand Lowering**   Score
   Describe movement:

   Score + if arm and hand lowers at least 6 inches
   by end of 10 seconds.   (1) _____

2. **Arm Rigidity**
   Describe movement:

   Score + if arm bends less than 2 inches by end
   of 10 seconds.   (2) _____

3 and 4. **Visual and Auditory Hallucination (TV)**
   Program preferred:
   (3) Visual
       Do you see it?
       Is picture clear?
       Is it black and white or color?
       What's happening? (detail of action)

   Score+ if child reports seeing a picture
   comparable to actual viewing.   (3) _____

   (4) Auditory
       Can you hear it?
       Is it loud enough?
       Sound reported (words, sound effects,
       music, etc.):

   Score + if child reports hearing some sound
   clearly.   (4) _____

5. **Dream**
   Verbatim account of dream:

   Score + if child has an experience comparable to
   a dream, with some action. This does not
   include vague, fleeting thoughts or feelings
   without accompanying imagery.   (5) _____

360

6. **Age Regression**   Score
   Target event:
   Where are you?
   What are you doing?

   How old are you?
   Look at yourself and tell me what you're
   wearing.
   How did it seem to be back there?

   Was it like being there, or did you just think
   about it?

   Did you feel smaller?
   Other:

   Score + if child gives appropriate responses and
   reports some experience of being there.   (6) ____

7. **Posthypnotic Response**
   Response to handclap:
   Did child close eyes?
   Appear to relax?
   Do you feel relaxed?
   As relaxed as before?
   Discussion of specific items:

   Response to handclap after suggestion removed:

   Score + if child closed eyes and relaxed at initial
   handclap   (7) ____

                              TOTAL SCORE   ____

Appendix C

Enuresis Questionnaire

Name of child _____   Date _____

Age of child   Filled out by _____
(years and months) _____

Birthdate _____

Please circle appropriate choice: Y= Yes; N= No; DK= Don't Know

Y N DK   1. Did your child ever have dry beds? If so, when
                    did he or she begin wetting the bed?

Y N DK   2. Did some frightening or upsetting event happen
                    before he or she began bedwetting? If so, what
                    and when?

_____   3. At what age did your child have complete bowel
                    control?

Y N DK   4. Is your child constipated frequently, or does he or
                    she have irregular, hard bowel movements?

Y N DK   5. Is there any stool soiling?

Y N DK   6. Does your child wet during the daytime now? If
                    so, how often?

Y N DK   7. Does your child have the feeling that he or she is
                    dribbling during the day?

Y N DK   8. Does your child have the feeling that he or she
                    must get to the bathroom immediately when he
                    or she feels the urge to go?

_____   9. How often does your child go to the bathroom
                    during the day?

_____	10.	How many nights a week does your child have dry beds?
Y N DK	11.	Is your child aware of any special time when he or she is certain that he or she will wet the bed? If so, when?
Y N DK	12.	Does anyone tease him or her about wet beds? If so, who?
Y N DK	13.	Do you punish him or her for bedwetting?
Y N DK	14.	Does your child have any allergies such as hay-fever, eczema, asthma, food or drug intolerance? If so, which one(s) and for how long?
Y N DK	15.	Did your child have any allergies when younger that have since disappeared? If so, which one(s), when, and for how long?
Y N DK	16.	Does your child take any medications at any time for any reason? If so, which one(s), when, and how often?
Y N DK	17.	Do either of the child's parents have allergies now or in the past? If so, who and which one(s)?
Y N DK	18.	Do any of the child's brothers and/or sisters wet the bed at night? If so, who and what age(s)?
Y N DK	19.	Do any of the child's brothers and/or sisters have allergies now or in the past? If so, who and which one(s)?
_____	20.	Who washes wet bedclothing?
Y N DK	21.	Have you tried any treatment plans to cure bed-wetting? If so, what were they?

Appendix D

Instruction Form for Parents—Bedwetting

Your child is practicing autosuggestion for control of bedwetting, and it is important that you enhance your child's self-confidence and learning in the following ways:

- You should ensure that there will be a quiet spot available every evening where your child can practice the relaxation exercise.
- In general, the best time for practice is shortly before bedtime; however, if your child is one who is exceedingly tired and ready to fall asleep as soon as he or she gets into bed, practice should be immediately after supper or at some other convenient time between suppertime and bedtime.
- Your child should practice while sitting on the bed, on the floor, or in a comfortable chair in the room designated for practice. Although it is perfectly all right to practice in bed he or she should not lie down.
- Ideally, a half-dollar—which can be a reminder to practice—should be available where your child is likely to see it.
- *You should not remind your child to practice!* This is hard for many parents to follow because we naturally remind our children to do many things. However, bladder control is entirely the child's responsibility, and we must recognize this. The only aid you can give is to provide a reminder—put the coin in a conspicuous spot or tie a colored string around a toothbrush.
- If your child does not practice, please tell his or her pediatrician, but not in the child's presence. Also let the pediatrician know if there are family stresses, such as the death of a pet, the absence of a parent, or anxiety over school.

(continued)

- Your child has been told to ask you to help draw a funny face on his or her thumbnail. This gives your child something to focus on during the relaxation exercise. If your child asks you to do this, please oblige. Don't remind him or her that it's "time to draw the face on the thumb now."

- Please encourage your child to make follow-up calls to the pediatrician as requested. We feel these are very important to successful outcome.

- Please don't put diapers or plastic pants on your child when he or she is practicing bladder-control, because doing so tells your child that you don't expect he or she will succeed.

- Please don't wake your child at night to use the bathroom.

- Praise your child when he or she tells you that the bed is dry and say something like, "That's fine. You really are showing that you can handle this problem yourself."

- Although we have told your child that he or she may show you the relaxation exercise, we suggest you wait until your child is ready to do so; don't plead with your child to share this special skill.

Author Index

Subject Index